New Frontiers in Hematology

New Frontiers in Hematology

Edited by Rylan Beckham

hayle
medical

New York

Hayle Medical,
750 Third Avenue, 9th Floor,
New York, NY 10017, USA

Visit us on the World Wide Web at:
www.haylemedical.com

ISBN: 978-1-63241-630-8

Cataloging-in-Publication Data

New frontiers in hematology / edited by Rylan Beckham.
      p. cm.
Includes bibliographical references and index.
ISBN 978-1-63241-630-8
1. Hematology. 2. Blood--Diseases. I. Beckham, Rylan.
RC633 .N49 2019
616.15--dc23

Table of Contents

Preface

Hematology is concerned with the treatment of diseases that affect blood production and its components. Some of these components include blood proteins, bone marrow, blood vessels, spleen, blood cells, platelets, hemoglobin, etc. Hematology is a distinct branch of medicine but sometimes it may overlap with oncology. A hematologist is a physician who specializes in hematology. Hematologists are concerned with the care and treatment of patients with blood disorders such as hematological malignancies, coagulopathies, sickle cell anemia, thalassemia, etc. This book is compiled in such a manner, that it will provide in-depth knowledge about hematology. From theories to research to practical applications, case studies related to all contemporary topics of relevance to this field have been included herein. With state-of-the-art inputs by acclaimed experts of this field, this book targets students and professionals.

This book has been the outcome of endless efforts put in by authors and researchers on various issues and topics within the field. The book is a comprehensive collection of significant researches that are addressed in a variety of chapters. It will surely enhance the knowledge of the field among readers across the globe.

It gives us an immense pleasure to thank our researchers and authors for their efforts to submit their piece of writing before the deadlines. Finally in the end, I would like to thank my family and colleagues who have been a great source of inspiration and support.

Editor

Haploidentical Hematopoietic Stem Cell Transplantation: Expanding the Horizon for Hematologic Disorders

Mohammad Faizan Zahid[1] and David Alan Rizzieri[2]

[1]*Aga Khan University, Karachi 74800, Pakistan*
[2]*Division of Hematologic Malignancies and Cellular Therapy, Duke Cancer Institute, Durham, NC 27710, USA*

Correspondence should be addressed to Mohammad Faizan Zahid; faizanzahid91@hotmail.com

Academic Editor: Suparno Chakrabarti

Despite the advent of targeted therapies and novel agents, allogeneic hematopoietic stem cell transplantation remains the only curative modality in the management of hematologic disorders. The necessity to find an HLA-matched related donor is a major obstacle that compromises the widespread application and development of this field. Matched unrelated donors and umbilical cord blood have emerged as alternative sources of donor stem cells; however, the cost of maintaining donor registries and cord blood banks is very high and even impractical in developing countries. Almost every patient has an HLA haploidentical relative in the family, meaning that haploidentical donors are potential sources of stem cells, especially in situations where cord blood or matched unrelated donors are not easily available. Due to the high rates of graft failure and graft-versus-host disease, haploidentical transplant was not considered a feasible option up until the late 20th century, when strategies such as "megadose stem cell infusions" and posttransplantation immunosuppression with cyclophosphamide showed the ability to overcome the HLA disparity barrier and significantly improve the rates of engraftment and reduce the incidence and severity of graft-versus-host disease. Newer technologies of graft manipulation have also yielded the same effects in addition to preserving the antileukemic cells in the donor graft.

1. Introduction

Today's age represents a truly unprecedented time in care of the patient with a hematologic malignancy with the advent of several targeted therapies and novel agents. These therapies have shown tremendous efficacy in treating several malignancies, yielding impressive response rates with limited toxicity profiles [1]. Despite substantial activity against different cancer types, relapse is often encountered at some point during the clinical course of most treated patients, with durable remissions being observed in only a certain percentage of patients. Allogeneic hematopoietic stem cell transplantation (allo-HSCT) is often the only treatment modality which can offer a cure to not only malignant but also benign hematological disorders [2]. A human leukocyte antigen- (HLA-) matched sibling donor is the preferred source of a stem cell graft in allo-HSCT. However, only 30% of patients requiring an allo-HSCT will have an HLA-matched sibling donor [3]. For patients not having a matched sibling donor, a matched unrelated donor (MUD) is an alternate source of stem cells,

the probability of finding which is up to 75% among Caucasians. However, these chances are much lower among non-Caucasian populations, with 40% chance in Hispanic individuals and less than 20% among Asian and African American individuals [3–5]. In addition, the cost of recruiting MUDs and maintaining donor registries is a major drawback, making this approach unaffordable and even impractical for developing countries. Hence, it is important to explore other possible stem cell sources.

Unrelated umbilical cord blood (UCB) represents another alternate source of stem cells, one which has been proven to be successful when performing allo-HSCT [6–10]. Key advantages include a comparatively quick donor search and a shorter time to proceed to transplant when compared with adult MUDs [11, 12]. This is especially important in the context of advanced/high-risk hematologic malignancies, where the risk of disease relapse is high and the goal is to proceed to a transplant while the patient is still in remission and has minimal disease burden after induction therapy [13]. In addition, UCB transplantation allows for a greater degree of HLA mismatch, most likely due to a lower number of activated alloreactive T lymphocytes present in cord blood [14, 15]. This accounts for very low and acceptable rates of graft-versus-host disease (GvHD) following UCB transplants [8, 12, 16]. One of the obstacles to UCB transplants is the nonavailability of a sufficient number of hematopoietic progenitor cells in an UCB unit [12]. Although this limitation can be overcome by using more than one unit of cord blood, it is daunted by the high cost of maintaining cord blood banks [17]. Delayed engraftment, increased time to hematopoietic recovery, and immune reconstitution lead to substantially increased risks of life-threatening infections and graft failure, often offsetting the advantages of using unrelated UCB as a stem cell source [5, 12]. Furthermore, due to a limited number of hematopoietic progenitor cells, posttransplant immune manipulation, such as donor lymphocyte infusions, is very difficult, which severely limits treatment options for patients who relapse after transplant [6, 12].

On the other hand, haploidentical related donors offer several key advantages over MUDs and UCB. Almost all patients have at least one haploidentical related donor in the family and the best donor amongst all candidate family members can be selected. Haploidentical related donors are readily available and are highly motivated to donate to a family member [18, 19]. Due to rapid availability of donors and substantially lower costs, patients can proceed to transplant fairly quickly (as early as 3 weeks) [18]. Another major advantage of haploidentical donors over UCB is easy access to the stem cell source that makes donor-derived cellular therapy, such as donor lymphocyte infusions and immune manipulation, available for use after transplant, if necessary [18].

The HLA mismatch between the haploidentical donor and the recipient offers a potent graft-versus-tumor (GvT) effect to completely eradicate malignant cells and offer a permanent cure [18]. Some studies have reported substantially reduced relapse rates with greater degree of HLA mismatches [20–22]. However, two immunological barriers need to be overcome: (1) graft rejection, or host-versus-graft effect, and (2) GvHD. In allo-HSCT studies involving myeloablative conditioning (MAC) regimens, HLA mismatches, either at the antigen level or at allele level, have been associated with inferior survival and poor outcomes after allo-HSCT, with greater degree of mismatch correlating with worse outcomes [21, 23, 24]. Since donor-recipient HLA histocompatibility is the most important independent predictor of outcomes after allo-HSCT, these two barriers are more difficult to overcome in haploidentical hematopoietic stem cell transplantation (haplo-HSCT) than in HLA-matched allo-HSCT. Although the lower risk of relapse due to HLA disparity supports the existence of a GvT effect, this positive aspect of haplo-HSCT is offset by markedly increased rates of GvHD, graft failure, and nonrelapse mortality [23, 25].

Several attempts to perform haplo-HSCT using T lymphocyte replete, unmanipulated grafts have been made. Since donor-derived T lymphocytes are the fundamental players in the pathogenesis of GvHD, these attempts have been associated with early and severe multiorgan failure and GvHD,

leading to alarming rates of transplant-related mortality despite pharmacological GvHD prophylaxis [26]. To reduce the risk of GvHD, a new approach of highly purified CD34+ stem cell grafts was adopted using ex vivo T lymphocyte depletion technologies [27]. With this strategy, almost no GvHD was observed in the recipients, despite the absence of posttransplant immunosuppressants for GvHD prophylaxis [28–30]. However, the small number of T lymphocytes transplanted using the highly purified CD34+ stem cell strategy does not allow for an efficient transfer of adoptive immunity, resulting in substantially delayed immune reconstitution and frequent, often fatal, infectious complications [18, 31]. Also, the risk of graft failure is also higher with T lymphocyte depleted haplo-HSCT [27, 32].

There is a key difference between positive selection of CD34+ progenitor cells and negative depletion of lymphocytes during graft manipulation. With CD34+ selection strategies, almost no cells other than the CD34+ stem cells are transplanted. On the other hand, negative depletion techniques (mainly CD3+ and CD19+ negative depletion) allows for other types of cells, such as dendritic cells, natural-killer (NK) cells, and monocytes, to be retained in the donor graft and transplanted with the CD34+ progenitors. Both graft manipulation techniques result in effective removal of B and T lymphocytes, leading to greatly reduced risks of developing posttransplant Epstein-Barr virus related lymphoproliferative disorders (B lymphocyte depletion) and GvHD (T lymphocyte depletion) [26, 33]. The detailed research and broad application of graft manipulation has provided insight into the biology of NK cells, lymphocytic constituents of the innate immune system, and their immunotherapeutic potential in allo- and haplo-HSCT [34].

NK cell activity is modulated by the interaction between killer cell immunoglobulin-like receptor (KIR) expressed on the surface of NK cells and cognate ligands (i.e., certain HLA alleles) to KIRs [35]. Engagement of KIRs by their corresponding ligands produces inhibitory signals and prevents NK cell activation. In the context of allo-HSCT, and especially haplo-HSCT, NK cells in the allograft can attack malignant cells in the recipient if there is a mismatch between the KIRs on the donor-derived NK cells and the HLA antigens on the recipient (and malignant) cells [36]. With so many haploidentical donors available for a vast majority of patients, the ideal donor can be picked based on the KIR haplotype on the donor NK cells to exploit their alloreactivity and induce powerful GvT effects [37, 38]. Additionally, the disparity between KIRs and HLA haplotypes does not increase the risk of developing GvHD [39].

Another fundamental difference between CD34+ selection and negative depletion of lymphocytes (CD3+/CD19+ depletion) is that the number of alloreactive lymphocytes "contaminating" the donor graft is approximately ten times higher in CD3+/CD19+ depletion. This necessitates the use of pharmacological GvHD prophylaxis after transplants using CD3+/CD19+ depleted grafts [33, 40]. However, a notable problem with the transplantation of T lymphocyte depleted grafts is the increased likelihood of relapse after transplantation [41, 42]. A more efficient approach is the depletion of T-cell receptor (TCR) $\alpha\beta$+ T lymphocytes and CD19+ cells

(TCR$\alpha\beta$+/CD19+ depletion) from donor grafts [43, 44]. This approach greatly increases the efficiency of alloreactive T lymphocyte removal (similar to that of CD34+ selection techniques), while retaining other cells such as NK cells and monocytes. In addition, this method also retains $\gamma\delta$+ T lymphocytes in the graft. $\gamma\delta$+ T lymphocytes constitute approximately 5% of circulating T lymphocytes. These cells are non-alloreactive and exhibit potent antitumor and anti-infectious properties [5, 44]. Since these cells are not activated by major histocompatibility complex (MHC) interactions, they do not react to alloantigens and hence do not contribute to GvHD [45, 46]. This is advocated by the fact that patients exhibiting high $\gamma\delta$+ T lymphocyte counts after allo-HSCT show better survival with reduced incidence of relapse and GvHD [47]. In contrast, the majority of circulating T lymphocytes (approximately 95%) are $\alpha\beta$+ T lymphocytes which act against alloantigens via MHC interactions and give rise to GvHD after allo-HSCT [48]. The TCR$\alpha\beta$+/CD19+ depletion technique allows for satisfactory removal of $\alpha\beta$+ T lymphocytes to prevent GvHD while retaining $\gamma\delta$+ T lymphocytes to ensure timely immune reconstitution and a robust GvT effect, especially after haplo-HSCT [47, 49, 50]. The most recent study [51] reporting the results of haplo-HSCT with TCR$\alpha\beta$+/CD19+ depletion in pediatric patients showed acceptable rates of GvHD (22%). In all but one patient, GvHD was grade 2 and responded to first-line therapy. Graft failure was observed in 27% of patients, all of whom were successfully retransplanted with different rescue protocols. The overall survival of patients from this study was 96.7%, advocating the efficacy of TCR$\alpha\beta$+/CD19+ depletion in improving outcomes after haplo-HSCT.

During the 1980s, outcomes of haplo-HSCT were discouraging due to severe GvHD and graft failure, often approaching rates as high as 90% [52, 53]. The introduction of graft manipulation and T lymphocyte depletion brought about notable improvements in outcomes of recipients of haplo-HSCT by dramatically reducing the incidence of GvHD [54]; however, the high incidence of graft failure remained a major obstacle to the application of haplo-HSCT [55, 56]. Graft failure is mediated by native cytotoxic T lymphocytes that persist in the recipient's system even after conditioning regimens are administered [57]. This barrier in histocompatibility was shown to be overcome in several animal-model studies [58] and, subsequently, in clinical studies [57, 59, 60] by infusing high doses of T lymphocyte depleted hematopoietic progenitor cells. Additional strategies to help engraftment included enhancing the ablative intensity of conditioning regimens and addition of anti-T lymphocyte agents [57, 59, 61]. Unfortunately, such intensive conditioning regimens result in extensive organ damage and toxicities which limit their use to younger and relatively healthier patients in comparison to individuals of older age groups [5]. Chemotherapeutic doses and total body irradiation used in MAC regimens cause extensive damage to host tissue and release of inflammatory cytokines, such as tumor necrosis factor alpha (TNFα) and interferon gamma (IFNγ). These inflammatory mediators, and several others, play an integral role in the pathophysiology of GvHD [62], which may be one of the reasons why MAC regimen transplants are frequently complicated by

GvHD [57, 63]. The problem with T lymphocyte depleted grafts is delayed immune reconstitution and significant period of immunodeficiency which predisposes to serious and often fatal infections [28, 57, 64].

Nonmyeloablative conditioning (NMAC) regimens are an attractive alternative for patients requiring an allo-HSCT who are not considered suitable candidates for MAC regimens due to advanced age, comorbidities, and/or increased risks of therapy-related adverse effects [65]. Using NMAC regimens also results in the decreased release of inflammatory mediators and cytokines and may consequently reduce the incidence and magnitude of GvHD, especially when used for haplo-HSCT. This significantly broadens the applicability of transplantation to patients who would otherwise be unfit to receive a transplant using standard protocols. Earlier studies applying haplo-HSCT with NMAC regimens showed discouraging patient outcomes, especially with alarming rates of graft failure [66, 67]. Rizzieri et al. [68] published the first large study on haplo-HSCT with fludarabine, cyclophosphamide, and alemtuzumab used as the preparatory NMAC regimen which demonstrated that the complications of GvHD and graft failure after haplo-HSCT could be overcome, making it a feasible treatment option in the therapy of patients with hematologic malignancies. 75% of the patients in this study achieved complete remission with only 10.2% transplant-related mortality in the first 100 days. Engraftment rate was high, with only 14% of patients suffering from graft failure, while only 8% of patients developed GvHD. However, relapse and infectious complications were major causes of mortality in this study (49% and 22%, resp.). One plausible reason for the high rate of relapse could be that the patients participating in this study harbored poor-risk hematologic malignancies which carry an inherent probability of relapse.

Cyclophosphamide is a highly immunosuppressive alkylating agent with an established role in anticancer chemotherapy and HSCT [69]. Historically, cyclophosphamide is commonly administered as part of several conditioning regimens prior to HSCT; however, as previously discussed, the cytotoxic effects of this agent lead to tissue damage and release of inflammatory mediators and increase the risk of GvHD [62]. Administration of cyclophosphamide between 48 and 72 hours after transplant has been shown to facilitate posttransplant immune-tolerance; however, this tolerance is not induced when the drug is administered at 24 or 96 hours after transplant [70]. Cyclophosphamide exploits the high cytotoxic sensitivity of alloreactive T lymphocytes (both host and donor) to DNA damage [71]; hence carefully timed administration of posttransplant cyclophosphamide inhibits GvHD and graft rejection [72, 73]. O'Donnell et al. [69] investigated the role of posttransplantation cyclophosphamide in patients receiving haplo-HSCT after NMAC conditioning. The results of their study concluded that this strategy substantially reduced the risks of GvHD and graft rejection and was able to produce long-lasting donor-recipient chimerism after transplant. Subsequently, Luznik et al. [64] reported their experience with using posttransplant cyclophosphamide after NMAC haplo-HSCT. The results of their study showed acceptable rates of graft failure (13%) and GvHD (grades 2–4: 34%, grades 3-4: 6%) with rapid achievement of donor-recipient chimerism after transplant. Administration of two doses of cyclophosphamide in the 48-to-72-hour window was associated with a lower risk of chronic GvHD than only one dose, further advocating that posttransplant cyclophosphamide is efficacious in inducing posttransplant tolerance. However, relapse of primary disease was a major cause of treatment failure and mortality (up to 51%). This study also recruited patients with poor-risk hematologic malignancies, which may explain the high incidence of relapse in this study group. Patients with lymphoid malignancies were at a lower risk of experiencing relapse than those with myeloid malignancies, indicating particular effectiveness of cyclophosphamide in treating lymphoid hematologic malignancies. Other studies have demonstrated similar findings, corroborating that this strategy depletes alloreactive T lymphocytes in the donor graft as well as the host immune system, dramatically reducing the risk of both GvHD and graft failure, which are much more difficult to control in the setting of haplo-HSCT and are substantial impediments [69]. While there is concern that posttransplant cyclophosphamide might damage or kill donor hematopoietic progenitors cells, these cells have high expression of aldehyde dehydrogenase enzymes which confer relative resistance to the cytotoxic effects of the drug [74].

A relatively newer strategy to increase the success rates of haplo-HSCT is the use of T regulatory cells (Tregs). Tregs are a specialized subset of CD4+ lymphocytes with concurrent expression of CD25 and FOXP3 genes which play crucial roles in antitumor immunity, posttransplant tolerance, and protection against autoimmunity [75–77]. In addition, they have low expression of CD127 [78]. The adoptive transfer of these specialized T lymphocytes limits graft and host alloreactivity, leading to reduced risks of GvHD and graft failure [79–82]. Tregs also preserve and maintain normal lymph node and thymus architecture from GvHD and allow for a quick posttransplant immune recovery while having no negative effects on the GvT responses of allo-HSCT [83]. Additional studies have also showed that Tregs become activated and proliferate by interaction with recipient antigen-presenting cells in the proinflammatory milieu after administration of conditioning regimens, attenuating alloreactive T lymphocyte activation while allowing nonalloreactive T lymphocyte expansion to ensure a timely immune recovery [82, 84–86].

Di Ianni et al. [87] performed the first human study evaluating the adoptive transfer of Tregs on posttransplantation outcomes in patients receiving haplo-HSCT. Early infusion of donor-derived Tregs on day −4 of transplant, followed by infusion of positively immunoselected CD34+ stem cells and conventional T lymphocytes on day 0, showed prevention of GvHD in the absence of any immunosuppressive GvHD prophylaxis and hastened posttransplant immune recovery and immunity against opportunistic pathogens and did not have any negative effects on GvT effects [87]. A follow-up study of these patients [84] showed successful engraftment in 26/28 (93%) patients. Only 2 (7.7%) of 26 evaluable patients developed grade 2–4 GvHD. Spectratyping analysis showed the rapid development of T lymphocyte repertoire within months after transplant. Naïve and memory T lymphocyte subpopulations showed rapid increase over the first year after

transplant, while CD4+ and CD8+ lymphocytes against opportunistic pathogens like *Aspergillus* and *Toxoplasma* appeared significantly earlier in comparison to historical controls comprising standard haplo-HSCT recipients. At a median follow-up of 21 months, 46.1% were alive and in remission [84].

Tregs can be isolated in vitro using standard donor-derived leukapheresis products using double negative selection with anti-CD8 and anti-CD19 monoclonal antibodies and positive selection for CD25 [88]. Expression of the FOXP3 gene represents the peripheral mature Tregs [89], while low CD127 expression correlates with exhibition of regulatory functions in this T lymphocyte subset [90]. Such cell-based transplantation and graft modifications prove to improve posttransplantation engraftment, allow quick immune reconstitution, and reduce GvHD; however, the expertise required for such cellular manipulations limits their clinical implementation to highly specialized medical centers.

With regard to Tregs, posttransplant GvHD prophylaxis may also play a role in selectively favoring the expansion of Tregs while suppressing mature effector T lymphocytes. Sirolimus is an immunosuppressant that demonstrates such properties [91]. Peccatori et al. [92] performed a recent study showing that a calcineurin inhibitor-free, sirolimus-based GvHD prophylaxis regimen promoted selective Treg expansion after haplo-HSCT. This strategy was well tolerated and a robust and rapid engraftment was observed in the majority of patients. While the incidence and severity of acute and chronic GvHD in this study were comparable to historical data from MUD allo-HSCT using peripheral blood stem cells [93, 94], they were much higher when compared with haplo-HSCT using bone marrow as the source of donor stem cells [64, 95, 96]. In addition, Tregs show a higher level of resistance to the cytotoxic effects of cyclophosphamide [97]. Future studies may be performed to ascertain the specific effects of GvHD prophylaxis in T lymphocyte dynamics to systematize the utility of regimens based on their effects on T lymphocyte dynamics to derive the maximum benefit, carefully weighing GvHD, GvT, engraftment, and immune recovery after transplant.

In conclusion, allo-HSCT remains the only treatment modality that offers a potential cure for some with hematologic disorders. HLA-matched donors are not always available, which has led to establishment of UCB and MUDs as alternative sources for stem cell transplantation. However, the high cost of maintaining donor registries and cord blood banks, limited size of the cord blood units, and high-risk nature of the ablative procedure limit the expansion of these donor sources as well. HLA haploidentical donors are an attractive choice for stem cells since nearly every patient has an available haploidentical donor from their family. In modern medicine, new strategies such as "megadose stem cell infusions" and posttransplantation immunosuppression with cyclophosphamide have shown the ability to overcome graft failure and GvHD, complications that occurred at overwhelmingly high rates and severely limited the application of haploidentical transplantation before the 21st century. Other strategies such as NMAC regimens prior to transplant and pretransplant graft manipulation have demonstrated similar survival rates when compared with HLA-matched allo-HSCT with MAC regimens, but with significantly reduced toxicities associated with HSCT and preservation of the antileukemic properties of immune cells in the donor graft. Future prospective studies to explore the biology of the GvT effects in this setting can provide more perspective on the advantages and drawbacks of haplo-HSCT over "traditional" allo-HSCT, suggest further enhancements of the process, and move this "now-controversial" modality into the standard of care for patients with limited options.

Conflict of Interests

The authors declare that there is no conflict of interests regarding the publication of this paper.

References

[1] S. Ciavarella, A. Milano, F. Dammacco, and F. Silvestris, "Targeted therapies in cancer," *BioDrugs*, vol. 24, no. 2, pp. 77–88, 2010.

[2] E. A. Copelan, "Hematopoietic stem-cell transplantation," *The New England Journal of Medicine*, vol. 354, no. 17, pp. 1813–1826, 2006.

[3] L. Gragert, M. Eapen, E. Williams et al., "HLA match likelihoods for hematopoietic stem-cell grafts in the U.S. registry," *The New England Journal of Medicine*, vol. 371, no. 4, pp. 339–348, 2014.

[4] J. Dehn, M. Arora, S. Spellman et al., "Unrelated donor hematopoietic cell transplantation: factors associated with a better HLA match," *Biology of Blood and Marrow Transplantation*, vol. 14, no. 12, pp. 1334–1340, 2008.

[5] M. Shabbir-Moosajee, L. Lombardi, and S. O. Ciurea, "An overview of conditioning regimens for haploidentical stem cell transplantation with post-transplantation cyclophosphamide," *American Journal of Hematology*, vol. 90, no. 6, pp. 541–548, 2015.

[6] K. K. Ballen, E. Gluckman, and H. E. Broxmeyer, "Umbilical cord blood transplantation: the first 25 years and beyond," *Blood*, vol. 122, no. 4, pp. 491–498, 2013.

[7] N. J. Chao, L.-P. Koh, G. D. Long et al., "Adult recipients of umbilical cord blood transplants after nonmyeloablative preparative regimens," *Biology of Blood and Marrow Transplantation*, vol. 10, no. 8, pp. 569–575, 2004.

[8] M. J. Laughlin, J. Barker, B. Bambach et al., "Hematopoietic engraftment and survival in adult recipients of umbilical-cord blood from unrelated donors," *The New England Journal of Medicine*, vol. 344, no. 24, pp. 1815–1822, 2001.

[9] G. D. Long, M. Laughlin, B. Madan et al., "Unrelated umbilical cord blood transplantation in adult patients," *Biology of Blood and Marrow Transplantation*, vol. 9, no. 12, pp. 772–780, 2003.

[10] D. A. Rizzieri, G. D. Long, J. J. Vredenburgh et al., "Successful allogeneic engraftment of mismatched unrelated cord blood following a nonmyeloablative preparative regimen," *Blood*, vol. 98, no. 12, pp. 3486–3488, 2001.

[11] J. N. Barker, T. P. Krepski, T. E. DeFor, S. M. Davies, J. E. Wagner, and D. J. Weisdorf, "Searching for unrelated donor hematopoietic stem cells: availability and speed of umbilical cord blood versus bone marrow," *Biology of Blood and Marrow Transplantation*, vol. 8, no. 5, pp. 257–260, 2002.

[12] J. Munoz, N. Shah, K. Rezvani et al., "Concise review: umbilical cord blood transplantation: past, present, and future," *Stem Cells Translational Medicine*, vol. 3, no. 12, pp. 1435–1443, 2014.

[13] U. D. Bayraktar, R. E. Champlin, and S. O. Ciurea, "Progress in haploidentical stem cell transplantation," *Biology of Blood and Marrow Transplantation*, vol. 18, no. 3, pp. 372–380, 2012.

[14] L. Garderet, N. Dulphy, C. Douay et al., "The umbilical cord blood $\alpha\beta$ T-cell repertoire: characteristics of a polyclonal and naive but completely formed repertoire," *Blood*, vol. 91, no. 1, pp. 340–346, 1998.

[15] E. W. Petersdorf, T. A. Gooley, C. Anasetti et al., "Optimizing outcome after unrelated marrow transplantation by comprehensive matching of HLA class I and II alleles in the donor and recipient," *Blood*, vol. 92, no. 10, pp. 3515–3520, 1998.

[16] J. E. Wagner, J. Rosenthal, R. Sweetman et al., "Successful transplantation of HLA-matched and HLA-mismatched umbilical cord blood from unrelated donors: analysis of engraftment and acute graft- versus-host disease," *Blood*, vol. 88, no. 3, pp. 795–802, 1996.

[17] T. Bart, M. Boo, S. Balabanova et al., "Impact of selection of cord blood units from the United States and Swiss registries on the cost of banking operations," *Transfusion Medicine and Hemotherapy*, vol. 40, no. 1, pp. 14–20, 2013.

[18] Y. Reisner, F. Aversa, and M. F. Martelli, "Haploidentical hematopoietic stem cell transplantation: state of art," *Bone Marrow Transplantation*, vol. 50, supplement 2, pp. S1–S5, 2015.

[19] J. A. Roth, M. E. Bensink, P. V. O'Donnell, E. J. Fuchs, M. Eapen, and S. D. Ramsey, "Design of a cost–effectiveness analysis alongside a randomized trial of transplantation using umbilical cord blood versus HLA-haploidentical related bone marrow in advanced hematologic cancer," *Journal of Comparative Effectiveness Research*, vol. 3, no. 2, pp. 135–144, 2014.

[20] C. Anasetti, P. G. Beatty, R. Storb et al., "Effect of HLA incompatibility on graft-versus-host disease, relapse, and survival after marrow transplantation for patients with leukemia or lymphoma," *Human Immunology*, vol. 29, no. 2, pp. 79–91, 1990.

[21] R. C. Ash, M. M. Horowitz, R. P. Gale et al., "Bone marrow transplantation from related donors other than HLA-identical siblings: effect of T cell depletion," *Bone Marrow Transplantation*, vol. 7, no. 6, pp. 443–452, 1991.

[22] Y. Kanda, S. Chiba, H. Hirai et al., "Allogeneic hematopoietic stem cell transplantation from family members other than HLA-identical siblings over the last decade (1991–2000)," *Blood*, vol. 102, no. 4, pp. 1541–1547, 2003.

[23] Y. Morishima, T. Yabe, K. Matsuo et al., "Effects of HLA allele and killer immunoglobulin-like receptor ligand matching on clinical outcome in leukemia patients undergoing transplantation with T-cell-replete marrow from an unrelated donor," *Biology of Blood and Marrow Transplantation*, vol. 13, no. 3, pp. 315–328, 2007.

[24] R. Szydlo, J. M. Goldman, J. P. Klein et al., "Results of allogeneic bone marrow transplants for leukemia using donors other than HLA-identical siblings," *Journal of Clinical Oncology*, vol. 15, no. 5, pp. 1767–1777, 1997.

[25] T. Kawase, Y. Morishima, K. Matsuo et al., "High-risk HLA allele mismatch combinations responsible for severe acute graft-versus-host disease and implication for its molecular mechanism," *Blood*, vol. 110, no. 7, pp. 2235–2241, 2007.

[26] L. Oevermann and R. Handgretinger, "New strategies for haploidentical transplantation," *Pediatric Research*, vol. 71, no. 4, part 2, pp. 418–426, 2012.

[27] Y. Reisner, I. Ben-Bassat, D. Douer, A. Kaploon, E. Schwartz, and B. Ramot, "Demonstration of clonable alloreactive host T cells in a primate model for bone marrow transplantation," *Proceedings of the National Academy of Sciences of the United States of America*, vol. 83, no. 11, pp. 4012–4015, 1986.

[28] F. Aversa, A. Terenzi, A. Tabilio et al., "Full haplotype-mismatched hematopoietic stem-cell transplantation: a phase II study in patients with acute leukemia at high risk of relapse," *Journal of Clinical Oncology*, vol. 23, no. 15, pp. 3447–3454, 2005.

[29] C. Peters, S. Matthes-Martin, G. Fritsch et al., "Transplantation of highly purified peripheral blood CD34+ cells from HLA-mismatched parental donors in 14 children: evaluation of early monitoring of engraftment," *Leukemia*, vol. 13, no. 12, pp. 2070–2078, 1999.

[30] Y. Reisner, N. Kapoor, D. Kirkpatrick et al., "Transplantation for severe combined immunodeficiency with HLA-A, B, D, DR incompatible parental marrow cells fractionated by soybean agglutinin and sheep red blood cells," *Blood*, vol. 61, no. 2, pp. 341–348, 1983.

[31] T. Klingebiel, J. Cornish, M. Labopin et al., "Results and factors influencing outcome after fully haploidentical hematopoietic stem cell transplantation in children with very high-risk acute lymphoblastic leukemia: impact of center size: an analysis on behalf of the Acute Leukemia and Pediatric Disease Working Parties of the European Blood and Marrow Transplant group," *Blood*, vol. 115, no. 17, pp. 3437–3446, 2010.

[32] N. A. Kernan, C. Bordignon, C. A. Keever et al., "Graft failures after T cell depleted marrow transplants for leukemia: clinical and in vitro characteristics," *Transplantation Proceedings*, vol. 19, no. 6, supplement 7, pp. 29–32, 1987.

[33] R. C. Barfield, M. Otto, J. Houston et al., "A one-step large-scale method for T- and B-cell depletion of mobilized PBSC for allogeneic transplantation," *Cytotherapy*, vol. 6, no. 1, pp. 1–6, 2004.

[34] W. Leung, "Use of NK cell activity in cure by transplant," *British Journal of Haematology*, vol. 155, no. 1, pp. 14–29, 2011.

[35] C. Bottino, L. Moretta, D. Pende, M. Vitale, and A. Moretta, "Learning how to discriminate between friends and enemies, a lesson from natural killer cells," *Molecular Immunology*, vol. 41, no. 6-7, pp. 569–575, 2004.

[36] A. Moretta, F. Locatelli, and L. Moretta, "Human NK cells: from HLA class I-specific killer Ig-like receptors to the therapy of acute leukemias," *Immunological Reviews*, vol. 224, no. 1, pp. 58–69, 2008.

[37] W. Leung, R. Iyengar, V. Turner et al., "Determinants of antileukemia effects of allogeneic NK cells," *The Journal of Immunology*, vol. 172, no. 1, pp. 644–650, 2004.

[38] L. Ruggeri, A. Mancusi, M. Capanni et al., "Donor natural killer cell allorecognition of missing self in haploidentical hematopoietic transplantation for acute myeloid leukemia: challenging its predictive value," *Blood*, vol. 110, no. 1, pp. 433–440, 2007.

[39] F. Locatelli, D. Pende, R. Maccario, M. C. Mingari, A. Moretta, and L. Moretta, "Haploidentical hemopoietic stem cell transplantation for the treatment of high-risk leukemias: how NK cells make the difference," *Clinical Immunology*, vol. 133, no. 2, pp. 171–178, 2009.

[40] R. Handgretinger, X. Chen, M. Pfeiffer et al., "Feasibility and outcome of reduced-intensity conditioning in haploidentical transplantation," *Annals of the New York Academy of Sciences*, vol. 1106, pp. 279–289, 2007.

[41] J. M. Goldman, R. P. Gale, M. M. Horowitz et al., "Bone marrow transplantation for chronic myelogenous leukemia in chronic phase: increased risk for relapse associated with T-cell depletion," *Annals of Internal Medicine*, vol. 108, no. 6, pp. 806–814, 1988.

[42] A. M. Marmont, M. M. Horowitz, R. P. Gale et al., "T-cell depletion of HLA-identical transplants in leukemia," *Blood*, vol. 78, no. 8, pp. 2120–2130, 1991.

[43] S. Chaleff, M. Otto, R. C. Barfield et al., "A large-scale method for the selective depletion of $\alpha\beta$ T lymphocytes from PBSC for allogeneic transplantation," *Cytotherapy*, vol. 9, no. 8, pp. 746–754, 2007.

[44] E. Rådestad, H. Wikell, M. Engström et al., "Alpha/beta T-cell depleted grafts as an immunological booster to treat graft failure after hematopoietic stem cell transplantation with HLA-matched related and unrelated donors," *Journal of Immunology Research*, vol. 2014, Article ID 578741, 14 pages, 2014.

[45] M. Bonneville, R. L. O'Brien, and W. K. Born, "$\gamma\delta$ T cell effector functions: a blend of innate programming and acquired plasticity," *Nature Reviews Immunology*, vol. 10, no. 7, pp. 467–478, 2010.

[46] S. Chiplunkar, S. Dhar, D. Wesch, and D. Kabelitz, "$\gamma\delta$ T cells in cancer immunotherapy: current status and future prospects," *Immunotherapy*, vol. 1, no. 4, pp. 663–678, 2009.

[47] K. T. Godder, P. J. Henslee-Downey, J. Mehta et al., "Long term disease-free survival in acute leukemia patients recovering with increased $\gamma\delta$ T cells after partially mismatched related donor bone marrow transplantation," *Bone Marrow Transplantation*, vol. 39, no. 12, pp. 751–757, 2007.

[48] J. L. M. Ferrara and P. Reddy, "Pathophysiology of graft-versus-host disease," *Seminars in Hematology*, vol. 43, no. 1, pp. 3–10, 2006.

[49] A. Q. Gomes, D. S. Martins, and B. Silva-Santos, "Targeting $\gamma\delta$ T lymphocytes for cancer immunotherapy: from novel mechanistic insight to clinical application," *Cancer Research*, vol. 70, no. 24, pp. 10024–10027, 2010.

[50] W. Scheper, S. Van Dorp, S. Kersting et al., "$\gamma\delta$ T cells elicited by CMV reactivation after allo-SCT cross-recognize CMV and leukemia," *Leukemia*, vol. 27, no. 6, pp. 1328–1338, 2013.

[51] D. Balashov, A. Shcherbina, M. Maschan et al., "Single-center experience of unrelated and haploidentical stem cell transplantation with TCR$\alpha\beta$ and CD19 depletion in children with primary immunodeficiency syndromes," *Biology of Blood and Marrow Transplantation*, vol. 21, no. 11, pp. 1955–1962, 2015.

[52] C. Anasetti, D. Amos, P. G. Beatty et al., "Effect of HLA compatibility on engraftment of bone marrow transplants in patients with leukemia or lymphoma," *The New England Journal of Medicine*, vol. 320, no. 4, pp. 197–204, 1989.

[53] P. G. Beatty, R. A. Clift, E. M. Mickelson et al., "Marrow transplantation from related donors other than HLA-identical siblings," *The New England Journal of Medicine*, vol. 313, no. 13, pp. 765–771, 1985.

[54] "The host barrier in animal models of T-cell depleted allogeneic bone marrow transplantation. T-cell depletion in allogeneic bone marrow transplantation," in *Serono Symposia Review*, Y. Reisner, T. Lapidot, T. S. Singer, and E. Schwartz, Eds., 1988.

[55] P. J. Martin, "The role of donor lymphoid cells in allogeneic marrow engraftment," *Bone Marrow Transplantation*, vol. 6, no. 5, pp. 283–289, 1990.

[56] R. J. Soiffer, P. Mauch, N. J. Tarbell et al., "Total lymphoid irradiation to prevent graft rejection in recipients of HLA non-identical T cell-depleted allogeneic marrow," *Bone Marrow Transplantation*, vol. 7, no. 1, pp. 23–33, 1991.

[57] F. Aversa, A. Tabilio, A. Velardi et al., "Treatment of high-risk acute leukemia with T-cell-depleted stem cells from related donors with one fully mismatched hla haplotype," *The New England Journal of Medicine*, vol. 339, no. 17, pp. 1186–1193, 1998.

[58] E. Bachar-Lustig, N. Rachamim, H.-W. Li, F. Lan, and Y. Reisner, "Megadose of T cell-depleted bone marrow overcomes MHC barriers in sublethally irradiated mice," *Nature Medicine*, vol. 1, no. 12, pp. 1268–1273, 1995.

[59] F. Aversa, A. Tabilio, A. Terenzi et al., "Successful engraftment of T-cell-depleted haploidentical 'three-loci' incompatible transplants in leukemia patients by addition of recombinant human granulocyte colony-stimulating factor-mobilized peripheral blood progenitor cells to bone marrow inoculum," *Blood*, vol. 84, no. 11, pp. 3948–3955, 1994.

[60] Y. Reisner and M. F. Martelli, "Bone marrow transplantation across HLA barriers by increasing the number of transplanted cells," *Immunology Today*, vol. 16, no. 9, pp. 437–440, 1995.

[61] E. Naparstek, M. Delukina, R. Or et al., "Engraftment of marrow allografts treated with Campath-1 monoclonal antibodies," *Experimental Hematology*, vol. 27, no. 7, pp. 1210–1218, 1999.

[62] J. L. M. Ferrara, R. Levy, and N. J. Chao, "Pathophysiologic mechanisms of acute graft-vs.-host disease," *Biology of Blood and Marrow Transplantation*, vol. 5, no. 6, pp. 347–356, 1999.

[63] N. A. Kernan, G. Bartsch, R. C. Ash et al., "Analysis of 462 transplantations from unrelated donors facilitated by the national marrow donor program," *The New England Journal of Medicine*, vol. 328, no. 9, pp. 593–602, 1993.

[64] L. Luznik, P. V. O'Donnell, H. J. Symons et al., "HLA-haploidentical bone marrow transplantation for hematologic malignancies using nonmyeloablative conditioning and high-dose, posttransplantation cyclophosphamide," *Biology of Blood and Marrow Transplantation*, vol. 14, no. 6, pp. 641–650, 2008.

[65] H. Ogawa, K. Ikegame, S. Yoshihara et al., "Unmanipulated HLA 2-3 antigen-mismatched (haploidentical) stem cell transplantation using nonmyeloablative conditioning," *Biology of Blood and Marrow Transplantation*, vol. 12, no. 10, pp. 1073–1084, 2006.

[66] S. Kreiter, N. Winkelmann, P. M. Schneider et al., "Failure of sustained engraftment after non-myeloablative conditioning with low-dose TBI and T cell-reduced allogeneic peripheral stem cell transplantation," *Bone Marrow Transplantation*, vol. 28, no. 2, pp. 157–161, 2001.

[67] J. R. Passweg, S. Meyer-Monard, M. Gregor et al., "Non-myeloablative stem cell transplantation: high stem cell dose will not compensate for T cell depletion in allogeneic non-myeloablative stem cell transplantation," *Bone Marrow Transplantation*, vol. 30, no. 5, pp. 267–271, 2002.

[68] D. A. Rizzieri, L. P. Koh, G. D. Long et al., "Partially matched, nonmyeloablative allogeneic transplantation: clinical outcomes and immune reconstitution," *Journal of Clinical Oncology*, vol. 25, no. 6, pp. 690–697, 2007.

[69] P. V. O'Donnell, L. Luznik, R. J. Jones et al., "Nonmyeloablative bone marrow transplantation from partially HLA-mismatched related donors using posttransplantation cyclophosphamide," *Biology of Blood and Marrow Transplantation*, vol. 8, no. 7, pp. 377–386, 2002.

[70] H. Mayumi, K. Himeno, N. Tokuda, and K. Nomoto, "Drug-induced tolerance to allografts in mice. VII. Optimal protocol and mechanism of cyclophosphamide-induced tolerance in an H-2 haplotype-identical strain combination," *Transplantation Proceedings*, vol. 18, no. 2, pp. 363–369, 1986.

[71] H. Mayumi, M. Umesue, and K. Nomoto, "Cyclophosphamide-induced immunological tolerance: an overview," *Immunobiology*, vol. 195, no. 2, pp. 129–139, 1996.

[72] L. Luznik, S. Jalla, L. W. Engstrom, R. Lannone, and E. J. Fuchs, "Durable engraftment of major histocompatibility complex-incompatible cells after nonmyeloablative conditioning with fludarabine, low-dose total body irradiation, and posttransplantation cyclophosphamide," *Blood*, vol. 98, no. 12, pp. 3456–3464, 2001.

[73] L. Luznik, L. W. Engstrom, R. Iannone, and E. J. Fuchs, "Post-transplantation cyclophosphamide facilitates engraftment of major histocompatibility complex-identical allogeneic marrow in mice conditioned with low-dose total body irradiation," *Biology of Blood and Marrow Transplantation*, vol. 8, no. 3, pp. 131–138, 2002.

[74] R. J. Jones, J. P. Barber, M. S. Vala et al., "Assessment of aldehyde dehydrogenase in viable cells," *Blood*, vol. 85, no. 10, pp. 2742–2746, 1995.

[75] S. Sakaguchi, N. Sakaguchi, M. Asano, M. Itoh, and M. Toda, "Immunologic self-tolerance maintained by activated T cells expressing IL-2 receptor α-chains (CD25): breakdown of a single mechanism of self-tolerance causes various autoimmune diseases," *The Journal of Immunology*, vol. 155, no. 3, pp. 1151–1164, 1995.

[76] Z. Fehérvari and S. Sakaguchi, "CD4+ Tregs and immune control," *The Journal of Clinical Investigation*, vol. 114, no. 9, pp. 1209–1217, 2004.

[77] C. I. Kingsley, M. Karim, A. R. Bushell, and K. J. Wood, "CD25+CD4+ regulatory T cells prevent graft rejection: CTLA-4- and IL-10-dependent immunoregulation of alloresponses," *The Journal of Immunology*, vol. 168, no. 3, pp. 1080–1086, 2002.

[78] J. Yu, X. Ren, F. Yan et al., "Alloreactive natural killer cells promote haploidentical hematopoietic stem cell transplantation by expansion of recipient-derived CD4+CD25+ regulatory T cells," *Transplant International*, vol. 24, no. 2, pp. 201–212, 2011.

[79] M. Edinger, P. Hoffmann, J. Ermann et al., "CD4+CD25+ regulatory T cells preserve graft-versus-tumor activity while inhibiting graft-versus-host disease after bone marrow transplantation," *Nature Medicine*, vol. 9, no. 9, pp. 1144–1150, 2003.

[80] A. Trenado, F. Charlotte, S. Fisson et al., "Recipient-type specific CD4+CD25+ regulatory T cells favor immune reconstitution and control graft-versus-host disease while maintaining graft-versus-leukemia," *The Journal of Clinical Investigation*, vol. 112, no. 11, pp. 1688–1696, 2003.

[81] S. C. Jones, G. F. Murphy, and R. Korngold, "Post-hematopoietic cell transplantation control of graft-versus-host disease by donor CD4+25+ T cells to allow an effective graft-versus-leukemia response," *Biology of Blood and Marrow Transplantation*, vol. 9, no. 4, pp. 243–256, 2003.

[82] K. Rezvani, S. Mielke, M. Ahmadzadeh et al., "High donor FOXP3-positive regulatory T-cell (T_{reg}) content is associated with a low risk of GVHD following HLA-matched allogeneic SCT," *Blood*, vol. 108, no. 4, pp. 1291–1297, 2006.

[83] V. H. Nguyen, S. Shashidhar, D. S. Chang et al., "The impact of regulatory T cells on T-cell immunity following hematopoietic cell transplantation," *Blood*, vol. 111, no. 2, pp. 945–953, 2008.

[84] M. Di Ianni, F. Falzetti, A. Carotti et al., "Immunoselection and clinical use of T regulatory cells in HLA-haploidentical stem cell transplantation," *Best Practice & Research: Clinical Haematology*, vol. 24, no. 3, pp. 459–466, 2011.

[85] A. M. Hanash and R. B. Levy, "Donor CD4+CD25+ T cells promote engraftment and tolerance following MHC-mismatched

hematopoietic cell transplantation," *Blood*, vol. 105, no. 4, pp. 1828–1836, 2005.

[86] P. Hoffmann and M. Edinger, "CD4$^+$CD25$^+$ regulatory T cells and graft-versus-host disease," *Seminars in Hematology*, vol. 43, no. 1, pp. 62–69, 2006.

[87] M. Di Ianni, F. Falzetti, A. Carotti et al., "Tregs prevent GVHD and promote immune reconstitution in HLA-haploidentical transplantation," *Blood*, vol. 117, no. 14, pp. 3921–3928, 2011.

[88] M. Di Ianni, B. Del Papa, D. Cecchini et al., "Immunomagnetic isolation of CD4$^+$CD25$^+$FoxP3$^+$ natural T regulatory lymphocytes for clinical applications," *Clinical & Experimental Immunology*, vol. 156, no. 2, pp. 246–253, 2009.

[89] L. M. Williams and A. Y. Rudensky, "Maintenance of the Foxp3-dependent developmental program in mature regulatory T cells requires continued expression of Foxp3," *Nature Immunology*, vol. 8, no. 3, pp. 277–284, 2007.

[90] D. J. Hartigan-O'Connor, C. Poon, E. Sinclair, and J. M. McCune, "Human CD4+ regulatory T cells express lower levels of the IL-7 receptor alpha chain (CD127), allowing consistent identification and sorting of live cells," *Journal of Immunological Methods*, vol. 319, no. 1-2, pp. 41–52, 2007.

[91] M. Battaglia, A. Stabilini, B. Migliavacca, J. Horejs-Hoeck, T. Kaupper, and M.-G. Roncarolo, "Rapamycin promotes expansion of functional CD4$^+$CD25$^+$FOXP3$^+$ regulatory T cells of both healthy subjects and type 1 diabetic patients," *The Journal of Immunology*, vol. 177, no. 12, pp. 8338–8347, 2006.

[92] J. Peccatori, A. Forcina, D. Clerici et al., "Sirolimus-based graft-versus-host disease prophylaxis promotes the in vivo expansion of regulatory T cells and permits peripheral blood stem cell transplantation from haploidentical donors," *Leukemia*, vol. 29, no. 2, pp. 396–405, 2014.

[93] C. Anasetti, B. R. Logan, S. J. Lee et al., "Peripheral-blood stem cells versus bone marrow from unrelated donors," *The New England Journal of Medicine*, vol. 367, no. 16, pp. 1487–1496, 2012.

[94] O. Ringdén, M. Labopin, D. W. Beelen et al., "Bone marrow or peripheral blood stem cell transplantation from unrelated donors in adult patients with acute myeloid leukaemia, an Acute Leukaemia Working Party analysis in 2262 patients," *Journal of Internal Medicine*, vol. 272, no. 5, pp. 472–483, 2012.

[95] A. M. Raiola, A. Dominietto, A. Ghiso et al., "Unmanipulated haploidentical bone marrow transplantation and posttransplantation cyclophosphamide for hematologic malignancies after myeloablative conditioning," *Biology of Blood and Marrow Transplantation*, vol. 19, no. 1, pp. 117–122, 2013.

[96] P. D. Bartolomeo, S. Santarone, G. De Angelis et al., "Haploidentical, unmanipulated, G-CSF-primed bone marrow transplantation for patients with high-risk hematologic malignancies," *Blood*, vol. 121, no. 5, pp. 849–857, 2013.

[97] C. G. Kanakry, S. Ganguly, M. Zahurak et al., "Aldehyde dehydrogenase expression drives human regulatory T cell resistance to posttransplantation cyclophosphamide," *Science Translational Medicine*, vol. 5, no. 211, Article ID 211ra157, 2013.

Burden of Sickle Cell Disease in Ghana: The Korle-Bu Experience

Eugenia V. Asare,[1,2] Ivor Wilson,[1] Amma A. Benneh-Akwasi Kuma ⓘ,[3] Yvonne Dei-Adomakoh ⓘ,[1,3] Fredericka Sey,[1] and Edeghonghon Olayemi ⓘ[1,3]

[1]Ghana Institute of Clinical Genetics, Korle-Bu, Accra, Ghana
[2]Department of Haematology, Korle-Bu Teaching Hospital, Accra, Ghana
[3]Department of Haematology, College of Health Sciences, University of Ghana, Accra, Ghana

Correspondence should be addressed to Edeghonghon Olayemi; eolayemi@ug.edu.gh

Academic Editor: Estella M. Matutes

In Africa, sickle cell disease (SCD) is a major public health problem with over 200,000 babies born per year. In Ghana, approximately 15,000 (2%) of Ghanaian newborns are diagnosed with SCD annually. A retrospective review of medical records of all SCD patients aged 13 years and above, who presented to the sickle cell clinic at Ghana Institute of Clinical Genetics (GICG), Korle-Bu, from 1st January 2013 to 31st December 2014, was carried out, using a data abstraction instrument to document their phenotypes, demographics, attendance/clinic visits, pattern of attendance, and common complications seen. During the period under review 5,451 patients were seen at the GICG, with 20,788 clinic visits. The phenotypes were HbSS (55.7%) and HbSC (39.6%) with other sickle cell phenotypes (4.7%). Out of the 20,788 clinic visits, outpatient visits were 15,802 (76%), and urgent care visits were 4,986 (24%), out of which 128 (2.6%) patients were admitted to the Teaching Hospital for further management of their acute complications. There were 904 patient referrals (out of 5,451 patients) for specialist care; the 3 specialties that had the most referrals were Obstetrics and Gynaecology (168 patients), Orthopaedics (150 patients), and Ophthalmology (143 patients). In 2014, complications seen at KBTH included 53 patients with avascular necrosis (AVN) and 61 patients with chronic leg ulcers. Our centre has a large number of patients living with sickle cell disease. From our experience, early recognition and referral of sickle cell related complications can reduce morbidity and mortality associated with this disease. A multidisciplinary approach to care of SCD patients is therefore important.

1. Introduction

Genetic diseases are very common; and it has been estimated that more than 7 million babies are born each year with a congenital genetic abnormality [1].

Sickle cell disease (SCD) is the most common haemoglobinopathy [1]; it is characterized by inheritance of 2 abnormal haemoglobins of which one is haemoglobin S (HbS). Haemoglobin S (HbS) is a structural variant of normal adult haemoglobin (HbA), inherited as an autosomal recessive Mendelian trait. The most common clinical phenotype is the homozygous form (HbSS or sickle cell anaemia). Compound heterozygous SCD include HbSC, HbSD, HbSO-Arab, and HbS/beta-thalassemia. Heterozygotes are generally less symptomatic compared to those who are homozygous [2].

Sickle cell disease is a major public health problem with over 200,000 babies born per year with SCD in Africa [3, 4]. Approximately 80% of all children born with SCD are in sub-Saharan Africa [1, 5]. In Ghana, 2% (about 15,000) of newborns have SCD, with 55% of them having the homozygous form [6].

Clinical features of SCD include acute pain episodes (which are the hallmark of the disease), anaemia, recurrent infections, and chronic end-organ damage [7, 8]. Newborn screening with early diagnosis and comprehensive care [9–16] has been shown to improve survival since the disease has a high mortality rate in the first few years of life. In 2010, Quinn et al. reported an increased life expectancy in the American SCD population, with over 90% of babies born with SCD currently reaching adulthood [17].

Despite the high prevalence of SCD in Ghana, the extent of the burden of the disease in adults is yet to be quantified and the life expectancy of the Ghanaian SCD patient is not known, though it is generally agreed that more children with the disease now survive into adulthood. Many of the newer modalities of management such as hydroxyurea are not widely used.

The Ghana Institute of Clinical Genetics (GICG) was established in Korle-Bu, Accra, Ghana, in 1974 and currently provides comprehensive outpatient care to both adolescents and adults with SCD, along with community education and research. The premier adult sickle cell clinic in Ghana is located in the institute with the largest number of registered adolescent and adult SCD patients in Ghana. The clinic receives patients (adolescents and adults) from all over Ghana but mainly from the southern part of the country.

This study was designed to outline the burden of sickle cell disease at the GICG and identify the common complications.

2. Materials and Methods

2.1. Study Design. A retrospective two-year chart review of all patient folders and records from January 1st, 2013, to December 31st, 2014, was carried out [2]. Institutional approval was obtained from GICG.

2.2. Study Sites. The GICG located on the campus of Korle-Bu Teaching Hospital renders outpatient services through an outpatient department and an urgent care unit. Referrals are received from other healthcare facilities all over Ghana. It has over 25,000 registered SCD patients. Every year, the clinic records between 10,000 and 15,000 clinic visits with an average daily attendance of almost 50 patients. Patients who need further specialist care are referred to the Teaching Hospital.

2.3. Study Population. The study population was made up of all SCD patients aged 13 years and above who presented to GICG and KBTH within the study period.

2.4. Data Collection. The demographic characteristics, clinical information, and pattern of attendance were obtained from the case files of all eligible patients. A data extraction form was used to document demographic characteristics and clinical information such as age, sex, sickle cell phenotypes, and sickle cell related complications (the data on SCD complications was extracted from the following departments at the Korle-Bu Teaching Hospital: Obstetrics and Gynaecology, Orthopaedics, Ophthalmology, and Urology). The World Health Organization (WHO) age group classification was used as follows: adolescents from 10 to 19 years, adults from 20 to 59 years (young adults from 20 to 39 years; middle age from 40 to 59 years), and elderly from 60 years and above [18]. The age group from 15 to 44 years is considered the reproductive age [18]. For the purposes of this study, our adolescent age group started from 13 to 19 years, because at our centre patients below 13 years are seen in the paediatric department.

2.5. Data Storage and Management. The data collected from the medical records was limited to only information that was necessary to the study. No personal identifiable data was collected. Only the authors had access to the data.

2.6. Data Analysis. Data were captured using Microsoft Access 2010 version, analysed using Excel (windows version 10), reported with simple descriptive statistics such as proportions, ratios, percentages, tables, and histograms.

3. Results

3.1. Phenotypic Patient Burden at GICG. Over the period of review, 5,451 adolescent and adult SCD patients were seen at the study site, with 20,788 clinic visits. The phenotypes were HbSS (55.7%), HbSC (39.6%), and other sickle cell phenotypes (4.7%). The male-to-female ratio was 1:1.6. The ages of patients seen at the clinic during the review ranged from 13 to 87 years with a higher proportion of young adults and middle-aged patients (Figure 1). A third (1,400) of the patients were in the reproductive age group. From age 13 to 44 years, there were more HbSS patients as compared to HbSC (ratio of 2:1). However, this was reversed after the age of 44 years.

3.2. Clinic Visits. Over the two-year study period, there were 20,788 clinic (GICG) visits made by the SCD patients. Approximately 27.5% of the patients made one clinic visit, 52.7% made 2 to 5 clinic visits, and 19.8% made >12 clinic visits per year (Figure 2).

Patients with HbSS phenotype were responsible for 61% of the clinic visits compared with 34% for HbSC and 5% for other phenotypes.

Clinic attendance was highest in January (approximately 1000) and lowest in December (approximately 700), with another increase seen from early May to late July (Table 1).

3.3. Proportion of SCD Patients Who Had Further Specialist Care at KBTH. During the study period, out of 5,451 patients seen, 904 (16.6%) were referred for specialist care at the Teaching Hospital (Table 2). The three specialties that had the most referrals were the Obstetrics and Gynaecology clinic (168 patients), the Orthopaedic clinic (150 patients), and the Ophthalmology clinic (143 patients).

3.4. Common Complications Confirmed in Patients Referred for Specialist Care. Records from the Orthopaedics department, KBTH, in 2014 showed that 53 (68.8%) out of 77 SCD patients seen were diagnosed with radiological evidence of avascular necrosis (AVN). Most patients were diagnosed between the ages of 20-24 years. Forty-nine (92.5%) of these had AVN of the femoral head and 4 (7.5%) had AVN of the humeral head. Only 4 of them had bilateral AVN of the femoral head.

At the Ophthalmology department, 16 (18.6%) out of the 86 patients seen in 2014 were diagnosed with sickle cell retinopathy. Twenty-eight (51.9%) of 54 patients seen by the urologists in 2014 had priapism.

TABLE 1: Pattern of attendance at GICG (2013-2014).

	2013						2014					
Month	HbSS	HbSC	Other	Total	New patients	D.A.A	HbSS	HbSC	Other	Total	New patients	DAA
January	620	350	56	1026	25	46.64	656	333	55	1044	16	47.45
February	540	294	48	888	24	44.40	492	299	33	825	12	41.25
March	514	240	38	790	36	41.58	517	296	29	854	19	42.70
April	330	173	27	530	7	29.44	468	275	39	783	16	39.15
May	551	275	42	868	20	41.33	532	324	41	898	14	44.90
June	537	311	69	919	16	45.95	488	312	46	849	16	40.43
July	621	364	29	1017	27	46.23	523	276	41	842	13	40.10
August	600	343	49	993	28	47.29	578	316	46	940	16	44.77
September	576	307	25	908	13	45.40	531	343	43	919	15	43.76
October	577	342	39	958	21	43.55	443	262	32	737	15	33.50
November	550	313	51	913	24	43.48	492	272	36	804	14	40.20
December	478	269	40	787	10	41.42	427	241	29	696	16	34.80
Total	6494	3581	513	10597	251	43.06	6147	3549	470	10191	182	41.08

DAA: Daily Average Attendance.

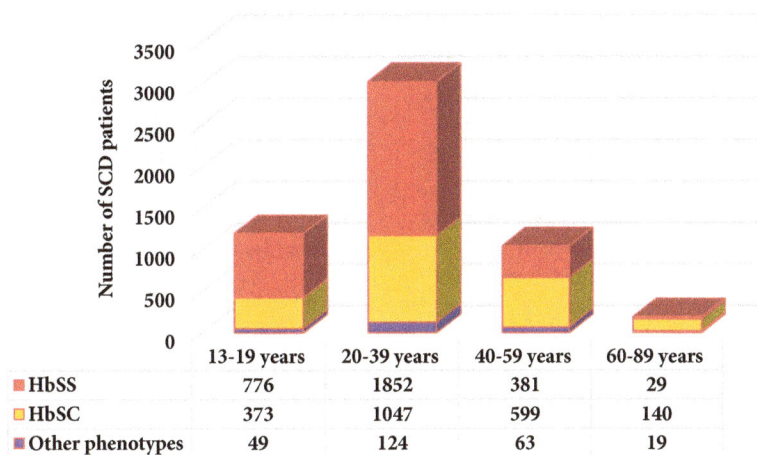

FIGURE 1: Age group and phenotypes of SCD patients.

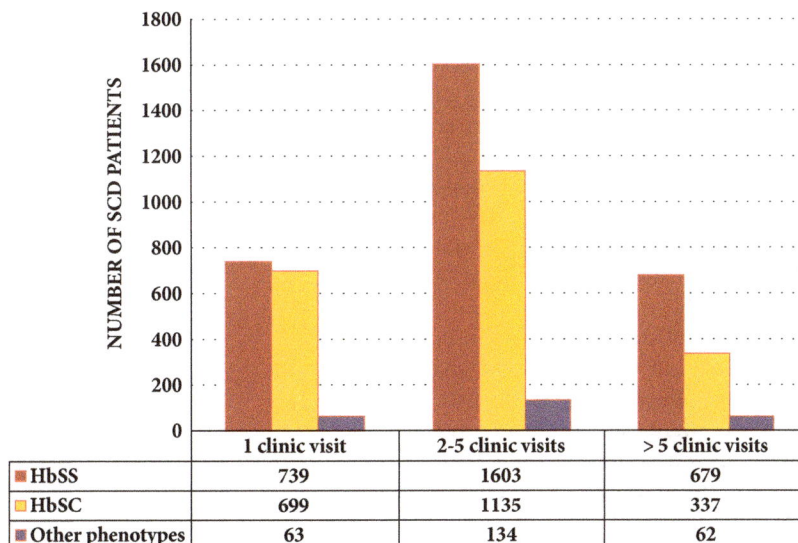

FIGURE 2: Clinic visits by phenotypes.

TABLE 2: SCD patients referred for specialist care.

Specialty	2013	2014	Total
Obstetrics	77	91	168
Orthopaedics	75	75	150
Ophthalmology	70	73	143
Plastics/general surgery	20	53	73
Urology	27	21	48
Nephrology	9	12	21
Others	153	148	301
Total	**431**	**473**	**904**

3.5. Proportion of SCD Patients Seen at GICG with Chronic Leg Ulcers. At the end of 2014, 61 SCD patients were seen at the GICG with chronic leg ulcers who were referred to either the general surgical or plastic surgery units. Chronic leg ulcers were more common in the male sex and phenotype SS and were mostly unilateral.

4. Discussion

Sickle cell disease is a major public health problem in Africa, where over 200,000 babies are born with the disease per year [3, 4]; and about 80% of all children born with SCD are in sub-Saharan Africa [1, 5]. There were more patients with HbSS compared to HbSC in our study (55.7% versus 39.6%) with a higher female-to-male ratio (1.6:1). This agrees with an earlier study by Ohene-Frempong et al. (2008) from Ghana, which showed that 55% of children born with SCD in Ghana had HbSS [6]. From ages of 13 to 44 years, the ratio of HbSS to HbSC was 2:1; this was reversed after 44 years possibly as a result of the higher mortality seen in HbSS patients who have been documented to have a more severe form of the disease [19].

The slightly higher female-to-male ratio in our study may be due to the better health seeking habits of females as compared to males [20] and the fact that in most populations women live longer than men [21]. It is therefore not surprising to see that the women in our cohort had better health maintenance, judging by their attendance. In Ghana, according to WHO data published in 2015, the life expectancy (in years) at birth for the Ghanaian male is 61.0 and the Ghanaian female is 63.9 [21]. This may also contribute to the male-to-female ratio of 1:1.6 seen in this cohort.

Expectedly, HbSS patients accounted for more clinic visits (61%) than other SCD phenotypes, since they are known to have a more severe form of SCD [19].

The effect of the Ghanaian climate was also seen in the pattern of clinic attendance by our patients. Ghana has a tropical climate; temperature in the country varies with season and elevation. In the Southern part of the country where Accra is located, two rainy seasons occur, from April to July and from September to November. The Harmattan, a dry desert wind, blows from the northeast from December to March. The Harmattan lowers humidity, creating hot days and cool nights in the north. In the south, the effects of the Harmattan are felt in January. In most parts of Ghana, the highest temperatures occur in March and the lowest in August [22].

Clinic attendance was lowest in December, probably because of the festive season, and highest after the festive season in January, which is often the peak of Harmattan season with cold, dry conditions, which predisposes SCD patients to developing crises. There was another peak from May to July as a result of the frequent rainfall, cold, and very humid weather conditions; these along with the increase in incidence of malaria [23] may also predispose our patients to ill-health and crises.

Unpublished data from KBTH shows that approximately 200 pregnant women with SCD are seen at the antenatal clinic each year. Despite the well-documented high rates of maternal and foetal morbidity and mortality in pregnant women with SCD [24], there is still a paucity of preconception care or family planning in this population [25, 26]. Given these pregnancy-associated problems for women with SCD, advice about both pregnancy planning and effective contraception is of paramount importance [27].

Our data showed that over 900 patients were referred for further specialist's care and that three specialties (Obstetrics and Gynaecology, Orthopaedics, and Ophthalmology) had over 50% of the referrals. With improved care, more children with SCD now survive into adulthood and are now prone to chronic complications which are more common in adults such as avascular necrosis and retinopathies.

5. Conclusions

Our study confirms that Ghana has a large burden of SCD; a pilot newborn screening program in one of the ten regions of Ghana has shown prevalence of 1.8%, which translates to about 15,000 babies with SCD being born in Ghana every year [6]. It is likely that, with appropriate use of basic medical facilities, more children with SCD now survive into adulthood with the oldest patient in our cohort now in her late 80s. It is almost certain that if Ghana and other African countries are to make an appreciable impact on the care of people living with SCD, more attention has to be paid to providing multidisciplinary care including adequate care at the primary level along with the development and implementation of a national sickle cell disease policy which will include but will not be limited to universal new born screening [28].

Conflicts of Interest

The authors declare that there are no conflicts of interest regarding the publication of this paper.

Authors' Contributions

Eugenia V. Asare and Edeghonghon Olayemi conceived the idea; Ivor Wilson and Eugenia V. Asare performed the data search; Eugenia V. Asare, Ivor Wilson, Amma A. Benneh-Akwasi Kuma, Yvonne Dei-Adomakoh, Fredericka Sey, and Edeghonghon Olayemi analysed the data. All authors participated in writing the article and reviewed and approved the final version before submission.

Acknowledgments

The authors acknowledge the help of the following: (i) Staff, Records Department, Ghana Institute of Clinical Genetics, Korle-Bu, Accra, Ghana; (ii) Dr. Amgbo Asare, Department of Trauma and Orthopaedics, Korle-Bu Teaching Hospital, Korle-Bu, Accra, Ghana; (iii) Dr. Samuel Antwi Oppong, Department of Obstetrics and Gynaecology, School of Medicine and Dentistry, University of Ghana, Accra, Ghana; and (iv) Ms. Mary Ampomah, Ghana Institute of Clinical Genetics, Korle-Bu, Accra, Ghana.

References

[1] B. Modell and M. Darlison, "Global epidemiology of haemoglobin disorders and derived service indicators," *Bulletin of the World Health Organization*, vol. 86, no. 6, pp. 480–487, 2008.

[2] D. C. Rees, T. N. Williams, and M. T. Gladwin, "Sickle-cell disease," *The Lancet*, vol. 376, no. 9757, pp. 2018–2031, 2010.

[3] Press Conference On Raising Awareness Of Sickle-Cell Anaemia—Meetings Coverage and Press Releases. http://www.un.org/press/en/2009/090619_Anaemia.doc.htm.

[4] D. Diallo and G. Tchernia, "Sickle cell disease in Africa," *Current Opinion in Hematology*, vol. 9, no. 2, pp. 111–116, 2002.

[5] F. B. Piel, A. P. Patil, R. E. Howes et al., "Global epidemiology of Sickle haemoglobin in neonates: a contemporary geostatistical model-based map and population estimates," *The Lancet*, vol. 381, no. 9861, pp. 142–151, 2013.

[6] K. Ohene-Frempong, J. Oduro, H. Tetteh, and F. Nkrumah, "Screening newborns for sickle cell disease in Ghana," *Pediatrics*, vol. 121, pp. S120–S121, 2008.

[7] T. N. Williams, S. Uyoga, A. Macharia et al., "Bacteraemia in Kenyan children with sickle-cell anaemia: a retrospective cohort and case-control study," *The Lancet*, vol. 374, no. 9698, pp. 1364–1370, 2009.

[8] J. A. G. Scott, J. A. Berkley, I. Mwangi et al., "Relation between falciparum malaria and bacteraemia in Kenyan children: A population-based, case-control study and a longitudinal study," *The Lancet*, vol. 378, no. 9799, pp. 1316–1323, 2011.

[9] C. J. Wang, P. L. Kavanagh, A. A. Little, J. B. Holliman, and P. G. Sprinz, "Quality-of-care indicators for children with sickle cell disease," *Pediatrics*, vol. 128, no. 3, pp. 484–493, 2011.

[10] M. P. Cober and S. J. Phelps, "Penicillin prophylaxis in children with sickle cell disease," *The Journal of Pediatric Pharmacology and Therapeutics*, vol. 15, no. 3, pp. 152–159, 2010.

[11] R. Hardie, L. King, R. Fraser, and M. Reid, "Prevalence of pneumococcal polysaccharide vaccine administration and incidence of invasive pneumococcal disease in children in Jamaica aged over 4 years with sickle cell disease diagnosed by newborn screening," *Annals of Tropical Paediatrics*, vol. 29, no. 3, pp. 197–202, 2009.

[12] A. M. Ellison, K. V. Ota, K. L. McGowan, and K. Smith-Whitley, "Pneumococcal bacteremia in a vaccinated pediatric sickle cell disease population," *The Pediatric Infectious Disease Journal*, vol. 31, no. 5, pp. 534–536, 2012.

[13] M. T. Lee, S. Piomelli, S. Granger et al., "Stroke prevention Trial in Sickle Cell Anaemia (STOP): extended Follow up and final results," *Blood*, vol. 108, no. 3, pp. 847–852, 2006.

[14] J. Malouf A.J., J. E. Hamrick-Turner, M. C. Doherty, G. S. Dhillon, R. V. Iyer, and M. G. Smith, "Implementation of the STOP protocol for stroke prevention in sickle cell anemia by using duplex power doppler imaging," *Radiology*, vol. 219, no. 2, pp. 359–365, 2001.

[15] S. Charache, "Hydroxyurea as treatment for sickle cell anemia," *Hematology/Oncology Clinics of North America*, vol. 5, no. 3, pp. 571–583, 1991.

[16] M. M. Heeney and R. E. Ware, "Hydroxyurea for Children with Sickle Cell Disease," *Hematology/Oncology Clinics of North America*, vol. 24, no. 1, pp. 199–214, 2010.

[17] C. T. Quinn, Z. R. Rogers, T. L. McCavit, and G. R. Buchanan, "Improved survival of children and adolescents with sickle cell disease," *Blood*, vol. 115, no. 17, pp. 3447–3452, 2010.

[18] Women's health [Internet]. World Health Organization. http://www.who.int/news-room/fact-sheets/detail/women-s-health.

[19] J. Kanter and R. Kruse-Jarres, "Management of sickle cell disease from childhood through adulthood," *Blood Reviews*, vol. 27, no. 6, pp. 279–287, 2013.

[20] A. E. Thompson, Y. Anisimowicz, B. Miedema, W. Hogg, W. P. Wodchis, and K. Aubrey-Bassler, "The influence of gender and other patient characteristics on health care-seeking behaviour: A QUALICOPC study," *BMC Family Practice*, vol. 17, no. 1, 2016.

[21] Global Health Observatory data repository—By category—Life expectancy and healthy life expectancy - Data by WHO region. WHO. http://apps.who.int/gho/data/view.main.SDG2016LEXREGv?lang=en.

[22] Ghana: Geography, Location, weather etc. https://www.ghanaweb.com/GhanaHomePage/geography/climate.php.

[23] T. A. Abeku, "Response to malaria epidemics in Africa," *Emerging Infectious Diseases*, vol. 13, no. 5, pp. 681–686, 2007.

[24] T. K. Boafor, E. Olayemi, N. Galadanci et al., "Pregnancy outcomes in women with sickle-cell disease in low and high income countries: A systematic review and meta-analysis," *BJOG: An International Journal of Obstetrics & Gynaecology*, vol. 123, no. 5, pp. 691–698, 2016.

[25] B. M. Ramesh, S. C. Gulati, and R. D. Retherford, "Contraceptive use in India, 1992-93," National Family Health Survey Subject Reports, International Institute for Population Sciences, October 1996.

[26] K. B. Parmar, S. L. Kantharia, N. R. Godara, H. M. Shah, and M. M. Patni, "A cross-sectional study to understand socio demographic profile of couples who adopted permanent sterilization in urban slums of Surat city," *National Journal of Community Medicine*, vol. 4, no. 3, pp. 443–448, 2013.

[27] A. A. Eissa, S. M. Tuck, K. Rantell, and D. Stott, "Trends in family planning and counselling for women with sickle cell disease in the UK over two decades," *Journal of Family Planning and Reproductive Health Care*, vol. 41, no. 2, pp. 96–101, 2015.

[28] N. Galadanci, B. J. Wudil, T. M. Balogun et al., "Current sickle cell disease management practices in Nigeria," *International Health*, vol. 6, no. 1, pp. 23–28, 2014.

Haploidentical Stem Cell Transplantation in Adult Haematological Malignancies

Kevon Parmesar[1,2] and Kavita Raj[1,3]

[1]*Department of Haematology, Kings College Hospital NHS Foundation Trust, Denmark Hill, London SE5 9RS, UK*
[2]*Kings College London, Kings College Hospital NHS Foundation Trust, Denmark Hill, London SE5 9RS, UK*
[3]*Department of Haematology, Guys and St. Thomas' NHS Foundation Trust, Great Maze Pond, London SE1 9RT, UK*

Correspondence should be addressed to Kevon Parmesar; kevon.parmesar@kcl.ac.uk

Academic Editor: Suparno Chakrabarti

Haematopoietic stem cell transplantation is a well-established treatment option for both hematological malignancies and nonmalignant conditions such as aplastic anemia and haemoglobinopathies. For those patients lacking a suitable matched sibling or matched unrelated donor, haploidentical donors are an alternative expedient donor pool. Historically, haploidentical transplantation led to high rates of graft rejection and GVHD. Strategies to circumvent these issues include T cell depletion and management of complications thereof or T replete transplants with GVHD prophylaxis. This review is an overview of these strategies and contemporaneous outcomes for hematological malignancies in adult haploidentical stem cell transplant recipients.

1. Introduction

Over 50 years ago, it was first demonstrated that total body irradiation (TBI) along with transplantation of genetically identical (syngeneic) bone marrow could induce remission in a minority of patients with end-stage leukaemia [1]. Whilst transplantation was initially limited to bone marrow obtained from an identical twin, later identification of HLA types made the process of allogeneic transplantation possible that is from nonidentical HLA-matched donors such as siblings [2]. Subsequently, allogeneic transplantation was shown to be curative in a small percentage of patients with acute leukaemia who, at that time, were deemed incurable [3]. This was an especially significant outcome, despite frequent setbacks such as aggressive leukaemia progression and posttransplant complications like infection and graft-versus-host disease (GVHD) [4].

Further efforts were therefore focused on exploring how the procedure could become more successful in a greater number of patients. It was later established that transplants were more effective during the first remission of leukaemia, when transplantation could achieve a cure in more than 50 percent of patients [3, 5]. It was also found that patients who suffered subsequent GVHD had a better leukaemia-free survival in the long term [6]. This has now been determined to be part of a graft-versus-tumour effect (graft-versus-leukaemia or GVL effect) in which allogeneic immune cells eliminate occult tumour cells which may have survived the initial conditioning [7, 8].

Even more recently, advances in transplantation techniques have led to improved survival rates and reduced incidence of complications such as GVHD, thus lowering rates of transplant-related morbidity and mortality [9]. These include improved preparative regimens such as reduced intensity conditioning (RIC), which causes less severe side effects whilst still ensuring transplant engraftment [10]. RIC has also enabled transplantation in older, more comorbid populations, where myeloablative (MA) conditioning would have led to more substantive harm. Other techniques used involve better informed measures to prevent or limit GVHD and techniques to reduce the risk of posttransplantation opportunistic infections [4].

Transplantation has now been extended successfully to include HLA-matched unrelated donors with the development of national bone marrow registries in over 50 countries worldwide [4]. Studies have shown that, in some cases, fully matched unrelated donor (MUD) transplants can be comparable with matched related donors (MRD) in terms of disease-free survival and overall survival [11, 12]. Umbilical cord blood has also been identified as a source of haematopoietic stem cells (HSCs) for transplantation [7].

Haematopoietic stem cell transplantation (HSCT) is now a well-established treatment option for conditions such as acute myeloid leukaemia (AML) and myelodysplastic syndromes (MDS), as well as a number of other blood disorders [13]. In European centres alone, close to 15,000 allogeneic transplants were performed in 2013 and this number is increasing annually [14].

2. Limitations of HLA-Matched Transplants

Unfortunately, as few as 30 to 35 percent of patients will have an HLA-identical matched sibling donor available for HSC donation [7]. Furthermore, despite an estimated 25 million HLA-typed potential volunteer donors on the worldwide register [15], it remains difficult for some patients to find timely unrelated donors. This problem is most significant for persons of ethnic backgrounds that vary from the donor pool and persons of mixed heritage. It has been estimated that the chance of success in finding a matched donor ranges from 79% of patients with Caucasian background to less than 20% for some ethnic groups [16]. This is due to a variety of factors, including greater HLA polymorphism among persons of ethnic minorities, a smaller pool of potential donors, and higher rates of attrition from donor registries [17, 18].

Additional difficulties arise when a transplant is needed urgently, for example, in the case of particularly aggressive or rapidly progressing disease. The search for a transplant can often be a lengthy process involving identification, typing, and collection of cells from the stem cell donor. The entire process has been estimated to take a median of 4 months [9]. Shockingly, retrospective data have shown that even after a matched donor is found, only 53% of transplants actually proceed with delays and resultant disease progression being a major factor preventing follow-through [19].

Umbilical cord donations can solve many of these issues, mainly through reduced search times and greater mismatch tolerance [7]. Unfortunately, cord blood produces very few HSCs and therefore double cords may be necessary to provide adequate HSCs in adult patient [20]. The availability of cords from accredited banks is also a significant limiting factor. Engraftment time may be prolonged compared to regular HSCT, leading to prolonged neutropenia and subsequent susceptibility to infection in the posttransplant period. UCBT therefore results in higher rates of posttransplant complications and higher overall transplant-related mortality [9, 21].

3. Haploidentical Transplants as an Option

An alternative option is the transplantation of stem cells from a related donor who is only partially HLA-matched [22].

The genes on chromosome 6, which encode HLA antigens, are very closely linked, and, as a result, a child is likely to inherit one full set of genes from each parent. Each set is referred to as a haplotype. Whilst there is only a 25% chance of siblings sharing the same two parental haplotypes, it is significantly easier for patients to find a family member who is matched fully with only one of the HLA haplotypes (with the other being different). A transplant of this type would be referred to as a haploidentical transplant [23].

Haploidentical transplants offer substantial benefit to patients who have difficulty finding a matching donor, as nearly all patients will have an available haploidentical parent, sibling, child, or other relatives [9]. Haploidentical transplants can therefore improve access to transplantation, especially in ethnic variant patients who may find it near impossible to secure a matching donor. One report has estimated that over 95% of patients can find at least one haploidentical donor, with the average patient having 2 options or more [24].

Haploidentical transplants may provide more choice in donor selection in terms of age, cytomegalovirus status, and ABO compatibility [25]. It also allows easy access to posttransplant cellular therapies like donor lymphocyte infusions, if necessary [21]. Importantly, in case of graft failure, it provides the opportunity for a second graft from the initial donor, or from another family member who is available as an alternative donor.

The immediate availability provided by haploidentical transplants can provide further benefit by reducing associated costs and delays of finding unmatched donors (as described above), thus helping patients who may need a transplant urgently and creating opportunities for many more. These transplants can have a special role in less wealthy countries, where volunteer donor registries may not exist or where cost might be a prohibitive factor for MUD transplants, which are typically more expensive [26].

4. Haploidentical Transplant Strategies

The effects of transplantation with HLA mismatch had been established very early, when researchers sought to determine the acceptable limits to which a mismatched transplant could still be completed successfully. It was found that, compared to patients who had fully matched donors available, patients who underwent haploidentical transplants after myeloablative conditioning (in the form TBI) had higher rates of graft rejection, with the extent of HLA mismatch predicting the incidence risk of graft failure [27]. Another noted complication was acute severe GVHD which developed more often and sooner after transplantation [28]. Mismatched patients had a higher (70 percent) chance of developing GVHD of grades II to IV, which occurred at a median of 14 days, compared to a 42 percent incidence at a median of 22 days for the fully matched control group.

Whilst the intense bidirectional alloreactivity to incompatible HLA molecules was clearly a major limitation to these transplants, it had been hypothesised at that point that the manipulation of donor T-lymphocytes in the transplanted marrow could alleviate some of the effects of graft rejection and GVHD. Prior studies had shown that T cell depleted transplantation reduced rates of GVHD but increased rates of graft failure, potentially due to immunologic rejection via residual recipient T-cytotoxic lymphocyte precursors with antidonor specificity [29]. On the other hand, transfusion of "buffy coat" peripheral lymphocytes reduced graft rejection but led to a higher incidence of chronic GVHD, likely due to activation of effector T cells against host tissue [30].

In order to circumvent these problems, strategies centred around two major modalities [21]. Firstly, the transplant could be depleted of T cells using one of several techniques, followed by various measures taken to improve engraftment rates and reduce infectious complications. Otherwise, the transplant could be T cell replete, but with measures taken to reduce the risk of GVHD. A number of these strategies and their corresponding biological rationales are detailed below.

4.1. T Cell Depleted Transplantation

4.1.1. T Cell Depletion with Megadose of Positively Selected CD34+ Progenitors. The earliest attempt focused on T cell depleted transplantation in patients with end-stage chemoresistant leukaemia and involved the use of an extremely myeloablative, immunosuppressive conditioning regimen (using 8 Gy unfractionated TBI, 50 mg/kg ×2 cyclophosphamide, rabbit anti-thymocyte globulin 25 mg/kg (ATG), and 10 mg/kg thiotepa) in order to assist engraftment [31, 32]. Key to overcoming the HLA mismatch was the infusion of a "megadose" of HSCs obtained by adding granulocyte colony stimulating factor (G-CSF) mobilised stem cells to bone marrow cells that were T cell depleted by soybean agglutinin and E-rosetting. This rationale was based on numerous preclinical studies that achieved high rates of engraftment using large doses of T cell depleted bone marrow. Preliminary follow-up showed a high engraftment rate (16 out of 17 patients engrafted successfully), and overall the regimen resulted in engraftment for 80 percent of patients with only 18% incidence of acute GVHD and no chronic GVHD reported.

Further modifications included the purification and positive immunoselection of CD34+ HSCs, in addition to further depletion of T cells and also B cells (to prevent EBV-related lymphoproliferative disorders) [33]. Fludarabine then replaced cyclophosphamide, the dose of TBI was reduced, and posttransplant G-CSF was removed from the protocol. Overall, 255 patients with acute leukaemia were treated, with engraftment rates of 95% and very low rates of both acute and chronic GVHD (only 5% of patients treated under the revised regimen suffered from acute GVHD grade II or higher).

These results confirmed that a megadose of CD34+ HSCs could overcome histocompatibility barriers by "veto activity," where a group of cells has the ability to specifically inhibit a cytotoxic T-lymphocyte precursor (CTLp) cell response, against antigens presented by those veto cells [21, 34]. It is thought that CD34+ cells, or a group of cells comprising part of the CD34+ megadose, could veto any residual antidonor CTLp activity that had previously acted to reject the graft. These carefully designed alterations to the graft demonstrated clearly that, by depleting T cells to less than 2×10^4/kg sufficiently, GVHD can be effectively prevented [33]. It is noteworthy that no posttransplant immunosuppression was

used in these patients, giving the added benefit of lower rates of leukaemia relapse.

The Achilles heel of this carefully constructed plan was delayed immune reconstitution resulting in nonrelapse mortality (NRM) as high as 57%, particularly due to opportunistic infections by viral and fungal pathogens. In response to this threat, donor T cell clones were raised in vivo against CMV and *Aspergillus* antigens, screened to be non-cross-reactive to the recipient, and were effective as posttransplant immunotherapy in doses up to 1×10^6/kg. Additional analyses of these patients highlighted that NK alloreactive donors impacted favourably upon the survival of patients with AML patients transplanted in CR with event-free survival of 67% compared to 18% in those without an NK alloreactive donor.

4.1.2. T Cell Depletion with Reduced Intensity Conditioning. RIC conditioning with reduced doses of fludarabine, thiotepa, and melphalan [35] and a CD3/CD19 depleted graft using anti-CD3 monoclonal antibody (OKT-3) was tried in a limited number of patients. Because of the less myeloablative conditioning and lack of a megadose, several modifications were necessary to promote engraftment. OKT-3 was chosen over ATG as it was thought to spare incoming donor NK cells, which could aid in engraftment. Additionally, a newer method of T cell depletion was developed involving the use of microbeads coated with anti-CD3 and anti-CD19 to negatively deplete B- and T-lymphocytes, whilst CD34+ stem cells, CD34– progenitor cells, NK cells, dendritic cells, and other engraftment-facilitating cells were spared. The graft contained a median of 7.8×10^6/kg CD34+ cells, 5×10^7/kg CD56+ cells, and less than 2×10^4/kg CD3+ cells.

This CD3/CD19 depleted haploidentical transplant was carried out on 61 adult patients with high-risk leukaemia. Rapid engraftment was observed with significant numbers of granulocytes and platelets present at 11 and 12 days after transplant, respectively. Overall TRM rates were comparable to the previous MA study [33], even in the older and higher-risk population used in this study. One limitation, however, was higher rates of grade II to IV acute and limited chronic GVHD (46% and 18%, resp.) when compared to the positively selected CD34+ transplants with cells probably as a result of higher doses of T cells being administered.

4.1.3. Other Selective T Cell Depletion Methods. Other methods of selective T cell depletion are also being investigated in smaller clinical trials [36, 37]. For example, one study sought to first activate donor T cells in vitro by culturing the cells with host cells (known as a mixed lymphocyte culture system). Activated alloreactive T cells proceed to express the CD25 membrane protein (interleukin 2Rα), allowing differentiation from nonalloreactive T cells. A CD25 immunotoxin was then used to selectively deplete these T cells whilst sparing those that assist in defence against infection [36].

Engraftment was achieved fully in 10 out of 16 paediatric patients in the study, with partial chimerism seen in five other patients. Early results indicated that there were no cases of GVHD above grade II, and importantly 12 patients showed signs of preserved immune responses.

Another study sought to use photodepletion to remove alloreactive T cells, which were found to selectively accumulate a photo-sensitizing compound known as 4,5-dibromorhodamine 123 (TH9402) [37]. Again, cells were stimulated in vitro and then selectively T cell depleted and infused into the patient. Of 24 patients who began the study, 11 patients survived for a median of 30 months. Incidence of grade III and IV GVHD was 13%, and six patients suffered relapse. Immune reconstitution, however, was still observed to be delayed.

4.1.4. CD45RA Depletion. A novel strategy used to circumvent issues commonly encountered in T cell depleted transplants, (namely, delayed immune reconstitution and graft failure) is the specific depletion of naïve T cells and terminal effector cells. The CD45RA cell marker can be found on naïve T cells, fully matured cells that have never encountered antigens specific to their T cell receptor [38]. These cells remain alloreactive and proliferate upon activation. Studies have suggested that these CD45RA+ naïve T cells are largely responsible for posttransplant GVH reactions and that infusions of memory T cells, lacking CD45RA+ cells, do not induce GVHD reactions [39–41]. Further study has shown that selective depletion of CD45RA+ cells is possible in donor leukapheresis products [42].

A trial at St. Jude Children's Research Hospital in Memphis, USA, was conducted to investigate the feasibility of CD45RA+ depletion in haploidentical transplantation, for paediatric patients with high-risk malignancy [43]. Eight patients with relapsed or refractory solid tumours received two cell product infusions, CD3+ depleted and CD45RA+ depleted, respectively, from KIR2DL1 mismatched donors. Infusions met a minimum CD34+ dose of 2×10^6 cells/kg and were below a maximum dose of 1×10^5 CD3+ cells/kg. All eight patients engrafted neutrophils successfully within 14 days. Despite high-risk disease and the high likelihood of TRM, the regimen was well tolerated with no cases of acute GVHD. It is also important to note that GVHD prophylaxis consisted solely of a brief course of sirolimus.

4.1.5. Treg/Tcon Haploidentical Transplants. Further attempts to manipulate transplants involve the use of combinations of regulatory T cells (Tregs) and conventional T cells (Tcons), working in tandem to provide substantial GVL effect whilst moderating the acute and chronic GVH effects. Thymus derived, naturally occurring Tregs are identified by CD4+ CD25+ FoxP3+ cell markers and are primarily involved in regulation of immune activity and maintenance of physiological self-tolerance [44, 45]. In animal models, these cells have been shown to suppress GVHD whilst maintaining the GVL effects of Tcons [46].

One study of 43 patients with high-risk acute leukaemia sought to investigate whether this Treg/Tcon coinfusion immunotherapy could replicate results seen in animal models [47]. Conditioning was MA and included TBI, thiotepa, and fludarabine, as well as either cyclophosphamide, alemtuzumab, or thymoglobulin. It is important to note that no GVHD prophylaxis was used. Overall results were encouraging, with a sustained engraftment rate of 95 percent and only 15 percent of patients developing acute GVHD (grades II to IV). The low rates of GVHD observed combined with the extremely low rates of relapse (cumulative incidence of 0.05) in a high-risk population suggest that the powerful Tcon derived GVL effect was maintained, despite Treg mediated GVHD suppression.

4.1.6. Graft Selection and NK Cell Alloreactivity. Although it would be expected that the extensive depletion of T cells would lead to loss of the GVL effect and a subsequent increase in posttransplantation leukaemia relapse rate, this was not observed in the T cell depleted studies. A potential reason for this is the alloreactivity of transplanted donor-derived natural killer (NK) cells [48]. NK cells have been found to possess inhibitory receptors known as "killer cell immunoglobulin-like receptors" or KIRs, which recognise KIR ligands shared by self-HLA molecules. On ligand presentation, these KIRs become "licensed" to react to allogeneic targets that do not express self-HLA KIR ligands. In haplotype-mismatched transplantation, NK cells develop in the bone marrow surrounded by cells of donor haplotype and thus become alloreactive to recipient leukaemia cells that lack the donor HLA KIR ligand.

A study of 112 patients who received haploidentical transplants demonstrated that transplantation from NK alloreactive donors, those who possessed HLA class I KIR ligands which were absent in the recipient as well as alloreactive NK cell clones, had a significantly lower incidence of leukaemia relapse (3% versus 47%) when transplanted in remission. Furthermore, transplantation from NK alloreactive donors led to overall better event-free survival rates and reduced risk of relapse or death. Maternal donation also provided protection from leukaemia relapse, additional to any benefit gained from NK alloreactive donation [49]. This is thought to be a result of maternal exposure to foetal antigens during pregnancy, leading to maternal memory T cell tolerance to the paternal HLA haplotype present in the foetus. This information can be useful in choosing the best potential donor when several are made available, as might be the case with haploidentical transplantation.

4.2. T Cell Replete Transplantation

4.2.1. High Dose Cyclophosphamide Posttransplantation. An alternative to complete T cell depletion is the selective depletion of T cells responsible for alloreactivity (leading to GVHD and graft rejection), whilst sparing the nonalloreactive T cell population which provides immune reconstitution and protection against infection (leading to a reduced TRM rate) [50, 51]. Cyclophosphamide (Cy) provides a unique way of achieving this. Cy has previously been used as part of a MA regimen, administered prior to transplantation to suppress the recipient immune system [52]. The effects of Cy are time dependent, and preclinical studies showed that when administered as a properly timed, high dose after transplantation (between 60 and 72 hours), it reduces incidence of both GVHD and graft rejection [53]. Cy is thought to affect both donor and recipient derived proliferating alloreactive T cells selectively, whilst sparing nonproliferating nonalloreactive T cells.

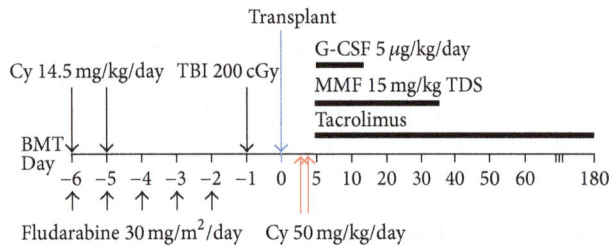

FIGURE 1: Conditioning regimen used for nonmyeloablative haplo-identical transplantation, using high dose cyclophosphamide (Cy) posttransplant for in vitro T cell depletion. Pretransplant conditioning involved Cy, fludarabine, and TBI, with administration of high dose Cy on day 3 (or days 3 and 4) after transplantation. GVHD prophylaxis consisting of tacrolimus and MMF was initiated after Cy. BMT: bone marrow transplantation, Cy: cyclophosphamide, TBI: total body irradiation, G-CSF: granulocyte colony stimulating factor, and MMF: mycophenolate mofetil.

It has also been observed to be less toxic to HSCs due to their high expression of its inactivating enzyme, aldehyde dehydrogenase (ALDH).

One study used a nonmyeloablative approach in order to reduce the likelihood of transplant-related mortality and also in the hope that, in case of graft rejection, autologous haematopoiesis could recommence [50]. Pretransplant conditioning involved Cy, fludarabine, and TBI, with administration of high dose Cy on day 3 (or days 3 and 4) after transplantation. GVHD prophylaxis consisting of tacrolimus and MMF was initiated after Cy. This regimen is illustrated in Figure 1. Whilst engraftment was sustained in a majority of patients (57 of 66), acute and chronic GVHD incidences were low (27% and 13% for grades II to IV) and NRM was relatively low (18%); incidence of relapse mortality was shown to be high (55%). This was thought to be partly due to a high-risk trial population and partly due to poor disease eradication by the nonmyeloablative conditioning used, in addition to the lack of GVL effect caused by depleting alloreactive T cells.

A similar procedure has also been carried out using peripheral blood stem cells (PBSCs) as opposed to bone marrow (BM) transplantation [54]. PBSCs are generally preferred in HLA-matched transplantation as they are easier to collect from donors, have higher yields of HSCs, and can lead to better short- and long-term survival. Due to their higher T cell content and increased risk of GVHD, they had previously been avoided in haploidentical transplants. Results have shown that RIC with posttransplant Cy can in fact lead to acceptable rates of GVHD, NRM, and relapse.

In another study, RIC with posttransplant Cy was also performed with conditioning consisting of thiotepa, busulfan, and fludarabine, or TBI plus fludarabine [55]. GVHD prophylaxis consisted of posttransplant Cy on days 3 and 5, ciclosporin, and MMF. Results showed low incidence of grade II to IV acute and chronic GVHD (12% and 10%, resp.) and low incidence of overall TRM (18%). Rate of relapse was also lower than that achieved by RIC in the previous study (26% in this study). Disease-free survival was also lower (68% for patients transplanted in remission and 37% for those transplanted in relapse).

One study has shown that haploidentical transplants using posttransplantation cyclophosphamide can achieve similar outcomes to MRD and MUD transplants [56]. Specifically, in 271 consecutive patients undergoing allogeneic transplantation for haematological malignancy, no significant difference in nonrelapse mortality, relapse, incidence of acute severe GVHD, and overall survival was found. This strategy has been lauded due to its relative success and has a major advantage over manipulated T cell depleted grafts as it can be performed in any centre performing HSCT and does not require specialist graft manipulation.

4.2.2. Posttransplant Rapamycin. An alternative conditioning to promote immune tolerization by increasing circulating TRegs employed treosulfan, fludarabine, ATG, and rituximab for T and B cell depletion and rapamycin/mycophenolate mofetil [57, 58]. Rapamycin was chosen for its activity in the promotion of natural regulatory T cells (Tregs), shown in preclinical models, in contrast with calcineurin inhibitors such as ciclosporin. Tregs play an important role in the induction of transplant tolerance and the prevention of autoimmune reactions [59]. Preclinical models have shown that adoptive transfer of purified natural Tregs can prevent GVHD whilst leaving the desirable graft-versus-leukaemia effect unaffected. Rapamycin also inhibits effector T cell action and has direct antineoplastic activity against haematological malignancies such as acute leukaemia and thus could provide additional benefit.

Fifty-nine patients were transplanted, with conditioning consisting of treosulfan, fludarabine, and ATG and rituximab for T and B cell depletion. GVHD prophylaxis consists of rapamycin and MMF. Engraftment occurred in all patients and was reported to result in fast immune reconstitution. Incidences of acute GVHD (grades II to IV) and chronic GVHD were 29% and 20%, respectively, and incidences of TRM and relapse were 25% and 44%, respectively. High levels of circulating Tregs were observed, which were found to suppress effector T cells when placed in vitro.

4.2.3. G-CSF Priming of Donor Bone Marrow. Another group of researchers sought to overcome the issues of T cell depletion via in vivo modulation of T cell function in the recipient and the donor [60]. The protocol they developed was termed GIAC, representing the four significant protocol adjustments: donor treatment with granulocyte colony stimulating factor (G-CSF), intensified immunologic suppression, infusion of ATG for GVHD prophylaxis, and use of a combination of PBSC and BM cells. Donors were treated with recombinant G-CSF for 5 to 6 consecutive days, with BM harvest occurring on the 4th day and PBSC collection occurring on the 5th day. Additional cells were collected on day 6 if the previous collections were insufficient. Cells were then infused into the recipient, unmanipulated, on the same day. The recipient was conditioned using cytosine arabinoside, busulfan, Cy, semustine, and ATG and treated after transplant with ciclosporin, MMF, and methotrexate as GVHD prophylaxis.

Two hundred and fifty patients with acute leukaemia underwent haploidentical transplantation using this regimen. Of these, 249 had sustained engraftment, with incidence of grade II to IV acute and chronic GVHD being 45.8% and

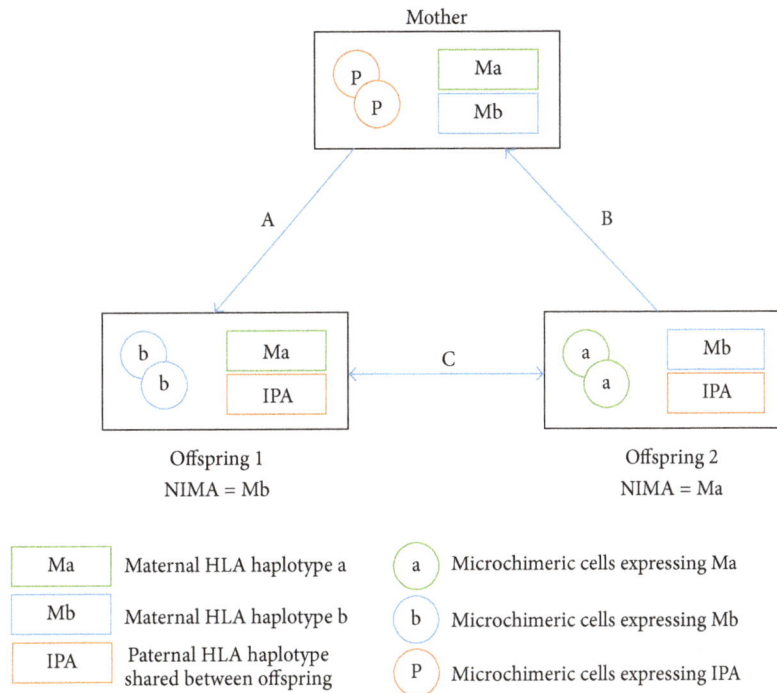

FIGURE 2: Illustration of three types of NIMA-complementary HLA haploidentical stem cell transplants: A, B, and C. Transplantation from mother to offspring (A) causes a graft versus host (GVH) reaction against the inherited paternal antigen (IPA) and a host versus graft (HVG) reaction against the NIMA of offspring 1 (Mb). Transplantation from offspring to mother (B) causes a GVH reaction against the NIMA of offspring 2 (Ma) and HVG reaction against the inherited paternal antigen (IPA). Transplantation between NIMA-mismatched siblings with a shared IPA (C) involves bidirectional mismatch for the NIMA and bidirectional GVH/HVG reactions. Adapted from Ichinohe et al. [63].

53.9%, respectively. Notably, the rates of GVHD were similar to those of HLA-identical allogeneic HSCT, in spite of the lack of extensive in vitro depletion of T cells. The mechanism for this is thought to be a combination of the effects of G-CSF priming of donor cells, in maintaining T cell hyporesponsiveness and encouraging the development of tolerant Th2 cells, as well as the in vivo effects of GVHD prophylaxis and ATG in the conditioning. Furthermore, probability of leukaemia-free survival for standard and high-risk AML was 70.7% and 55.9% and for ALL was 59.7% and 24.8%, which is comparable with previous studies.

Subsequently, another group of researchers has modified this protocol slightly, only using a G-CSF primed BM graft as opposed to combining it with HSCs [61]. Patients in this protocol either were conditioned with myeloablation using cytarabine and cyclophosphamide plus TBI, treosulfan, or busulfan or underwent RIC using fludarabine and melphalan. Extensive GVHD prophylaxis was also used via a combination of five drugs with differing mechanisms, ATG, ciclosporin, methotrexate (MTX), MMF, and basiliximab, an anti-CD25 monoclonal antibody.

80 patients with high-risk haematologic malignancies were transplanted using this protocol. An engraftment rate of 93% was achieved, with incidence of grade II to IV acute and chronic GVHD being 24% and 6%, respectively. Probability of overall survival at three years was 54% for standard risk patients (treated in first or second complete remission) and 33% for high-risk patients (treated in third or later remission, or in active disease).

The largest study done to date using the GIAC protocol involved 1210 consecutive patients transplanted between May 2002 and February 2013 at Peking University Institute of Hematology in China [62]. The study found that under this standardised protocol the degree of HLA mismatch did not significantly correlate with transplant outcomes. Rather, donor characteristics such as age, gender, family relationship, and microchimerism effects (expanded below) were more prognostic of favourable outcomes. Despite the large study number, experience and further data are limited outside of this institution.

4.2.4. Fetomaternal Microchimerism. Ichinohe and colleagues hypothesised that the rates of GVHD and graft rejection could be attenuated by transplanting T cell replete bone marrow or peripheral blood stem cells from mismatched family donors, such as sibling or children donors who were microchimeric for the noninherited maternal antigen (NIMA), or a mother who was microchimeric for the inherited paternal antigen (IPA) [63]. Prior exposure to either ingested or circulating mismatched antigen would have tolerised these donors; hence, T replete transplants with relatively shorter duration of immunosuppression would be possible, offsetting the risks of poor immune reconstitution. A summary of this is illustrated in Figure 2.

Ichinohe et al. reported the multicentre outcomes of 35 such transplants for haematological malignancies (AML 12, ALL 11, CML 7, and lymphoma 5) [63]. The transplants were T cell replete (30 patients received GCSF mobilised

PBSC harvests, four patients bone marrow harvests, and one patient a combination of both), predominantly myeloablative (21 patients/60%) transplant with tacrolimus/methotrexate GVHD prophylaxis in 63%. Posttransplant GCSF was administered in 28 patients. NIMA and IPA haplotypes were deduced based on tissue typing family members from 2 or 3 generations. The presence of recipient specific long-term microchimerism was confirmed by IPA or NIMA specific nested PCR with sequence specific primers. Fifteen donors were IPA mismatched (maternal donor) and 20 were NIMA mismatched (sibling or offspring). Engraftment occurred in 33 evaluable patients at a median of 14 days. The cumulative incidence of grades II–IV aGVHD was 56% (95% CI 38–71%) and III-IV 22% (95% CI 10–37%). The incidence of grades III-IV aGVHD in the NIMA mismatched group was 10% (95% CI 2–26%) and significantly lower than the IPA mismatched group 38% (95% CI 15%–60%). The incidence of cGVHD was 83%, six patients had limited cGVHD, and 13 had extensive cGVHD. Extensive cGVHD occurred in 4/9 patients (44%) in the IPA targeted group and 9/15 (66%) patients of the NIMA targeted group. The estimated probability of survival was 38% (95% CI 17–60%) for the whole cohort.

These results were encouraging but highlighted that in some individuals severe GVHD occurred despite fetomaternal chimerism, suggesting that whilst this was a relative indicator of hyporesponsiveness, it was not absolute. In particular, severe GVHD in the NIMA-complementary mismatch was associated with IPA mismatch in the GVH direction. Studies by Cai et al. [64] elucidated that the tolerance associated with long-term fetomaternal chimerism is determined by the balance between regulatory T cells (Tregs) and T effector cells (Teff) specific for IPAs or NIMAs. Tests to evaluate Treg versus Teff balance such as allopeptide-specific tetramer staining or trans vivo delayed type hypersensitivity assays (injection of cryopreserved human PBMCs into the footpad of a CB17 SCID mouse footpad with the relevant antigenic peptide and controlling or neutralising antibody) are available and may help in further clarifying the role of fetomaternal microchimerism in allospecific tolerance after mismatched haploidentical transplants.

4.2.5. The Role of HLA Matching in Donor Selection. The degree of HLA mismatching often predicts increased GVHD and lower relapse rates in the allogeneic transplant setting. In a retrospective analysis of 185 patients with haematological malignancies transplanted with the RIC posttransplant Cy protocol, no correlation was found between the number of HLA mismatches, the risk of acute grade II–IV GVHD, graft failure, and event-free survival [83]. The Peking group studied 1210 consecutive haploidentical transplants, treated on the GIAC protocol to identify the optimal donor, and found that HLA mismatching did not correlate with outcomes. Instead, lower NRM and better survival were evident with younger donors and male donors. Fathers demonstrated lower NRM and aGVHD than mothers, and children donors demonstrated lower aGVHD than siblings. For siblings with NIMA mismatches, the rates of aGVHD were lower compared with those with noninherited paternal antigen (NIPA) mismatches [62]. An EBMT registry study of 173 adults with AML and 93

with ALL transplanted with the T deplete megadose, CD34 approach confirmed that the degree of HAL mismatch did not correlate with outcomes in this setting [84].

5. Haploidentical Transplants for Haematological Malignancies

To date, a number of studies have been completed evaluating haploidentical transplants against several outcomes including rate of engraftment, relapse, and acute and chronic GVHD, as well as event-free survival and overall survival. In some cases, these transplants have been compared contemporaneously with MRD, MUD, mismatched unrelated donor, and cord blood transplants. Table 1 provides a summary of these studies, which are described in detail in the following.

5.1. Myelodysplastic Syndrome (MDS) and Acute Myeloid Leukaemia (AML). Single centre analyses of haploidentical transplant for MDS/AML report encouraging data for engraftment, acute and chronic GVHD, overall survival, and event-free survivals that are comparable to matched unrelated donor transplants [65–67]. Two studies focused on patients with acute leukaemia including AML [69, 70], and twelve other trials included one or more patients with AML or MDS among others [54, 56, 73–82].

Amongst these, a large CIBMTR retrospective study compared 192 haploidentical (predominantly bone marrow graft and posttransplant Cy) with 1982 8/8 matched unrelated donor (predominantly peripheral blood grafts) transplants for AML [65]. The study demonstrated that, for MA transplants, neutrophil engraftment was at 90% for haploidentical transplants but 97% for MUD, whereas for RIC haploidentical transplant and MUD it was 93% and 96%, respectively. Reassuringly, aGVHD, grades II to IV, at 3 months for MA haploidentical transplant was low at 16% with this being doubled at 33% with MUD transplants ($p < 0.001$). Similarly, cGVHD at three years was 30% in MA haploidentical transplant and 53% for MUD ($p < 0.001$). This pattern is replicated with RIC transplants with aGVHD grades II to IV being 19% compared to 28% ($p = 0.05$) with MUD, and cGVHD at 3 years being 34% versus 52% ($p = 0.002$). These translate into comparable probabilities of overall survival (OS) of 45% (95% CI 36–54) and 50% (95% CI 47–53%) with haploidentical transplant and MUD MA transplants and 46% (95% CI 35–56) and 44% (95% CI 40–47) for haploidentical transplant and MUD RIC transplants, respectively. Although this retrospective analysis is not powered to detect small differences, these data are reassuring that mismatched family donors afford equivalent results.

A Chinese study also compared outcomes of patients with AML transplanted with a T replete low dose ATG conditioned transplant [85]. Of these, 90 patients had matched sibling donors (MSD), 116 had unrelated donors, and 99 haploidentical related donors (HRD). With this conditioning, the rates of aGVHD grades II–IV were 42.4% and grades III-IV were 17.2%, which resulted in a higher nonrelapse mortality (NRM) of 30.5%. This seems however to lead to a lower risk of relapse at 5 years in HRD of 15.4% in comparison with 28.2% with URD and 49.9% with MSD ($p = 0.002$).

TABLE 1: Summary of studies evaluating use of haploidentical transplantation, along with reported outcomes.

Study	Indications for transplant	HSC manipulation	Study group	N	Conditioning	HSC source	Engraft rate (%)	aGVHD II-IV (%)	cGVHD (%)	Relapse (%)	PFS/DFS/EFS (%)	OS (%)
[65]	2174 AML	Unmanipulated (T cell replete)	Haplo	192	104 myeloablative CNI, MMF, and PTCy	85 BM, 19 PB	90*	16*	30*	44	24*	3 yr OS 45
					88 RIC CNI, MMF, and PTCy	77 BM, 11 PB	93	19	34*	58*	18	3 yr OS 46
			MUD (8/8)	1982	1245 myeloablative CNI + MMF/MTX	231 BM, 1014 PB	97*	33*	53*	39	12*	3 yr OS 50
					737 RIC CNI + MMF/MTX	80 BM, 657 PB	96	28	52*	42*	10	3 yr OS 44
[66]	227 AML/MDS	Unmanipulated (T cell replete)	MRD	87	Fludarabine, melphalan, tacrolimus, and mini-MTX	2 BM, 23 PB	99	31	43	28	36	56
			MUD	108	Fludarabine, melphalan, tacrolimus, mini-MTX, and ATG	10 BM, 16 PB	96	29	30	23	27	
			Haplo	32	Fludarabine, melphalan, thiotepa, PTCy, tacrolimus, and MMF	18 BM, 1 PB	97	29	19	33	30	66
[67]	450 AML	Unmanipulated (T cell replete)	Haplo	231	Cytarabine, busulfan, Cy, Me-CCNU, and ATG; CsA, MMF, and MTX	Combined	100	36*	42*	15	74	79
			MRD (Sib)	219	Hydroxycarbamide, cytarabine, busulfan, Cy, Me-CCNU, and ATG; CsA, MMF, and MTX	14 BM, 81 PB, 124 combined	100	13*	15*	15	78	82
[68]	82 ALL	Unmanipulated (T cell replete)	MRD/MUD	35	TBI, Cy, MMF, CsA, and MTX ± imatinib	Not specified	***	26*	26*	45*	46*	63
			Haplo	47	Ara-C, Cy, ATG, MMF, CsA, and MTX ± imatinib			51*	49*	19*	60*	64
[69]	918 AML	Unmanipulated (T cell replete)	CB	558	Various (276 MAC, 280 RIC)	558 cord	84*	31	24	(NS)***	38	***
			Haplo	360	Various (219 MAC, 141 RIC)	171 BM, 175 PB, 14 combined	91*	27	29		32	
	528 ALL		CB	370	Various (261 MAC, 108 RIC)	370 cord	80*	31	25		28	
			Haplo	158	Various (111 MAC, 43 RIC)	65 BM, 78 PB, 15 combined	94*	33	31		34	
[70]	7874 AML, 2805 ALL	T cell depleted	MRD	297	Various				30*	31	48	
		Unmanipulated (T cell replete)	MRD	9518	Various	1585 BM, 8174 PB, 56 combined	***	24	37*	32	52	***
		T cell depleted	Haplo	268	Various			25	17*	25	21	
		Unmanipulated (T cell replete)	Haplo	596	Various	284 BM, 544 PB, 36 combined			27*	40	30	
[71]	90 HL	Unmanipulated (T cell replete)	MRD	38	Various: TBI ± fludarabine, MMF, or CsA + tacrolimus	38 PBSC	95	50	50	56	23	53
			MUD/mmUD	24		24 PBSC	99	50	63	63	29	58
			Haplo	28	Nonmyeloablative: Cy, fludarabine, TBI, PTCy, tacrolimus, and MMF	28 BM	100	43	35	40*	51*	58
[72]	718 NHL, 199 HL	Unmanipulated (T cell replete)	MUD	241	Various (fludarabine + busulfan/Cy/melphalan ± TBI) + ATG	26 NM, 279 PBSC	97	49	33*	36	38*	50*
			MUD	491	Various (fludarabine + busulfan/Cy/melphalan ± TBI) without ATG	31 BM, 460 PBSC	97	40	51*	28	49*	62*
			Haplo	185	RIC (fludarabine, Cy, TBI, and PTCy)	172 BM, 13 PBSC	94	27	13*	36	47*	60*

TABLE 1: Continued.

Study	Indications for transplant	HSC manipulation	Study group	N	Conditioning	HSC source	Engraft rate (%)	aGVHD II-IV (%)	cGVHD (%)	Relapse (%)	PFS/DFS/EFS (%)	OS (%)
[55]	26 HL	Unmanipulated (T cell replete)	Haplo	26	(RIC) Cy, fludarabine, low dose TBI, PTCy, tacrolimus/CsA, and MMF	26 BM	96	24	9	31	63	77
[56]	91 AML, 44 NHL, 41 ALL, 26 CML/MPD, 22 MDS, 17 HL, 15 CLL, 13 MM, and 2 others	Unmanipulated (T cell replete)	MRD	117	Various	7 BM, 108 PB, 2 combined	98	8	54*	34	53	76
			MUD	101	Various	6 BM, 92 PB	98	11	54*	34	52	67
			Haplo	53	35 nonmyeloablative: fludarabine, TBI, Cy, PTCy, tacrolimus, and MMF. 18 myeloablative: fludarabine, busulfan, Cy, PTCy, tacrolimus, and MMF	32 BM, 21 PB	98	11	38*	33	60	64
[73]	170 AML, 62 ALL, 70 NHL, 53 MDS, 29 HL, 29 CML, 26 CLL, 21 MPD, and 15 MM	Unmanipulated (T cell replete)	MRD	181	Various. Tacrolimus and MTX for GVHD prophylaxis	2 BM, 179 PBSC	98	21*	58	30	56	72*
			MUD	178	Various. Tacrolimus and MTX for GVHD prophylaxis	32 BM, 146 PBSC	98	48	62	34	50	59
			Haplo	116	Nonmyeloablative (fludarabine, TBI, Cy, and PTCy) or myeloablative (fludarabine, busulfan, Cy, PTCy or fludarabine, TBI, and PTCy)	64 BM, 52 PBSC	97	41	38*	29	54	57
[74]	42 AML, 30 NHL, 22 MDS, 17 MM, 10 ALL, 10 CLL, 4 MPD, 3 HL, and 3 CML	Unmanipulated (T cell replete)	MRD	47	RIC (fludarabine, busulfan, ATG, CsA, and MMF)	47 PB	100	21	35*	25	64	78
			MUD/MMUD	63	RIC (fludarabine, busulfan, ATG, CsA, and MMF)	3 BM, 60 PB	100	44	24	31	38*	51
			Haplo	31	Initially nonmyeloablative (Cy, fludarabine, and TBI) increased if necessary to RIC (Cy/thiotepa, fludarabine, and busulfan) + PTCy, CsA, and MMF	4 BM, 27 PB	97	23	13*	23	67*	70
[75]	29 HL, 24 NHL, 4 CLL, 4 AML/MDS, 4 MM, and 2 ALL	Unmanipulated (T cell replete)	Haplo BM	46	(RIC) Cy, fludarabine, low dose TBI, PTCy, tacrolimus/CsA, and MMF	46 BM	87	25	13	***	62**	68**
			Haplo PB	23		23 PB	95	33	13	***		
[76]	38 AML, 20 ALL, 11 NHL, 7 MDS/MPD, and 1 SAA	Fixed CD3 DLI, positive CD34 selection	MRD	27	TBI, Cy, tacrolimus, and MMF	27 DLI	100	8*	12	27	70	71
			Haplo	50	TBI, Cy, tacrolimus, and MMF	50 DLI	96	4077*	19	21	68	70
[77]	16 AML, 4 ALL, 3 NHL, 2 MDS, 1 SAA, and 1 other	Fixed CD3 DLI w/OKT3	Haplo	27	TBI, Cy, tacrolimus, and MMF	27 PB	85	59	16	32	***	48
[78]	15 AML, 10 ALL, 2 NHL, and 1 MDS	Fixed CD3 DLI, positive CD34 selection	Haplo	28	TBI, Cy, tacrolimus, and MMF	28 PB	100	39	22	***	2 yr DFS 74	2 yr OS 77
[79]	15 AML, 2 ALL, 2 MDS, and 1 CML	Unmanipulated (T cell replete)	Haplo 1 × PTCy	9	Fludarabine, cytarabine, ATG, busulfan/melphalan, and PTCy	9 PB	95	56	10	***	35	44*
			Haplo 2 × PTCy	11	Fludarabine, cytarabine, ATG, busulfan/melphalan, and PTCy × 2	11 PB		64				64*
[80]	25 AML, 12 ALL, 5 HL/NHL, 4 MF, 3 CML, and 1 MPD	Unmanipulated (T cell replete)	Haplo	50	Thiotepa, busulfan, and fludarabine; PTCy, CsA, and MMF; or TBI, fludarabine, PTCy, CsA, and MMF	50 BM	90	12	26	26	51	62

TABLE 1: Continued.

Study	Indications for transplant	HSC manipulation	Study group	N	Conditioning	HSC source	Engraft rate (%)	aGVHD II–IV (%)	cGVHD (%)	Relapse (%)	PFS/DFS/EFS (%)	OS (%)
			MRD (Sib)	176	Various myeloablative or RIC. GvHD prophylaxis CsA, MTX	156 BM, 20 PB		31*	29	40	32	45
			MUD	43	Various myeloablative or RIC. GvHD prophylaxis CsA, MTX, and ATG	26 BM, 17 PB		21*	22	23	36	43
[81]	232 AML/ALL, 59 HL/NHL, 74 MPD, 81 MDS, and 13 others	Unmanipulated (T cell replete)	MMUD	43	Various myeloablative or RIC. GvHD prophylaxis CsA, MTX, and ATG	28 BM, 15 PB	***	42*	19	30	34	40
			CB	105	Various myeloablative or RIC. GvHD prophylaxis CsA, MMF, and ATG	105 cord		19*	23	30	33	34
			Haplo	92	Thiotepa, busulfan, and fludarabine; PTCy, CsA, and MMF; or TBI, fludarabine, PTCy, CsA, and MMF	92 BM		14*	15	35	43	52
[54]	16 AML, 12 NHL, 9 HL, 5 MDS, 4 SAA, 4 CLL, 3 CML, and 2 ALL	Unmanipulated (T cell replete)	Haplo	55	RIC (fludarabine, Cy, TBI, PTCy, tacrolimus, and MMF)	55 PB	96	61	18	28	51	48
[82]	12 AML, 3 CML, 2 ALL, 2 NHL, and 1 HL	Unmanipulated (T cell replete)	Haplo	20	Fludarabine, busulfan ± Cy and PTCy, tacrolimus, and MMF	20 PB	100	30	35	40	50	69

* $p < 0.05$, ** no statistical comparison available, and *** data not reported.
AML: acute myeloid leukaemia, ALL: acute lymphoblastic leukaemia, HL: Hodgkin's lymphoma, NHL: non-Hodgkin's lymphoma, CLL: chronic lymphocytic leukaemia, CML: chronic myeloid leukaemia, MM: multiple myeloma, SAA: severe aplastic anaemia, MDS: myelodysplastic syndrome, MPD: myeloproliferative disorder, SCD: sickle cell disease, Haplo: haploidentical transplant, MUD: matched unrelated donor transplant, MRD: matched related donor transplant, Sib: matched sibling donor transplant, MMUD: mismatched unrelated donor transplant, RIC: reduced intensity conditioning, MAC: myeloablative conditioning, CNI: calcineurin inhibitor, MMF: mycophenolate mofetil, PTCy: posttransplant cyclophosphamide, Cy: cyclophosphamide, MTX: methotrexate, Me-CCNU: methyl chloride hexamethylene urea nitrate, ATG: antithymocyte globulin, CsA: ciclosporin A, TBI: total body irradiation, OKT3: muromonab CD3, BM: bone marrow, PB: peripheral blood stem cell, CB: cord blood transplant, DLI: donor leucocyte infusion, aGVHD: acute graft-versus-host disease, cGVHD: chronic graft-versus-host disease, TRM: transplant-related mortality, PFS: progression-free survival, DFS: disease-free survival, EFS: event-free survival, and OS: overall survival.

The 5-year disease-free survival (DFS) for those undergoing transplant with the three donors was 63.6% for MSD, 58.4% for URD, and 58.3% for HRD. This group then prospectively compared consecutive transplants between 2010 and 2013 for AML in CR1 with intermediate or high-risk disease who had either MSD (219 patients) or HRD (231 patients) transplanted with very similar conditioning, including ATG for haploidentical transplants and Cy/MTX for MSD [67]. Whilst the haploidentical group tended to be younger, the results for both groups were similar in terms of aGVHD and cGVHD with NRM in HRD being 10% (similar to that seen with posttransplant Cy, 7% at 1 year). These GVHD rates were also comparable to those with posttransplant Cy. Additional MRD monitoring and preemptive DLI or therapeutic DLI resulted in low relapse rates of 15% with both donors. The 3-year probabilities of leukaemia-free survival were 76% (95% CI 64–87) and 80% (95% CI 70–91) for HRD and MSD, respectively. Three-year probabilities of OS were 79% (95% CI 73–85) and 82% (95% CI 76–88) for HRD and MSD, respectively. Features of the underlying leukaemia including cytogenetics and white cell count $>50 \times 10^9$/L at presentation were independent predictors of outcome on multivariate analysis.

As patients with AML and MDS are older, the comparison of transplant outcomes by donor type in the older recipient is relevant. Blaise et al. [74] compared outcomes of 31 patients older than 55 years (predominantly MDS/AML) transplanted with RIC PB Cy haploidentical transplants with MSD and MUD conditioned with ATG and cyclosporine (CsA) ± MMF in the same age group. Whilst GVHD rates were comparable (CI 23% Haplo, 21% MSD) for related donors, it was higher (CI 44%) for MUD. No patient with HRD developed cGVHD whereas 16% of MSD and 14% of MUD developed this. Importantly, the cumulative incidence of relapse (CIR) was similar in all the groups but NRM after an MUD was threefold higher compared to a related donor. Thus, 2-year OS was 70%, progression-free survival (PFS) was 67%, and severe cGVHD-free survival was 67% after HRD transplant. Similar outcomes were seen with MSD (78%, 64%, and 51%) whereas the results in this small cohort for URD transplants were 51% ($p = 0.08$), 38% ($p = 0.02$), and 31% ($p = 0.007$), respectively.

These reports build a case for HRD to be considered where a MSD is unavailable. They may be preferred over MUD, in the older patient particularly with posttransplant Cy due to reduced side effects of transplant and in all recipients where an 8/8 MUD is not available.

5.2. Acute Lymphoblastic Leukaemia (ALL). There are fewer reports of the efficacy of modern platforms of T cell replete haploidentical stem cell transplantation for ALL. A report from southwest China studied 82 patients with Philadelphia chromosome positive ALL, transplanted with MSD in 35 patients and HRD in 47 patients [68]. The conditioning regimen consisted of 9–10.5 Gy TBI and cyclophosphamide 60 mg/kg for two days in the MSD group, with the addition of 6 g/m² ATG IV for 3 days in the haploidentical transplant group and reduction of Cy to 45 mg/kg/day for 2 days. GVHD prophylaxis in the MSD consisted of CsA, MTX, and MMF to day 30 whereas the haploidentical transplant

group received additional ATG and MMF to 90 days. Most patients were transplanted in molecular remission but *bcr-abl* was detectable at circa 2% in 7 MSD and 10 HRD before transplant. Imatinib was commenced after transplant when *bcr-abl* was detected molecularly. The cumulative incidence of GVHD both acute (51% HRD versus 26% MSD) and chronic (49% HRD versus 26% MSD) was higher in the HRD and appeared to exert a GVL effect with a CIR at 9.1% being lower than that for MSD 19.1%, HR 0.413 (95% CI 0.178–0.958). Transplantation in CR > 1 was predictive of relapse. The study provides encouraging data for a HRD in the absence of MUD.

Two further studies considered acute leukaemia including ALL [69, 70]. In particular, EBMT registry data compared the outcomes of haploidentical transplant with UCBT for 918 acute myeloid leukaemia patients (HRD 360 patients and UCBT 558 patients) and 528 acute lymphoblastic leukaemia patients (HRD 158 patients and UCBT 370 patients). For ALL, although the HRD had significantly more patients with advanced stage disease (48% versus 34%, $p = 0.02$) and poor risk cytogenetics (26% versus 14%, $p = 0.03$), OS and DFS were similar to both graft sources whereas the incidence of cGVHD was lower with UCBT. Nonengraftment was higher with UCBT but did not translate into a higher NRM. Transplant conditioning regimens were heterogeneous and cGVHD rates were higher for HRD than those reported from single centre studies. The deleterious effect of RIC on relapse and advanced disease on transplant outcomes was seen in LFS, NRM, and relapse ($p < 0.001$). Notwithstanding these criticisms, results from this large dataset suggest that both sources of stem cells would be appropriate in the absence of a suitable matched donor. Further twelve studies with mixed patient groups all included patients with ALL among others [54, 56, 73–82].

5.3. Hodgkin's Lymphoma (HL). Burroughs et al. [71] transplanted patients with Hodgkin's lymphoma with relapsed or refractory disease, treated with a median of five chemotherapy regimens, with MRD (38 patients), MUD (24 patients), or HRD (28 patients with the RIC BM, posttransplant Cy). Whilst OS was similar at 2 years (53% MRD, 58% MUD, and 58% HRD), relapse was less frequent with HRD 40% versus 63% with MUD and 56% with MRD resulting in a PFS of 51% with HRD compared to 29% with MUD and 23% with MRD. These were the initial set of data where a HRD transplant resulted in outcomes superior to conventional donor, paving the way for further such comparisons. A number of mixed studies also included patients with HL [54, 56, 73–75, 81, 82] or unspecified lymphoma [80].

A recent study published by Kanate et al. [72] compared 917 adult patients with both Hodgkin and non-Hodgkin lymphoma, undergoing either haploidentical ($n = 185$) or MUD ($n = 732$) transplants. The MUD transplant group was further divided into conditioning regimens with additional ATG as GVHD prophylaxis and those without. The study found the haploidentical group to be at significantly reduced risk of severe acute GVHD (grades III and IV) compared to ATG and non-ATG groups (8% versus 12% and 17%, resp., $p = 0.01$ and 0.001). There was also significantly reduced risk of chronic GVHD (13% versus 51% and 33%, $p < 0.0001$).

The study also demonstrated no significant differences in OS between both MUD groups and the haploidentical group and showed no overall difference in NRM, relapse, and PFS. These results provide further evidence that haploidentical transplants may be an acceptable option for lymphoma patients lacking an HLA-identical donor and can be safely chosen over MUD donors without compromising survival outcomes.

5.4. Non-Hodgkin's Lymphoma (NHL) and Chronic Lymphocytic Leukaemia (CLL).

Ten of the twelve studies with mixed patient groups included patients with NHL [54, 56, 73–78, 81, 82] whilst five of these also included patients with CLL [54, 56, 73–75]. None of these studies reported outcomes for these diseases separately.

In one of the bigger comparative studies, Bashey et al. [56] retrospectively looked at 271 consecutive transplant patients at their centre in Atlanta, USA. Fifty-three patients underwent haploidentical transplants, 117 underwent MRD, and 101 underwent MUD transplants. Several different conditioning regimens were used for the MRD and MUD groups. In the haploidentical group, 35 patients underwent non-myeloablative conditioning with fludarabine (30 mg/m^2), 2 Gy TBI, and Cy (14.5 mg/kg before transplant and 50 mg/kg after transplant), whilst 18 patients underwent myeloablative conditioning involving fludarabine (25 mg/m^2), busulfan (110–130 mg/m^2), and Cy (14.5 mg/kg before transplant and 50 mg/kg after transplant). Tacrolimus, MMF, and G-CSF were also used in all patients. Rates of relapse, NRM, aGVHD, cGVHD, 2-year OS, and DFS for MRD, MUD, and haploidentical transplants were nonsignificant across all groups.

In a later study, Bashey et al. [73] retrospectively analysed further 475 consecutive transplant patients at their centre, with a longer follow-up period than the previous study. Transplants were either MRD (181 patients), MUD (178 patients), or haploidentical (116 patients) with a heterogeneous mixture of conditions including 70 NHL and 26 CLL patients as well as 170 AML and 62 ALL among others. Conditioning for MRD and MUD groups varied whilst a posttransplant Cy regimen was used for haploidentical transplants. At 2-year follow-up, OS was comparable in haploidentical and MUD groups (57% versus 59%, resp., $p > 0.05$), as well as DFS (54% versus 50%), NRM (17% versus 16%), and acute GVHD (41% versus 48%). Rates for moderate to severe cGVHD were observed to be lower in the haploidentical group (31% versus 47%, $p = 0.004$), and haploidentical transplants were less likely to receive systemic immunosuppressive treatment (19% versus 42%, $p = 0.007$). Results for MRD were significantly superior for OS and aGVHD only. The study went on to suggest that haploidentical transplants are an appropriate alternative in patients lacking a fully matched related donor. Fully HLA-matched unrelated donors (10/10 HLA alleles) have been previously shown to be superior to mismatched unrelated donor transplants (>1 mismatched allele); hence, it was suggested that haploidentical transplants may in fact be a more appropriate alternative than mismatched transplants.

Raiola et al. [81] conducted a study of 459 consecutive patients with a variety of malignancies including 232 patients with acute leukaemia (AML/ALL) and 59 patients with lymphoma (HL/NHL). Transplants were categorised as being either a matched sibling donor (MSD), MUD, mismatched unrelated donor (mmUD), unrelated cord blood donor (UCD), or haploidentical donor. Haploidentical transplants were either myeloablative using thiotepa, busulfan, and fludarabine or nonmyeloablative using TBI and fludarabine. Regimens also included posttransplant Cy, CsA, and MMF. Acute GVHD was significantly lower in the haploidentical group (14%) compared to the MSD and mmUD groups (31% and 42%, $p < 0.001$), and there was a similar but not statistically significant pattern for chronic GVHD ($p = 0.053$). Haploidentical transplant recipients had the highest 4-year OS (52%), which was nonsignificant across all groups ($p = 0.10$) but comparable with MSD transplants in multivariate analysis (45%, $p = 0.80$). Again, results suggested that haploidentical transplants could be a valid option, comparable to MUD transplants, in the absence of an HLA-identical related donor.

Castagna et al. [75] sought to compare the use of PBSC and BM in haploidentical patients. Sixty-nine consecutive patients (46 BM and 23 PBSC) were analysed in this retrospective study, including 29 patients with HL, 24 with NHL, and 4 with CLL among others. A nonmyeloablative regimen with posttransplant Cy was used in both groups of patients. Results showed similar rates of acute and chronic GVHD in PBSC and BM groups (33% versus 25%, $p = 0.43$, and 13% versus 13%, $p = 0.21$) as well as similar NRM (12% versus 22%, $p = 0.96$), suggesting that PBSC transplants using this regimen were not inferior to BM transplants for this regimen used. A major limitation of this study was the small number of patients included; the limited data nonetheless suggest that PBSCs are a valid option in haploidentical transplants compared to BM transplants.

5.5. Multiple Myeloma (MM).

Few haploidentical transplants for multiple myeloma with posttransplant Cy have been included in studies [56, 73–75]; however, outcomes are not reported separately. A single series reported on 10 patients transplanted with the RIC PBSC posttransplant Cy haploidentical transplant with TBI doses between 2 Gy and 4 Gy [86]. The median age of patients was 53 years (range 28–61 years) who had relapsed or were refractory after autograft. Fludarabine 30 mg/m^2 was added to the protocol if CD4 counts before transplant were greater than 200×10^9/L. Bone marrow graft was used in six patients and PBSC in four patients. Engraftment kinetics of neutrophils and platelets were similar to those reported from other posttransplant Cy RIC studies. Median neutrophil engraftment occurred by day 18 and platelet engraftment occurred by day 17. The median OS was 443 days; OS at 1 year was 61.7% and at 2 years was 46.3%. Causes of death included sepsis in one patient and disease progression in two patients. Grade II–IV aGVHD occurred in 8/10 patients and five developed cGVHD. Relapse occurred in five patients with a median time to progression of 7.8 months: of these, two patients were salvaged with chemotherapy and DLI. More data are needed.

5.6. Myeloproliferative Neoplasms/Disorders (MPD).

Raiola et al. [80] transplanted 50 patients with a variety of high-risk haematologic malignancies, which included four patients with primary myelofibrosis and one patient with MPD. Myeloablative conditioning consisted of either thiotepa (5 mg/kg/day ×2), fludarabine (50 mg/m^2/day ×3), or busulfan (3.2 mg/kg/day ×3). The F-TBI regime consisted of 3.3 Gy TBI/day ×3 and fludarabine (30 mg/m^2/day ×4). Posttransplantation Cy, CsA, and MMF were also used. Neutrophil engraftment occurred in 90% of patients in a median of 18 days. Incidence of acute GVHD was 12% and limited to grades II to III. Ten patients (26%) developed chronic GVHD of which six were mild. Overall incidence of relapse, TRM, and OS were 26%, 18%, and 68%, respectively. Results for patients with myelofibrosis were not reported individually.

One of the largest studies involving patients with MPD was by Raiola et al. [81] described previously. Studies by Raj et al. [54] and Solomon et al. [82] both included three patients each with CML; however, results were not reported separately. A number of other studies also included patients with CML [56, 73, 74, 79, 80] or unspecified myeloproliferative disorder (MPD) [73, 74, 76, 80, 81].

6. Conclusion and Future of Haploidentical Transplants

Undoubtedly, the techniques now used in haploidentical transplantation have had a positive impact on several outcome measures, namely, overall survival, disease-free progression, and survival free from acute or chronic GVHD. The studies described above are just a selection of cases where haploidentical transplants can feasibly be conducted on patients without an available HLA-matched donor. Recent retrospective analyses are beginning to assert that the paradigm for donor selection is changing, with haploidentical donors vying with MUD. Early data from China would suggest that these donors perform as well as MRD but this needs to be validated in further studies.

The ease of posttransplant Cy has led to its adoption across the world with data from EBMT showing an increasing trend for haploidentical transplants as opposed to stagnant levels of UCB transplantation [14]. With disease risk stratification, the role of the underlying disease on subsequent relapse has become clearer. It is increasingly clear that for patients with disease risk index, low/intermediate disease outcomes with haploidentical transplants are encouraging due to intrinsically lower relapse rates and low rates of acute GVHD and cGVHD. However, strategies to overcome high-risk disease with all types of donors remain to be identified. In this respect, engineered grafts with NK alloreactive donors may come to the fore.

It is important to note, however, that the majority of clinical data currently gathered for haploidentical transplants come from nonrandomised trials with retrospective comparison. Because of this, it is difficult to interpret data and compare and declare definitively whether one method is superior to another. Bearing this in mind, current recommendations are based on the expertise of the centre performing the transplantation and the facilities available, for example, for accommodating manipulation of grafts.

More studies, particularly randomised trials, are most certainly necessary before haploidentical transplants can be more readily used and their numerous benefits can be substantiated. Particularly, comparisons between donor sources (such as MRD, MUD, umbilical cord, and haploidentical donor) would be useful, as well as comparisons between various conditioning regimens and graft manipulation (or lack thereof). Studies can also be improved by recruiting more patients, focusing on specific conditions to remove confounding by disease variables and following-up patients for longer. Based on these, it may then be possible for haploidentical transplantation to fulfil its potential in providing substantial benefit to the field of allogeneic haematopoietic stem cell transplantation.

Competing Interests

The authors declare that there are no competing interests regarding the publication of this paper.

Acknowledgments

This paper was funded by Kings College London.

References

[1] E. D. Thomas, H. L. Lochte Jr., J. H. Cannon, O. D. Sahler, and J. W. Ferrebee, "Supralethal whole body irradiation and isologous marrow transplantation in man," *The Journal of Clinical Investigation*, vol. 38, no. 10, pp. 1709–1716, 1959.

[2] R. A. Gatti, H. J. Meuwissen, H. D. Allen, R. Hong, and R. A. Good, "Immunological reconstitution of sex-linked lymphopenic immunological deficiency," *The Lancet*, vol. 2, no. 7583, pp. 1366–1369, 1968.

[3] E. D. Thomas, C. D. Buckner, M. Banaji et al., "One hundred patients with acute leukemia treated by chemotherapy, total body irradiation, and allogenic marrow transplantation," *Blood*, vol. 49, no. 4, pp. 511–533, 1977.

[4] F. R. Appelbaum, "Hematopoietic-cell transplantation at 50," *The New England Journal of Medicine*, vol. 357, no. 15, pp. 1472–1475, 2007.

[5] E. D. Thomas, C. D. Buckner, R. A. Clift et al., "Marrow transplantation for acute nonlymphoblastic leukemia in first remission," *The New England Journal of Medicine*, vol. 301, no. 11, pp. 597–599, 1979.

[6] P. L. Weiden, N. Flournoy, E. D. Thomas et al., "Antileukemic effect of graft-versus-host disease in human recipients of allogeneic-marrow grafts," *The New England Journal of Medicine*, vol. 300, no. 19, pp. 1068–1073, 1979.

[7] E. A. Copelan, "Hematopoietic stem-cell transplantation," *The New England Journal of Medicine*, vol. 354, no. 17, pp. 1813–1826, 2006.

[8] T. I. Mughal and K. Raj, "Port-wine-flavour bone-marrow sandwiches and beyond," *The Lancet Oncology*, vol. 10, no. 9, p. 926, 2009.

[9] L.-P. Koh and N. Chao, "Haploidentical hematopoietic cell transplantation," *Bone Marrow Transplantation*, vol. 42, no. 1, pp. S60–S63, 2008.

[10] S. Giralt, "Reduced-intensity conditioning regimens for hematologic malignancies: what have we learned over the last 10 years?" *ASH Education Book*, vol. 2005, no. 1, pp. 384–389, 2005.

[11] W. Saber, S. Opie, J. D. Rizzo, M.-J. Zhang, M. M. Horowitz, and J. Schriber, "Outcomes after matched unrelated donor versus identical sibling hematopoietic cell transplantation in adults with acute myelogenous leukemia," *Blood*, vol. 119, no. 17, pp. 3908–3916, 2012.

[12] W. Saber, C. S. Cutler, R. Nakamura et al., "Impact of donor source on hematopoietic cell transplantation outcomes for patients with myelodysplastic syndromes (MDS)," *Blood*, vol. 122, no. 11, pp. 1974–1982, 2013.

[13] M. Pasquini and X. Zhu, *Current Use and Outcome of Hematopoietic Stem Cell Transplantation: CIBMTR Summary Slides*, 2014, http://www.cibmtr.org.

[14] J. R. Passweg, H. Baldomero, P. Bader et al., "Hematopoietic SCT in Europe 2013: recent trends in the use of alternative donors showing more haploidentical donors but fewer cord blood transplants," *Bone Marrow Transplantation*, vol. 50, no. 4, pp. 476–482, 2015.

[15] BMDW—Bone Marrow Donors Worldwide, Bone Marrow Donors Worldwide (BMDW), http://www.bmdw.org/.

[16] L. Gragert, M. Eapen, E. Williams et al., "HLA match likelihoods for hematopoietic stem-cell grafts in the U.S. registry," *The New England Journal of Medicine*, vol. 371, no. 4, pp. 339–348, 2014.

[17] G. E. Switzer, J. G. Bruce, L. Myaskovsky et al., "Race and ethnicity in decisions about unrelated hematopoietic stem cell donation," *Blood*, vol. 121, no. 8, pp. 1469–1476, 2013.

[18] P. G. Beatty, M. Mori, and E. Milford, "Impact of racial genetic polymorphism on the probability of finding an HLA-matched donor," *Transplantation*, vol. 60, no. 8, pp. 778–783, 1995.

[19] J. Pidala, J. Kim, M. Schell et al., "Race/ethnicity affects the probability of finding an HLA-A,-B,-C and-DRB1 allele-matched unrelated donor and likelihood of subsequent transplant utilization," *Bone Marrow Transplantation*, vol. 48, no. 3, pp. 346–350, 2013.

[20] J. N. Barker, D. J. Weisdorf, T. E. DeFor et al., "Transplantation of 2 partially HLA-matched umbilical cord blood units to enhance engraftment in adults with hematologic malignancy," *Blood*, vol. 105, no. 3, pp. 1343–1347, 2005.

[21] Y. Reisner, D. Hagin, and M. F. Martelli, "Haploidentical hematopoietic transplantation: current status and future perspectives," *Blood*, vol. 118, no. 23, pp. 6006–6017, 2011.

[22] *Library of Medicine. HLA Gene Family - Genetics Home Reference*, US National, URL http, 2015.

[23] T. Spitzer, "Haploidentical stem cell transplantation: the always present but overlooked donor," *ASH Education Program Book*, vol. 2005, no. 1, pp. 390–395, 2005.

[24] E. J. Fuchs, "Haploidentical transplantation for hematologic malignancies: where do we stand?" *ASH Education Book*, vol. 2012, no. 1, pp. 230–236, 2012.

[25] F. Patriarca, L. Luznik, M. Medeot et al., "Experts' considerations on HLA-haploidentical stem cell transplantation," *European Journal of Haematology*, vol. 93, no. 3, pp. 187–197, 2014.

[26] S. O. Ciurea and U. D. Bayraktar, "'No donor'? Consider a haploidentical transplant," *Blood Reviews*, vol. 29, no. 2, pp. 63–70, 2015.

[27] C. Anasetti, D. Amos, P. G. Beatty et al., "Effect of HLA compatibility on engraftment of bone marrow transplants in patients with leukemia or lymphoma," *The New England Journal of Medicine*, vol. 320, no. 4, pp. 197–204, 1989.

[28] P. G. Beatty, R. A. Clift, E. M. Mickelson et al., "Marrow transplantation from related donors other than HLA-identical siblings," *The New England Journal of Medicine*, vol. 313, no. 13, pp. 765–771, 1985.

[29] P. J. Martin, J. A. Hansen, C. D. Buckner et al., "Effects of in vitro depletion of T cells in HLA-identical allogeneic marrow grafts," *Blood*, vol. 66, no. 3, pp. 664–672, 1985.

[30] R. Storb, K. C. Doney, E. D. Thomas et al., "Marrow transplantation with or without donor buffy coat cells for 65 transfused aplastic anemia patients," *Blood*, vol. 59, no. 2, pp. 236–246, 1982.

[31] F. Aversa, A. Tabilio, A. Velardi et al., "Treatment of high-risk acute leukemia with T-cell-depleted stem cells from related donors with one fully mismatched hla haplotype," *The New England Journal of Medicine*, vol. 339, no. 17, pp. 1186–1193, 1998.

[32] F. Aversa, A. Tabilio, A. Terenzi et al., "Successful engraftment of T-cell-depleted haploidentical 'Three-Loci' incompatible transplants in leukemia patients by addition of recombinant human granulocyte colony-stimulating factor-mobilized peripheral blood progenitor cells to bone marrow inoculum," *Blood*, vol. 84, no. 11, pp. 3948–3955, 1994.

[33] F. Aversa, Y. Reisner, and M. F. Martelli, "The haploidentical option for high-risk haematological malignancies," *Blood Cells, Molecules, and Diseases*, vol. 40, no. 1, pp. 8–12, 2008.

[34] N. Rachamim, J. Gan, H. Segall et al., "Tolerance induction by "mega-dose" hematopoietic transplants: donor-type human CD34 stem cells induce potent specific reduction of host anti-donor cytotoxic T lymphocyte precursors in mixed lymphocyte culture," *Transplantation*, vol. 65, no. 10, pp. 1386–1393, 1998.

[35] W. A. Bethge, M. Haegele, C. Faul et al., "Haploidentical allogeneic hematopoietic cell transplantation in adults with reduced-intensity conditioning and CD3/CD19 depletion: fast engraftment and low toxicity," *Experimental Hematology*, vol. 34, no. 12, pp. 1746–1752, 2006.

[36] I. André-Schmutz, F. Le Deist, S. Hacein-Bey-Abina et al., "Immune reconstitution without graft-versus-host disease after haemopoietic stem-cell transplantation: a phase 1/2 study," *The Lancet*, vol. 360, no. 9327, pp. 130–137, 2002.

[37] S. Mielke, Z. A. McIver, A. Shenoy et al., "Selectively T cell-depleted allografts from hla-matched sibling donors followed by low-dose posttransplantation immunosuppression to improve transplantation outcome in patients with hematologic malignancies," *Biology of Blood and Marrow Transplantation*, vol. 17, no. 12, pp. 1855–1861, 2011.

[38] N. Chao, "Memory T cells," *Biology of Blood and Marrow Transplantation*, vol. 14, no. 1, supplement 1, pp. 17–22, 2008.

[39] B. J. Chen, X. Cui, G. D. Sempowski, C. Liu, and N. J. Chao, "Transfer of allogeneic CD62L—memory T cells without graft-versus-host disease," *Blood*, vol. 103, no. 4, pp. 1534–1541, 2004.

[40] B. E. Anderson, J. McNiff, J. Yan et al., "Memory CD4+ T cells do not induce graft-versus-host disease," *The Journal of Clinical Investigation*, vol. 112, no. 1, pp. 101–108, 2003.

[41] E. Distler, A. Bloetz, J. Albrecht et al., "Alloreactive and leukemia-reactive T cells are preferentially derived from naïve precursors in healthy donors: implications for immunotherapy with memory T cells," *Haematologica*, vol. 96, no. 7, pp. 1024–1032, 2011.

[42] D. Teschner, E. Distler, D. Wehler et al., "Depletion of naive T cells using clinical grade magnetic CD45RA beads: a new approach for GVHD prophylaxis," *Bone Marrow Transplantation*, vol. 49, no. 1, pp. 138–144, 2014.

[43] D. R. Shook, B. M. Triplett, P. W. Eldridge, G. Kang, A. Srinivasan, and W. Leung, "Haploidentical stem cell transplantation augmented by CD45RA negative lymphocytes provides rapid engraftment and excellent tolerability," *Pediatric Blood & Cancer*, vol. 62, no. 4, pp. 666–673, 2015.

[44] D. A. A. Vignali, L. W. Collison, and C. J. Workman, "How regulatory T cells work," *Nature Reviews Immunology*, vol. 8, no. 7, pp. 523–532, 2008.

[45] M. Miyara and S. Sakaguchi, "Human FoxP3⁺ CD4⁺ regulatory T cells: their knowns and unknowns," *Immunology and Cell Biology*, vol. 89, no. 3, pp. 346–351, 2011.

[46] M. Edinger, P. Hoffmann, J. Ermann et al., "CD4⁺CD25⁺ regulatory T cells preserve graft-versus-tumor activity while inhibiting graft-versus-host disease after bone marrow transplantation," *Nature Medicine*, vol. 9, no. 9, pp. 1144–1150, 2003.

[47] M. F. Martelli, M. Di Ianni, L. Ruggeri et al., "HLA-haploidentical transplantation with regulatory and conventional T-cell adoptive immunotherapy prevents acute leukemia relapse," *Blood*, vol. 124, no. 4, pp. 638–644, 2014.

[48] L. Ruggeri, A. Mancusi, M. Capanni et al., "Donor natural killer cell allorecognition of missing self in haploidentical hematopoietic transplantation for acute myeloid leukemia: challenging its predictive value," *Blood*, vol. 110, no. 1, pp. 433–440, 2007.

[49] M. Stern, L. Ruggeri, A. Mancusi et al., "Survival after T cell–depleted haploidentical stem cell transplantation is improved using the mother as donor," *Blood*, vol. 112, no. 7, pp. 2990–2995, 2008.

[50] L. Luznik, P. V. O'Donnell, H. J. Symons et al., "HLA-haploidentical bone marrow transplantation for hematologic malignancies using nonmyeloablative conditioning and high-dose, posttransplantation cyclophosphamide," *Biology of Blood and Marrow Transplantation*, vol. 14, no. 6, pp. 641–650, 2008.

[51] A. Munchel, C. Kesserwan, H. J. Symons et al., "Nonmyeloablative, HLA-haploidentical bone marrow transplantation with high dose, post-transplantation cyclophosphamide," *Pediatric Reports*, vol. 3, supplement 2, 2011.

[52] O. Alpdogan, D. Grosso, and N. Flomenberg, "Recent advances in haploidentical stem cell transplantation," *Discovery Medicine*, vol. 16, no. 88, pp. 159–165, 2013.

[53] L. Luznik, R. J. Jones, and E. J. Fuchs, "High-dose cyclophosphamide for graft-versus-host disease prevention," *Current Opinion in Hematology*, vol. 17, no. 6, pp. 493–499, 2010.

[54] K. Raj, A. Pagliuca, K. Bradstock et al., "Peripheral blood hematopoietic stem cells for transplantation of hematological diseases from related, haploidentical donors after reduced-intensity conditioning," *Biology of Blood and Marrow Transplantation*, vol. 20, no. 6, pp. 890–895, 2014.

[55] A. Raiola, A. Dominietto, R. Varaldo et al., "Unmanipulated haploidentical BMT following non-myeloablative conditioning and post-transplantation CY for advanced Hodgkin's lymphoma," *Bone Marrow Transplantation*, vol. 49, no. 2, pp. 190–194, 2014.

[56] A. Bashey, X. Zhang, C. A. Sizemore et al., "T-cell-replete HLA-haploidentical hematopoietic transplantation for hematologic malignancies using post-transplantation cyclophosphamide results in outcomes equivalent to those of contemporaneous HLA-matched related and unrelated donor transplantation," *Journal of Clinical Oncology*, vol. 31, no. 10, pp. 1310–1316, 2013.

[57] F. Ciceri, M. Bregni, and J. Peccatori, "Innovative platforms for haploidentical stem cell transplantation: the role of unmanipulated donor graft," *Journal of Cancer*, vol. 2, no. 1, pp. 339–340, 2011.

[58] J. Peccatori, D. Clerici, and A. Forcina, "In-vivo T-regs generation by rapamycin-mycophenolate-ATG as a new platform for GVHD prophylaxis in T-cell repleted unmanipulated haploidentical peripheral stem cell transplantation: results in 59 patients," *Bone Marrow Transplantation*, vol. 45, supplement 2, p. S3, 2010.

[59] M. Di Ianni, F. Falzetti, A. Carotti et al., "Tregs prevent GVHD and promote immune reconstitution in HLA-haploidentical transplantation," *Blood*, vol. 117, no. 14, pp. 3921–3928, 2011.

[60] X.-J. Huang, D.-H. Liu, K.-Y. Liu et al., "Treatment of acute leukemia with unmanipulated HLA-mismatched/haploidentical blood and bone marrow transplantation," *Biology of Blood and Marrow Transplantation*, vol. 15, no. 2, pp. 257–265, 2009.

[61] P. D. Bartolomeo, S. Santarone, G. De Angelis et al., "Haploidentical, unmanipulated, G-CSF-primed bone marrow transplantation for patients with high-risk hematologic malignancies," *Blood*, vol. 121, no. 5, pp. 849–857, 2013.

[62] Y. Wang, Y.-J. Chang, L.-P. Xu et al., "Who is the best donor for a related HLA haplotype-mismatched transplant?" *Blood*, vol. 124, no. 6, pp. 843–850, 2014.

[63] T. Ichinohe, T. Uchiyama, C. Shimazaki et al., "Feasibility of HLA-haploidentical hematopoietic stem cell transplantation between noninherited maternal antigen (NIMA)-mismatched family members linked with long-term fetomaternal microchimerism," *Blood*, vol. 104, no. 12, pp. 3821–3828, 2004.

[64] J. Cai, J. Lee, E. Jankowska-Gan et al., "Minor H antigen HA-1-specific regulator and effector CD8⁺ T cells, and HA-1 microchimerism, in allograft tolerance," *The Journal of Experimental Medicine*, vol. 199, no. 7, pp. 1017–1023, 2004.

[65] S. O. Ciurea, M.-J. Zhang, A. A. Bacigalupo et al., "Haploidentical transplant with posttransplant cyclophosphamide vs matched unrelated donor transplant for acute myeloid leukemia," *Blood*, vol. 126, no. 8, pp. 1033–1040, 2015.

[66] A. Di Stasi, D. R. Milton, L. M. Poon et al., "Similar transplantation outcomes for acute myeloid leukemia and myelodysplastic syndrome patients with haploidentical versus 10/10 human leukocyte antigen-matched unrelated and related donors," *Biology of Blood and Marrow Transplantation*, vol. 20, no. 12, pp. 1975–1981, 2014.

[67] Y. Wang, Q.-F. Liu, L.-P. Xu et al., "Haploidentical vs identical-sibling transplant for AML in remission: a multicenter, prospective study," *Blood*, vol. 125, no. 25, pp. 3956–3962, 2015.

[68] L. Gao, C. Zhang, L. Gao et al., "Favorable outcome of haploidentical hematopoietic stem cell transplantation in Philadelphia chromosome-positive acute lymphoblastic leukemia: a multicenter study in Southwest China," *Journal of Hematology and Oncology*, vol. 8, article 90, 2015.

[69] A. Ruggeri, M. Labopin, G. Sanz et al., "Comparison of outcomes after unrelated cord blood and unmanipulated haploidentical stem cell transplantation in adults with acute leukemia," *Leukemia*, vol. 29, no. 9, pp. 1891–1900, 2015.

[70] O. Ringdén, M. Labopin, F. Ciceri et al., "Is there a stronger graft-versus-leukemia effect using HLA-haploidentical donors compared with HLA-identical siblings?" *Leukemia*, vol. 30, no. 2, pp. 447–455, 2016.

[71] L. M. Burroughs, P. V. O'Donnell, B. M. Sandmaier et al., "Comparison of outcomes of HLA-matched related, unrelated, or HLA-haploidentical related hematopoietic cell transplantation following nonmyeloablative conditioning for relapsed or refractory Hodgkin lymphoma," *Biology of Blood and Marrow Transplantation*, vol. 14, no. 11, pp. 1279–1287, 2008.

[72] A. S. Kanate, A. Mussetti, M. A. Kharfan-Dabaja et al., "Reduced-intensity transplantation for lymphomas using haploidentical related donors vs HLA-matched unrelated donors," *Blood*, vol. 127, no. 7, pp. 938–947, 2016.

[73] A. Bashey, X. Zhang, K. Jackson et al., "Comparison of outcomes of hematopoietic cell transplants from T-replete haploidentical donors using post-transplantation cyclophosphamide with 10 of 10 HLA-A, -B, -C, -DRB1, and -DQB1 allele-matched unrelated donors and HLA-identical sibling donors: a multivariable analysis including disease risk index," *Biology of Blood and Marrow Transplantation*, vol. 22, no. 1, pp. 125–133, 2016.

[74] D. Blaise, S. Fürst, R. Crocchiolo et al., "Haploidentical T cell–replete transplantation with post-transplantation cyclophosphamide for patients in or above the sixth decade of age compared with allogeneic hematopoietic stem cell transplantation from an human leukocyte antigen–matched related or unrelated donor," *Biology of Blood and Marrow Transplantation*, vol. 22, no. 1, pp. 119–124, 2016.

[75] L. Castagna, R. Crocchiolo, S. Furst et al., "Bone marrow compared with peripheral blood stem cells for haploidentical transplantation with a nonmyeloablative conditioning regimen and post-transplantation cyclophosphamide," *Biology of Blood and Marrow Transplantation*, vol. 20, no. 5, pp. 724–729, 2014.

[76] S. Gaballa, N. Palmisiano, O. Alpdogan, M. Carabasi, J. Filicko-O'Hara, M. Kasner et al., "A two-step haploidentical versus a two-step matched related allogeneic myeloablative peripheral blood stem cell transplantation," *Biology of Blood and Marrow Transplantation*, vol. 22, no. 1, pp. 141–148, 2016.

[77] D. Grosso, M. Carabasi, J. Filicko-O'Hara et al., "A2-step approach to myeloablative haploidentical stem cell transplantation: a phase 1/2 trial performed with optimized T-cell dosing," *Blood*, vol. 118, no. 17, pp. 4732–4739, 2011.

[78] D. Grosso, S. Gaballa, O. Alpdogan et al., "A two-step approach to myeloablative haploidentical transplantation: low nonrelapse mortality and high survival confirmed in patients with earlier stage disease," *Biology of Blood and Marrow Transplantation*, vol. 21, no. 4, pp. 646–652, 2015.

[79] H. Nakamae, H. Koh, T. Katayama et al., "HLA haploidentical peripheral blood stem cell transplantation using reduced dose of posttransplantation cyclophosphamide for poor-prognosis or refractory leukemia and myelodysplastic syndrome," *Experimental Hematology*, vol. 43, no. 11, pp. 921.e1–929.e1, 2015.

[80] A. M. Raiola, A. Dominietto, A. Ghiso et al., "Unmanipulated haploidentical bone marrow transplantation and posttransplantation cyclophosphamide for hematologic malignancies after myeloablative conditioning," *Biology of Blood and Marrow Transplantation*, vol. 19, no. 1, pp. 117–122, 2013.

[81] A. M. Raiola, A. Dominietto, C. di Grazia et al., "Unmanipulated haploidentical transplants compared with other alternative donors and matched sibling grafts," *Biology of Blood and Marrow Transplantation*, vol. 20, no. 10, pp. 1573–1579, 2014.

[82] S. R. Solomon, C. A. Sizemore, M. Sanacore et al., "Haploidentical transplantation using T cell replete peripheral blood stem cells and myeloablative conditioning in patients with high-risk hematologic malignancies who lack conventional donors is well tolerated and produces excellent relapse-free survival: results of a prospective phase II trial," *Biology of Blood and Marrow Transplantation*, vol. 18, no. 12, pp. 1859–1866, 2012.

[83] Y. L. Kasamon, L. Luznik, M. S. Leffell et al., "Nonmyeloablative HLA-haploidentical bone marrow transplantation with high-dose posttransplantation cyclophosphamide: effect of HLA disparity on outcome," *Biology of Blood and Marrow Transplantation*, vol. 16, no. 4, pp. 482–489, 2010.

[84] F. Ciceri, M. Labopin, F. Aversa et al., "A survey of fully haploidentical hematopoietic stem cell transplantation in adults with high-risk acute leukemia: a risk factor analysis of outcomes for patients in remission at transplantation," *Blood*, vol. 112, no. 9, pp. 3574–3581, 2008.

[85] Y. Luo, H. Xiao, X. Lai et al., "T-cell-replete haploidentical HSCT with low-dose anti-T-lymphocyte globulin compared with matched sibling HSCT and unrelated HSCT," *Blood*, vol. 124, no. 17, pp. 2735–2743, 2014.

[86] P. McKiernan, D. Vesole, D. Siegel et al., "Haploidentical allogeneic transplantation as salvage in relapsed multiple myeloma," *Blood*, vol. 124, no. 21, p. 5918, 2014.

4

A Novel Approach for Objective Assessment of White Blood Cells Using Computational Vision Algorithms

Cesar Mauricio Rodríguez Barrero,[1] **Lyle Alberto Romero Gabalan,**[1] **and Edgar Eduardo Roa Guerrero** ⓘ [1,2]

[1]*KINESTASIS Seedlings of Research, University of Cundinamarca, Fusagasugá, Colombia*
[2]*GITEINCO Research Group, University of Cundinamarca, Fusagasugá, Colombia*

Correspondence should be addressed to Edgar Eduardo Roa Guerrero; eeduardoroa@ucundinamarca.edu.co

Academic Editor: Erwin Strasser

In the field of medicine, the analysis of blood is one of the most important exams to determine the physiological state of a patient. In the analysis of the blood sample, an important process is the counting and classification of white blood cells, which is done manually, being an exhaustive, subjective, and error-prone activity due to the physical fatigue that generates the professional because it is a method that consumes long laxes of time. The purpose of the research was to develop a system to identify and classify blood cells, by the implementation of the networks of Gaussian radial base functions (RBFN) for the extraction of its nucleus and subsequently their classification through the morphological characteristics, its color, and the distance between objects. Finally, the results obtained with the validation through the coefficient of determination showed an overall accuracy of 97.9% in the classification of the white blood cells per individual, while the precision in the classification by type of cell evidenced results in 93.4% for lymphocytes, 97.37% for monocytes, 79.5% for neutrophils, 73.07% for eosinophils, and a 100% in basophils with respect to the professional. In this way, the proposed system becomes a reliable technological support that contributes to the improvement of the analysis for identification of blood cells and therefore would benefit the low-level hematology establishments as well as to the processes of research in the area of medicine.

1. Introduction

The complete blood count (CBC) is a test that provides information relevant to the pathologic diagnosis of a patient; by the analysis the professionals in hematology observe the sample and make cell counts with the purpose to find morphological alterations of interest [1]. Within the analysis of the leucogram or count of leukocytes (white blood cells), this procedure is to determine the number of white blood cells in a given unit of blood volume of total and differential form. This test it is essential to know the values of concentration and morphology of blood cells, providing information associated with a wide range of diseases that are present in the body [2] as the estimate of malaria parasites [3].

At present, the hematology laboratories and centers of high level carried out a large number of analyses of blood per day, using automated techniques [4], in order to reduce the amount of time at each examination. However, this technique requires sophisticated and expensive equipment with technology imported from difficult access to low-level hematology establishments, as well as requiring the constant calibration by specialists [5]. For this reason, health centers or hematologists opt to perform the analysis manually, incorporating high levels of subjectivity and measurement error.

In recent years research in the field of computer vision has been developed, which has made it possible to remove and recognize patterns or objects in images little perceptible to the human vision. In [6] an efficient method for the automatic segmentation through the use of active contour techniques is posed. On the other hand, in [7] neural networks are used for the classification of the white blood cells in a blood smear. Other authors in [8] propose the segmentation of the nucleus in the white blood cell through the use of automatic thresholding classical techniques as OTSU [9, 10]. In [11] an iterative method of region growing is applied, to get better segmentation in images that have degeneration in the sample. Although in Colombia there is no presence of commercial systems, there is already significant progress in that present research [12].

The purpose of this research was to develop a system for the identification and classification of white blood cells, which decreases the subjective errors in the manual analysis through the development of a system that uses image processing techniques, in order to provide technological support reliable with repeatability in the results.

For its development, the acquisition of images from the peripheral blood smears was made, which are adapted using the YCbCr color space and in this way extract the regions belonging to the white blood cell count using the technique of the networks of Gaussian radial base functions; later a graphical interface to assist the professional in hematology during the procedure of identification of white blood cells was designed. Finally, the results of the classification of the white blood cells with respect to the manual analysis were validated.

In the present research work, we present the results of the development, implementation, and validation of a computational tool for the classification of blood cells from microscopic images of blood smears obtained from 13 different individuals.

2. Materials and Methods

In the first place, the preparation of blood samples was carried in accordance with the protocols laid down in the manual of clinical rationale in hematology [13], which define a series of steps for the preparation of the smears of blood samples, then the blood is drawn by a venous puncture; later a drop of blood is placed on a microscope slide and the spread of the same. Subsequently, it applies the dye type Wright in order to differentiate between white blood cells with respect to the substance of the sample. Finally, using a binocular microscope LEICA DM500 with digital camera led WiFi model ICC50W, later the capture made 260 microscopic images in JPG format with a resolution of 1200x1600, from a set of 13 blood smears of different individuals, previously analyzed by specialists in a specialized blood center in the city of Fusagasugá, Colombia.

The methodology proposed for the identification of blood cells is divided into 4 stages, with different processes as shown in Figure 1. At the stage of preprocessing the image RGB is converted to YCbCr color space for an improvement in the contrast of the nuclei of cells with respect to the background. In the stage of segmentation they are extracted from the nuclei of cells using the technique of the networks of Gaussian radial base functions (RBFN). After the extraction process, in the third stage the classification was made according to the morphological characteristics and color present in the cells. Later, in the fourth stage the results obtained with the system in comparison with specialists in hematology are validated. Finally, through a graphical user interface, the results obtained in the identification are displayed. The

following describes each of the techniques implemented in the stages described above.

2.1. Preprocessing of Images. Once the microscopic images are obtained from the blood smears, they are converted from the RGB color space to YCbCr [14], which allows better highlighting the nuclei of the globules present in the image with respect to other color spaces.

2.2. Networks of Gaussian Radial Base Functions. For the extraction of the white blood cells the average value of the pixels present in the nucleus of the cell obtained, according to a database of 260 images of 13 individuals. Following this, the criterion of the Euclidean distance using equation 1 is applied, in order to represent the difference between each pixel value in the image, with respect to the pixel average found in the database.

$$D = \sqrt{\left(R_i - R_{pm}\right)^2 + \left(G_i - G_{pm}\right)^2 + \left(B_i - B_{pm}\right)} \quad (1)$$

where Ri, Gi, and Bi represent the levels of red, green, and blue color of each pixel in the image and Rpm, gpm, and bpm represent the levels of red, green, and blue color of the pixel average previously obtained of the white blood cells in in the image.

Following this evaluates the distance D in a Gaussian radial basis function [7] for each pixel using (2), where α is the number of values that each pixel can have in this case 255. This provides a value between 0 to 1, where 0 indicates that the pixel analyzed does not look like the average pixel belonging to the object, while 1 indicates that they are identical; in this way the image is thresholdized through the use of a bell curve [15].

$$E = e^{-D/\alpha} \quad (2)$$

In this way we take the values with a very low coefficient of deviation with respect to the central value of the neuron in the campaign, in order to segment the objects of interest in this case, the nuclei of the white blood cells with greater accuracy.

After obtaining the thresholded image, the method of objects (n) connected was applied to determine whether two pixels are adjacent to each other in a binary image [14]. In the image each group of pixels connected corresponds to the nuclei of the cells, because platelets present in the images which have pixel values very similar to those of the nuclei are also removed. To do this, morphological operations were used in order to eliminate small areas belonging to unwanted objects in the image.

2.3. Morphological Descriptors. To measure the properties of the objects morphological descriptors were used which allowed finding a relationship between shape and size to perform the classification [14]. Among the measures that stand out the eccentricity, solidity, elongation, among others

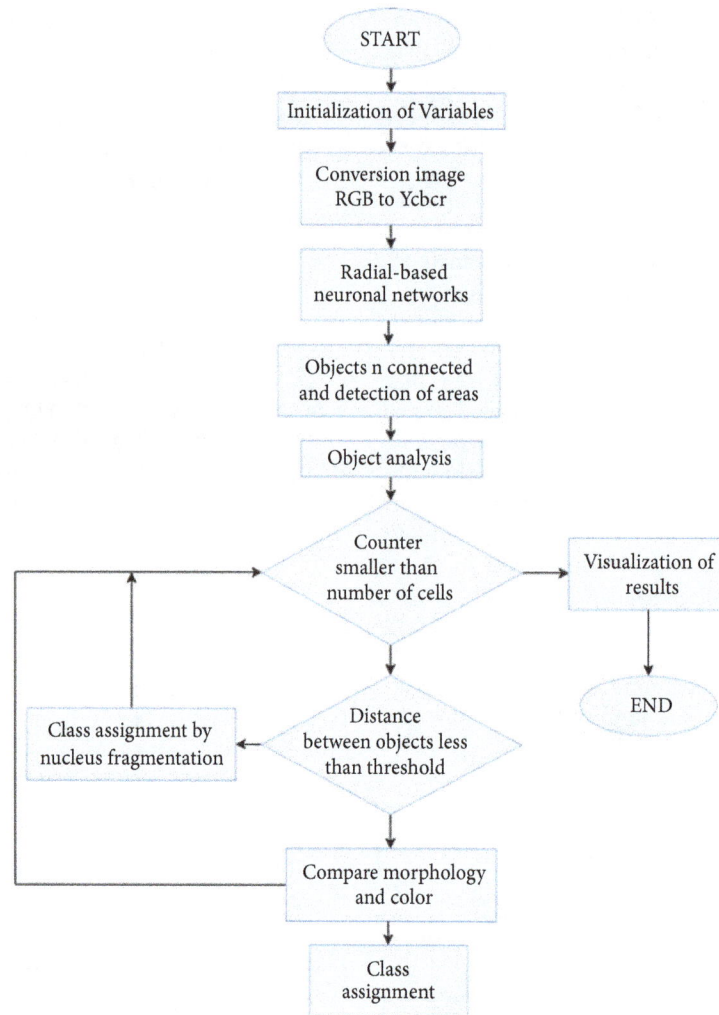

FIGURE 1: Proposed methodology.

were found. In addition, they allowed knowing the centroid or coordinates of the nucleus center of the cell on the image. According to the different measurements, an analysis of the morphological characteristics of each cell type was carried out, in order to find the characteristic that would allow differentiating the classes of globules, with the solidity being the characteristic with the most variation between each type of cell. This feature made it possible to differentiate the nucleus of the cell as follows: if the object segmented is compact, its value is close to 1 and in the case that the object is not compact its value is close to 0.

In addition of the use of morphological descriptors in the classification, A measurement of the color belonging to the nucleus and cytoplasm of the cell was also implemented, in order to make the system more robust at the time of classifying, allowing differentiating monocytes and eosinophils, which are two types of cells that have very similar characteristics in the shape of the nucleus but with variation of color.

2.4. Distance between Objects. It consists of finding a distance value between two coordinates that represent two objects found in the image. This is done by a mathematical process based on the Pythagorean theorem equation (3) where the value of the hypotenuse is interpreted as distance.

$$c^2 = a^2 + b^2 \qquad (3)$$

To apply this concept, you must know the coordinates of the center of the object in the image; once these values are obtained, a right triangle is drawn between these two points in order to apply the Pythagorean theorem and determine the separation between the objects. In the system, this distance is necessary to determine if it is a fragmented nucleus, since neutrophils can be found in embedded or fragmented. With the value below a certain distance threshold between two objects in the image, the system determines what type of nucleus is present at the time of classifying the cells.

3. Results

3.1. Image Preprocessing. The conversion to other color spaces applied to the original image in RGB was carried out in order to see their impact on the definition of the nuclei with respect to the fund to improve the stage of segmentation. It was noted in the YCbCr color space an improvement in the contrast of the nuclei of cells with respect to the background which makes the segmentation by networks of radial basis functions; in Figures 2(a) and 2(b), there is evidence of improvement in the definition of the nuclei with respect to the background.

3.2. Segmentation of White Blood Cell. Figure 2(c) shows the process of segmentation of the nuclei of white blood cells, through which its shape and size are preserved. At the same time, small particles were extracted that are present in the blood platelets because they have the same shade of color. The image resulting from the segmentation process contains binary values (1 white and 0 black), which allows the use of morphological operators to remove small particles generated by platelets whose area is less than 1500 pixels for images with a spatial resolution of 1200x1600 pixels, because a nucleus of a cell presents major areas to this value. Followed this an operator of dilatation with a structuring element of type disk with a radius of 3 pixels was implemented, and finally it fills in gaps of the nuclei in order to give uniformity as may be evidenced in Figure 2(d).

3.3. Classification of White Blood Cell. Once the images are obtained with the objects belonging to the nuclei of the cells, the value of the centroids is found, in order to identify the position of each of these cells in order to subsequently perform an analysis of the morphological characteristics, distance between objects, and the color of the cytoplasm, allowing the classification according to each type of white blood cell. Initially, there was a sweep through the entire image by calculating the values of the morphological descriptors of each object present in it as shown in Figure 2(d).

Subsequently, Table 1 describes the most relevant features that are used by the algorithm in the identification of the cells. Objects 1 and 2 according to the specialists belong to two different types of cells such as neutrophil and eosinophil, but these present values in its morphology very similar making it impossible for their identification by applying only this analysis, so it was necessary to perform an analysis of the tonality of the cytoplasm of the cell as evidenced in Figure 2(e); this analysis was performed by knowing the coordinates of objects in order to determine the values of the different components of color in the image on the periphery of the nucleus of the cell in order to make the correct identification of the cell.

Some white blood cells present fragmented nuclei as shown in Figure 2(e), where a neutrophil with a nucleus divided into two was found. To prevent the algorithm taking objects segmented as two different cells, the calculation is made of the distance of the centroids of each one. The calculation is based on the Pythagorean theorem where

Table 1: Values obtained with the morphological descriptors.

	1 object	2 objects	3 objects
Centroid	X=266	X=866	X=1202
	Y=1054	Y=394	Y=563
Strength	0.778	0.777	0.965
Area	9127	8549	8257
Perimeter	523.361	600.605	340.583

the hypotenuse of the triangle formed by the coordinates represents the distance measured in pixels. This measurement between the objects allows determining if these belong to the same cell, if it is below a threshold of 115 pixels away.

Applying a joint analysis of the different methods mentioned above, the algorithm performs the identification of the cells, classifying them in the 5 different populations (neutrophils, basophils, monocytes, eosinophils, and lymphocytes) effectively having a good performance with very similar cell populations, as evidenced in Figure 2(f).

4. Discussion

The purpose of the system is to contribute to the identification of white blood cells in a semiautomatic manner, based on the images obtained from the blood smear. This identification was made through an analysis of the different characteristics of each of the cells, in order to achieve a classification in each of their populations. The validation was carried out by comparing the results obtained with the system with respect to the results issued by a specialist in hematology, finding thus a correlation index between the two measurements to corroborate the accuracy of the system; for this purpose 20 images per individual were used. Table 2 shows the analysis performed by the professional in hematology and by the computational tool, respectively, for the 13 individuals.

The validation of the results of the system with respect to the analysis carried out by a professional in hematology presented a coefficient of determination $R2 = 0.979$, as shown in Figure 3, indicating a high correlation between the measurements per individual.

On the other hand, a correlation analysis was made between the hematology professional and the developed tool, in which it was evidenced that the obtained data follow the trend of the results from the analysis of the hematology professional; as shown in Figure 4, it shows the trend of the results obtained by the algorithm against the results obtained by the expert, evidencing high correlation between the two measurements to identify the cells of white blood cells in its 5 different populations. Therefore, it is possible to say that the implementation of this segmentation algorithm based on networks of radial basis functions and classification by morphological characteristics had a good performance in the identification of white blood cells.

On the other hand, the validation of the computational tool with respect to the professional in hematology for each class of white blood cell is present in the blood. Table 3 shows the percentages of correlation for each class. For the

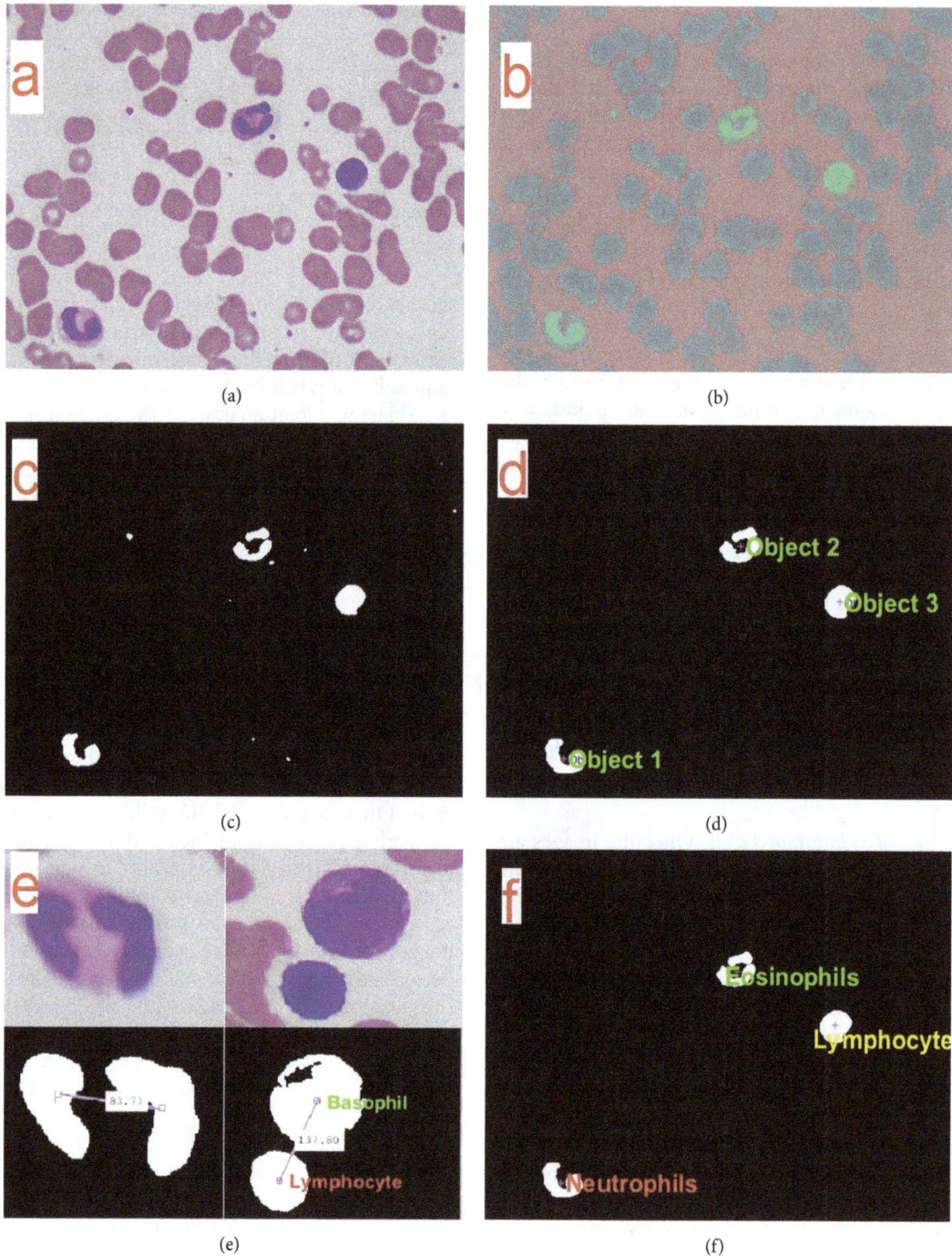

FIGURE 2: (a) Original Image. (b) Image in YCbCr. (c) Segmentation based on networks of Gaussian radial base functions. (d) Application of morphological operators. (e) Analysis of morphological characteristics. (f) Classification of white blood cells.

class of basophils, a high percentage of correlation (100%) was presented due to the low number of cells; according to [16], the percentage of basophils in an adult sample is 0.4% compared to the total number of cells in the sample, while for eosinophils it is 2.3%, for monocytes it is 5.3%, for lymphocytes it is 30%, and for neutrophils it is 62%.

The accuracy of the tool to identify the types of cells was also determined, achieving high percentages of success with respect to what was established by the professional in hematology. For basophils it was 100%, while the lowest evidence in the eosinophils has a value of 73.07% as shown in Figures 5(a) and 5(b), respectively, and for lymphocytes a percentage of 93.42% was determined, as shown in Figure 5(c). In the same way a percentage of 97.37% for the cells belonging to the population of monocytes was obtained as seen in Figure 5(d). Finally, for the population of neutrophils

TABLE 2: Analysis of the smears of blood performed by the professional in hematology versus computational tool.

individuals	Analysis of professional expert in hematology versus Tool									
	Neutrophil		Lymphocyte		Basophil		Monocyte		Eosinophilic	
	Expert	Tool	Expert	Tool	Expert	Tool	Expert	Tool	Expert	Tool
1	23	21	13	14	2	2	1	1	2	3
2	16	14	7	8	0	0	0	0	0	0
3	14	18	13	14	0	0	0	0	1	1
4	17	13	13	17	0	0	0	0	1	1
5	24	23	16	17	1	1	1	1	0	0
6	15	14	7	7	1	1	1	1	1	2
7	14	12	10	12	0	0	0	0	0	0
8	23	20	9	11	0	0	0	0	0	1
9	14	12	7	8	1	1	2	2	0	1
10	24	21	7	9	0	0	0	0	0	1
11	14	13	5	7	0	0	4	3	0	0
12	19	17	11	13	0	0	0	0	0	0
13	21	19	6	7	0	0	1	1	1	2

TABLE 3: Percentages of correlation by type of white blood cell.

correlation percentage	Lymphocyte	Neutrophil	Basophil	Monocyte	Eosinophilic
	93.42%	79.52%	100%	97.37%	73.07%

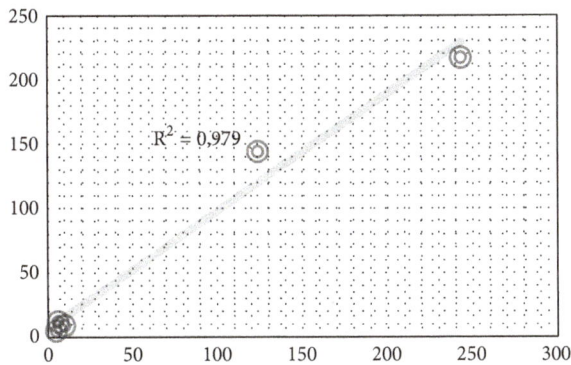

FIGURE 3: Validation of the tool versus analysis of professional in hematology.

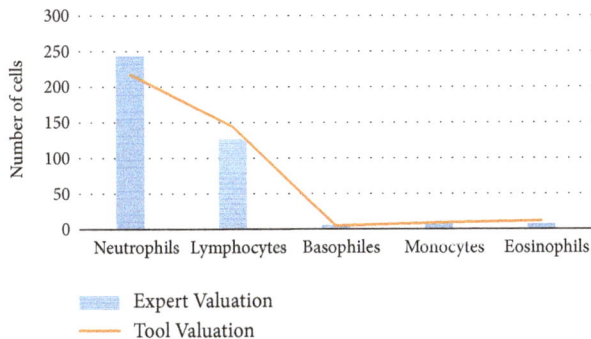

FIGURE 4: Comparison of results of the identification of white blood cells, carried out by the professional in hematology and the computational tool.

a percentage of 79.52% was obtained, as evidenced in the correlation of Figure 5(e).

On the other hand, using the Bland-Altman test which represents the difference between two measurements shown in the Figure 5(f), there was significant variability between the identification of white blood cells by the professional in hematology using the manual technique and by the computational tool developed. The results obtained show the differences with a ratio of 0.923 in a confidence interval of 95% (2.68 to 2.77), indicating that the two measurements were similar. If the two methodologies were the same the expected proportion would be 1. Finally, we compared the accuracy of the results and the characteristics of the system developed with regard to the current semiautomatic systems, as shown in Table 4. The proposed system was implemented in MatLab, obtaining percentages of accuracy higher than 79% indicating that there was no significant variability between the two measurements.

5. Conclusions

Research in the area, it demonstrated the importance of the computer vision to automate repetitive processes that are carried out manually through observation, by providing an objective analysis with high precision, in short periods of time.

The process of obtaining blood samples was carried out by means of the protocol stipulated in the manuals for the hematologic analysis, in which the staining plays a significant role since it highlights the white blood cells of other objects, allowing for the correct identification of the white blood cells through images. Although there were problems with some

TABLE 4: Comparison between systems semiautomatic versus developed algorithm.

Author	Techniques	Results
[7]	Segmentation by OTSU and classification by neural networks.	Average performance of 65% and 95% after training.
[12]	Algorithm based on gram-Schmidt orthogonalization.	Average performance of 85.4%.
[11]	Iterative method of increasing region.	Effectiveness was obtained to identify the cells of 76.47% for Basophils, 95.5% for neutrophils.
[17]	Contrast adjustment in RGB and complex-value neural networks.	To precision in complex value of 99.3% and 97.5% in real value was obtained.
[18]	Image segmentation with contrast adjustment and filtering in grayscale.	An accuracy of 80.04%, 69.3%, 86.3%, 80.3% and 83.8% was obtained for basophils, eosinophils, monocytes, neutrophils and lymphocytes.
[19]	Classification by PCA and Dendrodendritic.	The average efficiency of the process was 77.2%.
[20]	The overlapped Detection of red blood cells in microscopic images of blood smear.	Sensitivity and specificity percentages were obtained higher than 96%
[21]	Classification of different types of white blood cells by global threshold and features geometrics.	Percentages of classification were obtained higher than 98%, 92% and 95% for lymphocyte, monocyte and neutrophil respectively.
[22]	Leukocyte nucleus segmentation and recognition by K-Means clustering.	Was obtained to precision of 98% for Basophil, 98% Eosinophil, 84.3% 93.3% Lymphocyte, monocyte and neutrophil 81.3.
[23]	Leukocytes Classification In Blood Smear by support vector machines (SVM).	Was obtained to accuracy of 98.5%, 99.9% Neutrophil for Eosinophil, 98.8% 93.7% Lymphocyte and Monocyte.
[16]	WBC Segmentation and Classification by Fuzzy C-Mean.	The accuracy of the process was 91% for the 5 types of cells.
Proposed System	Classification of cells by networks of Gaussian radial basis functions (RBFN) and morphological descriptors.	Was obtained to 100% accuracy of 73.07%, 93.42%, 97.37% and 79.52% for Basophiles, Eosinophil's, lymphocytes, monocytes and neutrophils respectively and 98.2%.

samples during the acquisition of the images, they must take into account the space of the extended you are observing with the objective of the microscope, given that the identification of the white blood cells is carried out in the fields where the cells are not clustered.

The implementation of the networks of Gaussian radial base functions in conjunction with morphological descriptors and the distance between objects yielded better results in the segmentation of the nuclei with regard other segmentation techniques used, due to that highlights and extracts which completely removed the nuclei while retaining its shape on images directly in the color space.

The results obtained in the validation of the tool expose the good performance that was achieved in comparison with the results obtained from the analysis of a specialist. However, when the individual suffers from some types of infectious process or a type of pathology, it causes alterations directly in the white blood cells, thus hindering the precise identification of the cell type. However, the correlation index presented percentages higher than 95% for the individuals; on average the tool presented 98.09% accuracy in the classification of white blood cells with respect to the manual method performed by the professional in hematology.

Finally, the system developed for the analysis of blood cells allowed the technological support to the specialist, with the ability to reduce the errors generated by the subjectivity presented in the interpretation on the part of the specialist and in this way it provides reliable results. In Colombia, this tool would provide an economic alternative accessible for analysis in future research. In addition, it is proposed to expand the study to perform the complete count and classification of white blood cells, in addition to diagnose diseases associated with the reference test ranges, thus contributing to the processes of interdisciplinary research in the University of Cundinamarca.

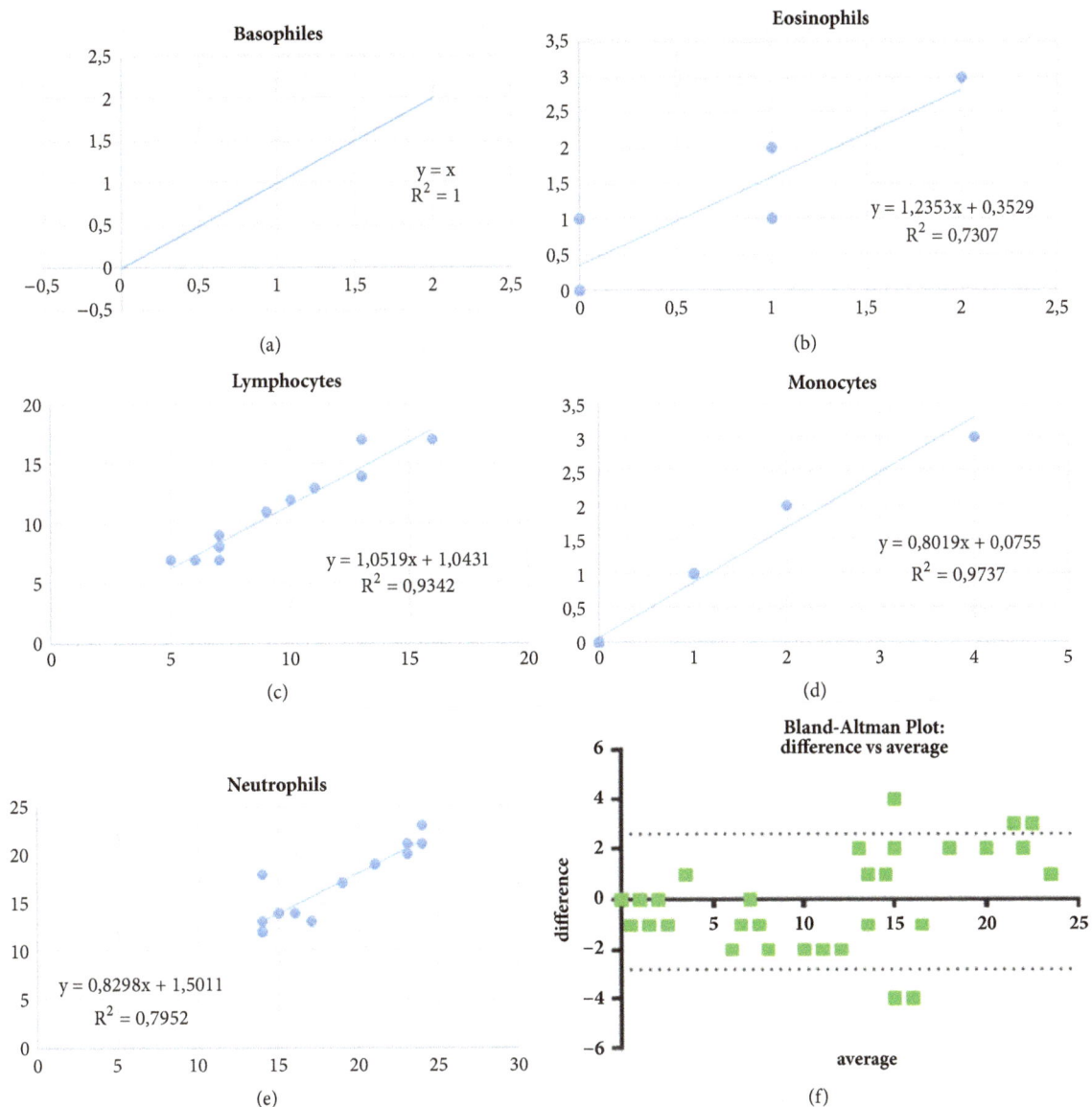

FIGURE 5: The coefficient of determination for each class of white blood cells. (a) Basophils, (b) eosinophils, (c) lymphocytes, (d) monocytes, (e) neutrophils, and (f) the Bland-Altman test between the professional in hematology and the tool.

Conflicts of Interest

The authors declare that there are no conflicts of interest.

Acknowledgments

The authors thank the expert staff of the Hematology Laboratory led by the Doctor Nancy Magally Santos, for the support in the acquisition of images and assistance in the detection and classification of white blood cell.

References

[1] D. M. T. P. clinical interpretation of the hemogram, Las Condes Clinic Magazine, 2015.

[2] G. Maya Campuzano, "The complete blood count (CBC) manual to the fourth generation," *Medical & Laboratory*, vol. 13, no. 11-12, pp. 511–550, 2007.

[3] H. Liu, G. Feng, W. Zeng et al., "A more appropriate white blood cell count for estimating malaria parasite density in Plasmodium vivax patients in northeastern Myanmar," *Acta Tropica*, vol. 156, pp. 152–156, 2016.

[4] M. d. C. S. Garcia and M. J. G. Bermejo, "Technical Manual of clinical analysis laboratory," Tech. Rep., Mad S.L, Spain, 2004.

[5] M. Freitas and L. Fernandez, "Evaluation of the Differential Leukocyte count performed with the Coulter STKS and Coulter MAXM," *RFM*, vol. 25, no. 2, pp. 189–201, 2002.

[6] J. Theerapattanakul, J. Plodpai, and C. Pintavirooj, "An efficient method for segmentation step of automated white blood cell classifications," in *Proceedings of the IEEE TENCON 2004 - 2004 IEEE Region 10 Conference: Analog and Digital Techniques in Electrical Engineering*, pp. A191–A194, Chiang Mai, Thailand, November 2004.

[7] E. Silva, *Methods of reducing neural redec RBF using the decomposition QLP for applications of data and classification [Ph.D. thesis]*, The Editorial Board of the University of Granada, 2007.

[8] A. Gautam and H. Bhadauria, "Classification of white blood cells based on morphological features," in *Proceedings of the 3rd International Conference on Advances in Computing, Communications and Informatics, ICACCI 2014*, pp. 2363–2368, New Delhi, India, September 2014.

[9] S. Nazlibilek, D. Karacor, T. Ercan, M. H. Sazli, O. Kalender, and Y. Ege, "Automatic segmentation, counting, size determination and classification of white blood cells," *Measurement*, vol. 55, pp. 58–65, 2014.

[10] K. K. Jha, B. K. Das, and H. S. Dutta, "Detection of abnormal blood cells on the basis of nucleus shape and counting of WBC," in *Proceedings of the 2014 IEEE International Conference on Green Computing, Communication and Electrical Engineering, ICGCCEE 2014*, Coimbatore, India, March 2014.

[11] S.-F. Lin and Y.-B. Hong, "Differential count of white blood cell in noisy normal blood smear," in *Proceedings of the 2012 7th IEEE Conference on Industrial Electronics and Applications, ICIEA 2012*, pp. 1784–1789, Singapore, Singapore, July 2012.

[12] M. M. A. Mohamed and B. Far, "A fast technique for white blood cells nuclei automatic segmentation based on gram-schmidt orthogonalization," in *Proceedings of the 2012 IEEE 24th International Conference on Tools with Artificial Intelligence, ICTAI 2012*, pp. 947–952, Athens, Greece, November 2012.

[13] *Rodak's Hematology Clinical Principles and Applications*, Pan American Health Care, Buenos Aires, Argentina, 5th edition, 2015.

[14] R. C. Gonzalez and R. E. Woods, *Digital Image Processing*, Prentice Hall, New Jersey, NJ, USA, 2008.

[15] Excel Total, "How to make a bell curve in Excel," https://exceltotal.com/como-hacer-una-campana-de-gauss-en-excel/.

[16] J. Prinyakupt and C. Pluempitiwiriyawej, "Segmentation of white blood cells and comparison of cell morphology by linear and naïve Bayes classifiers," *Biomedical Engineering Online*, vol. 14, no. 1, article 63, 2015.

[17] M. Mohamed, B. Far, and A. Guaily, "An efficient technique for white blood cells nuclei automatic segmentation," in *Proceedings of the 2012 IEEE International Conference on Systems, Man, and Cybernetics, SMC 2012*, pp. 220–225, Seoul, South Korea, October 2012.

[18] S. Nazlibilek, D. Karacor, K. L. Ertürk, G. Sengul, T. Ercan, and F. Aliew, "White blood cells classifications by SURF image matching, PCA and dendrogram," *Biomedical Research*, vol. 26, no. 4, pp. 633–640, 2015.

[19] M. F. Romero-Rondón, L. M. Sanabria-Rosas, L. X. Bautista-Rozo, and A. Mendoza-Castellanos, "Algorithm for detection of overlapped red blood cells in microscopic images of blood smears," *DYNA*, vol. 83, no. 198, pp. 188–195, 2016.

[20] P. Hiremath, P. Bannigidad, and S. Geeta, "Automated identification and classification of white blood cells (leukocytes) in digital microscopic images," in *Recent Trends in Image Processing and Pattern Recognition*, pp. 1–5, 2010.

[21] D.-C. Huang, K.-D. Hung, and Y.-K. Chan, "A computer assisted method for leukocyte nucleus segmentation and recognition in blood smear images," *The Journal of Systems and Software*, vol. 85, no. 9, pp. 2104–2118, 2012.

[22] O. Sarrafzadeh, H. Rabbani, A. Talebi, and H. U. Banaem, "Selection of the best features for leukocytes classification in blood smear microscopic images," in *Proceedings of the Medical Imaging 2014: Digital Pathology*, San Diego, Calif, USA, February 2014.

[23] S. Ravikumar and A. Shanmugam, "WBC image segmentation and classification using RVM," *Applied Mathematical Sciences*, no. 45-48, pp. 2227–2237, 2014.

5

Frequency of Red Blood Cell Alloimmunization in Patients with Sickle Cell Disease in Palestine

Fekri Samarah ![ORCID],[1] **Mahmoud A. Srour**,[2] **Dirgham Yaseen**,[3] **and Kamal Dumaidi** ![ORCID][1]

[1]Department of Medical Technology, Faculty of Allied Health Sciences, Arab American University in Jenin, State of Palestine
[2]Department of Biology and Biochemistry, Faculty of Science, Birzeit University, Birzeit, State of Palestine
[3]Rafidia Governmental Hospital, Ministry of Health, Nablus, State of Palestine

Correspondence should be addressed to Fekri Samarah; fekri.samarah@aauj.edu

Academic Editor: Maria Rios

Background. Transfusion of red blood cells (RBC) is an essential therapeutic tool in sickle cell disease (SCD). Repeated RBC transfusions can cause alloimmunization which causes difficulty in cross-matching and finding compatible blood for transfusions. This study aimed to investigate the frequency of RBC alloimmunization and related risk factors among Palestinian SCD patients. *Materials and Methods.* A multicenter cross-sectional study on 116 previously transfused SCD patients from three centers in West Bank, Palestine. Demographic, medical data and history of transfusion were recorded. Blood samples were collected from transfused consenting SCD patients. Gel card method was used for antibody screening and identification. In all patients, autocontrol and direct antiglobulin (DAT) test were performed using polyspecific (anti-IgG + C3d) anti-human globulin (AHG) gel cards for the detection of autoantibodies. *Results.* Of the SCD patients, 62 (53.4%) patients were HbSS and 54 (46.6%) patients were sickle β-thalassemia (S/β-thal). There were 53 (45.7%) females and 63 (54.3%) males. Mean age was 18.8 years (range 3-53 years). The frequency of RBC alloimmunization among SCD patients was 7.76%, with anti-K showing the highest frequency (33.3%) followed by anti-E (22.2%), anti-D (11.1%), anti-C (11.1%), and anti-c (11.1%). All reported IgG alloantibodies were directed against antigens in the Rh (66.7%) and Kell (33.3%) systems. Older ages of patients, increased number of blood units transfused, and splenectomy were the commonest risk factors for alloimmunization in our study. *Conclusions.* RBC alloimmunization rate among Palestinian SCD patients is low compared to neighboring countries and countries all over the world but still warrants more attention. Phenotyping of donors/recipients' RBC for Rh antigens and K_1 (partial phenotype matching) before their first transfusion may reduce the incidence of alloimmunization.

1. Introduction

Of all inherited diseases of human, sickle cell disease (SCD) is remarkable due to its pathology and disease complications and challenges it provides compared to other diseases. Factors that contribute to the unique character of SCD include its wide geographic distribution, chronicity, and poor response to therapy. SCD results from genetic mutations in the β-globin gene. The control of SCD, as well as its cure, still eludes physicians, research workers, and social scientists [1]. In Palestine, β-thalassemia and SCD are among the most common inherited abnormalities of hemoglobin synthesis. The prevalence of sickle cell trait in West Bank region of Palestine is estimated to be 1.2% based on the documentation of 116 cases of homozygote sickle cell anemia (HbSS) in the West Bank region [2] with a population of three million [3]. While the prevalence of β-thalassemia trait in West Bank region is 3.5% [4]. Analysis of the β^S-globin gene cluster haplotypes in a cohort of Palestinian patients homozygotes, for HbS [β6(A3)Glu→Val, GAG>GTG], revealed that these patients had low levels of HbF and severe clinical course, which contributes to a shortened lifespan. The β^S-mutation present in Palestine has been traced back to the Benin region and has been probably brought to Palestine along the slave trade routes [5]. Complications of SCD are attributed mainly to chronic hemolysis and painful crises due to vasooclusions, ischemia, and inflammations [6]. SCD includes all genotypes of homozygous HbSS as well as cases of compound heterozygotes with other hemoglobinopathies such as β-thalassemia (β^0 or β^+), with varying degrees of severity influenced by the amount of HbA production [7]. The last three decades have witnessed improvements in the management and treatment of SCD [8]. Hydroxyurea administration has improved SCD patient outcomes and morbidity [9]. Packed red blood cell (RBC) transfusion is an essential therapeutic component in the management of SCD, in both acute and chronic episodes like splenic sequestration crisis, acute chest syndrome (ACS), and many others [10]. Blood transfusion improves the oxygen-carrying capacity of patient's blood by reducing the level of HbS and increasing its hemoglobin concentration [11]. However, alloimmunization to RBC group antigens is a major complication of allogeneic blood transfusion and generally presents significant challenges in the management of SCD patients [12]. The frequency of RBC alloimmunization in SCD patients was reported to range from 7 to 47% [13]. In the United States, the Cooperative Study of Sickle Cell Disease revealed that more than 50% of alloimmunized SCD patients showed multiple antibodies [14]. The high frequency of alloimmunization in patients with SCD is not clearly understood. One of the most important mechanisms responsible for the development of alloimmunization is the RBC genetic disparity between donors and recipients due to racial differences [15]. Additional risk factors may include older age and sex, increased number and timing of blood transfusions, use of nonleukoreduced RBC, pregnancy, use of long-term stored blood products, patient's diagnosis, and genetic factors [9, 10, 13–17]. Alloimmunization has been associated with increased morbidity in SCD, due to the difficulty in cross-matching to find compatible blood for future transfusion, autoantibody formation, hemolysis, and delayed transfusion reactions [15, 18]. The most frequently reported alloantibodies identified in SCD are those directed against antigens of the Rh and Kell systems, followed by the Kidd and Duffy systems [9, 10, 13–16, 19]. Blood transfusion in Palestine takes place in both public and private hospitals, which are all governed by the guidelines and directions of the Palestinian Ministry of Health (MOH) on blood bank issues. To the best of our knowledge, no similar previous studies are available in Palestine. Therefore the aim of this study was to determine the frequency of RBC alloimmunization and the related risk factors among Palestinian SCD patients.

2. Materials and Methods

2.1. Study Design and Population. This was a multicenter cross-sectional study. SCD patients from three major governmental hospitals in Nablus, Jenin, and Tulkarem in West Bank region were included in this study. A total of 116 SCD patients were recruited between January and December 2017. Of these, 62 patients have sickle cell anemia (HbSS) and 54 patients have sickle β-thalassemia. The inclusion criteria included all transfusion dependent SCD patients as well as those that have had a history of at least two transfusions of ABO- and RhD-matched RBC during their lifespan.

The study was approved by the Palestinian MOH and the principles of Helsinki Declaration were implemented. Written informed consent was obtained from patients or their guardians in case of minors. A special questionnaire was used to collect demographic and medical data including patient's age, sex, age on first RBC transfusion, ABO and Rh blood group, hemoglobin concentration, history of splenectomy, number of blood units transfused, transfusion reactions, frequency, and specificity of alloantibodies by direct interview of patients or their guardians and from medical files. Clinical files and transfusion records were analyzed in all SCD patients for the presence of alloantibodies in SCD patients.

2.2. Laboratory Investigations. The diagnosis of SCD patients included in this study was based on clinical (stated in their medical records) and laboratory investigation including hemoglobin electrophoresis as well as B-globin gene mutation analysis. Complete blood count (CBC) including hemoglobin concentration and mean cell volume (MCV) was measured using Nihon Kohden (MEK-6510K) (Diamond Diagnostics, Japan) cell counter. Sickle cell phenotypes were diagnosed by conventional electrophoresis methods (cellulose acetate at alkaline and acid pH) [20]. Homozygosity for the β^S-mutations was determined by RFLP-PCR using the restriction enzyme DdeI as described earlier [21]. S/β^0-thal resembles HbSS clinically, but here S/β^0-thal cases were differentiated from HbSS by the presence of heterozygous β^S-mutations, elevated HbA2 concentrations, low MCV, and family history [7].

2.3. Alloantibody Testing. SCD patients enrolled in this study were transfused with ABO- and RhD-matched packed RBC at the three healthcare centers included in this study. This was the transfusion policy adopted at all government hospitals in West Bank until 2014. From 2014 and on, a new pretransfusion strategy for patients was applied including antibody screening and identification tests.

In this study, pretransfusion blood samples were obtained from each patient in two separate tubes, K2-EDTA tube for direct globulin test (DAT) and autocontrol (for detection of autoantibodies) and the second tube without anticoagulant (plain) (for cross-matching, antibody screening, and identification). All immunohematological tests were performed using the gel card method (Diamed ID, Switzerland), according to the manufacturer's instructions. Pretransfusion blood samples from all SCD patients were tested for the presence of alloantibodies by gel technology using commercial 3-cell panel (Diacell, Diamed ID, Switzerland), with polyspecific (anti-IgG + C3d) anti-human globulin (AHG) and homozygous expression of the antigens. All samples testing positive for alloantibody screening were further tested to identify the antibody specificity using an extended panel of 11 cells (Diacell, Diamed ID, Switzerland). Autocontrol was performed with each sample to detect autoantibodies (patient's RBC with patient's serum). Direct antiglobulin test (DAT) was also performed for each sample. In cases with a positive DAT, elution and adsorption methods were employed. Specific reagents to detect IgG, IgM, or complement were carried out using standard laboratory techniques. The alloimmunization state was ascertained by the presence of antibodies to one or more RBC antigens.

TABLE 1: SCD patients' demographic and transfusion characteristics in Palestine.

Variable	SCD alloimmunized	SCD nonimmunized	Total	P-value
n (%)	9 (7.76%)	107 (92.24%)	116 (100)	- -
Age (years), (Mean ± SD)	24.0 ± 10.99	18.4 ± 9.66	- -	- -
Number of transfused units, (Mean ± SD)	53.3 ± 22.2	27.7 ± 17.6	29.7 ± 19.1	0.019 (S)
Sex, n (%):				0.73 (NS)
Male	4 (6.3)	59 (93.7)	63 (100)	
Female	5 (9.4)	48 (90.6)	53 (100)	
Age distribution in years, n (%):				0.001 (S)
Child (< 14)	1 (1.4%)	72 (98.6%)	73 (100%)	
Adult (> 14)	8 (18.6)	35 (81.4)	43 (100%)	
Type of hemoglobin, n (%):				0.73 (NS)
HbSS	4 (6.45)	58 (93.55)	62 (100)	
S/B-thal	5 (9.26)	49 (90.74)	54 (100)	
Splenomegaly, n (%):				0.009 (S)
Yes	7 (28)	18 (72)	25 (100)	
No	2 (2.2)	89 (97.8)	91 (100)	

2.4. Statistical Analysis. Descriptive statistics and Chi-square analysis were performed using IBM SPSS statistics (version 23). Data were recorded as mean ±SD. A p value less than 0.05 was considered statistically significant.

3. Results

A total of 116 SCD patients, attending three thalassemia governmental units in Palestine (Nablus, Jenin, and Tulkarem) were included in the study. The group of SCD patients included in this study was phenotypically distributed as follows: 62 patients (53.4%) with HbSS and 54 (46.6%) patients with S/β-thal. Of the S/β-thal patients, 39 (72.2%) were S/β^0-thal and 15 (27.8%) were S/β^+-thal. The study population included 53 (45.7%) females and 63 (54.3%) males. Mean age was 18.8 ± 9.83 (range of 3-53 years) for all patients. Nine patients (7.76%) developed alloantibodies and 107 (92.24%) did not. The mean age of the alloimmunized and nonalloimmunized participants was 24 (range, 8-48) years and 18.4 (range, 3-53) years, respectively (Table 1). Our data indicated that there was no association between gender and the rate of alloimmunization (P=0.73). The rates of alloimmunization among female and male SCD patients were 9.4% (5/53) and 6.3% (4/63), respectively (Table 1).

To investigate the association between age and risk of alloimmunization, patients were categorized into two age groups. As shown in Table 1, there was a statistically significant association between age and rate of alloimmunization (P=0.001). Most SCD patients are young patients, where children (<14 years) accounted for 62.9% (n=73/116) of all patients. Most alloimmunized SCD patients (8 out of 9) were adult patients, while only one alloimmunized patient was observed among the child SCD patients. Thus our data indicated that the rate of alloimmunization increased with increasing age. Alloimmunization was more frequent in S/β-thal (9.26%) than in HbSS (6.45%) patients but was statistically insignificant (P=0.73). Splenectomy was more

TABLE 2: Alloantibody specificity and frequency in 116 Palestinian SCD patients.

Alloantibody specificity	Frequency and percentage of alloantibody, n (%)
Anti-K	3 (33.3%)
Anti-E	2 (22.2%)
Anti-D	1 (11.1%)
Anti-C	1 (11.1%)
Anti-c	1 (11.1%)
Anti-D, -C	1 (11.1%)
Total	9 (100%)

common in alloimmunized than nonalloimmunized patients and the difference was statistically significant (P=0.009).

In our study, the patients were transfused with a total of 3441 units of blood (mean= 29.7 ± 19.1; range 4-98) (Table 1). A total of 40 SCD patients were on the chronic transfusion regimen, 15 patients with homozygous HbSS and 25 patients with HbS/B-thal. All the alloimmunized SCD patients were on chronic transfusion regimen. Our data indicated that there was a statistically significant difference in the number of blood transfusion units between the alloimmunized group compared to nonalloimmunized group (P=0.019), with the alloimmunized group having a higher number of transfusions (Table 1).

Data presented in Table 2 shows the type and frequency of alloantibodies reported in our study. IgG alloantibodies against RBC antigens were detected in nine (7.76%) of the 116 SCD patients who received blood transfusions. All reported IgG alloantibodies were directed against antigens in the Rh (66.7%) and Kell (33.3%) systems. Alloantibody against K had the highest frequency (33.3%) followed by E (22.2%), D (11.1%), C (11.1%), and c (11.1%), respectively. One case (0.86%) of 116 SCD patients in the nonalloimmunized

TABLE 3: Characteristics of alloimmunized SCD patients (HbSS and HbS/β-thal.).

Patient No.	Sex	Age(years)	Hemoglobinopathy	No. of blood units transfused	Alloantibody detected	Indication for transfusion	Transfusion reaction
1	F	20	HbSS	73	Anti-K	Anemia, Hb< 7g/dl	No
2	M	48	HbSS	98	Ant-C + D	Painful crisis, anemia	DHTR[1], jaundice
3	F	31	HbSS	57	Anti-K	Painful crisis, anemia	DHTR, jaundice
4	M	24	HbSS	48	Anti-C	Joint pain, painful crisis Anemia	No
5	M	8	HbS/ β-Thal.	20	Anti-D	Anemia, Hb< 8g/dl	IHTR[2], jaundice
6	F	18	HbS/ β-Thal.	42	Anti-E	Anemia, joint pain	No
7	F	26	HbS/ β-Thal.	51	Anti-K	Anemia, Hb< 6g/dl	Jaundice
8	M	22	HbS/ β-Thal.	54	Anti-E	Anemia, painful crisis	No
9	M	19	HbS/ β-Thal.	37	Anti-c	Anemia, painful crisis	Jaundice

[1]DHTR: delayed hemolytic transfusion reactions; [2]IHTR: immediate hemolytic transfusion reaction.

patients developed autoantibody as revealed by positive polyclonal autocontrol and direct antiglobulin tests.

Table 3 shows the profile of patients who developed RBC alloantibodies in our study. All the RBC alloimmunized SCD patients were on chronic blood transfusion and received a higher rate of transfusion (53.3 ± 22.2 RBC units). The most frequent indications for blood transfusion in all patients were anemia and vasooclussive crisis. Transfusion reactions ranged between immediate hemolytic transfusion reaction (IHTR) in one patient, asymptomatic in 3 patients, and delayed hemolytic transfusion reactions (DHTR) in the rest.

4. Discussion

The high prevalence of the β^S mutation in Africa, the Middle East, India, and parts of the Mediterranean has a relation to the selective protective effect of HbS against malaria. Its spread to other regions of the world may be due to the slave trade and/or population migration [7]. RBC transfusion is an essential therapeutic component in the management of acute and chronic complications in SCD patients, where 90% of patients will have been transfused at least once in their life [22]. Despite the importance of RBC transfusions in improving SCD patients' outcomes and morbidity, alloimmunization to RBC group antigens is one of the major adverse effects of allogeneic blood transfusion [12]. Alloimmunization is a multifactorial process, but at least three elements are most important: the antigenic differences between the donor and recipient, the immune status of the recipient, and the immunomodulatory effect of the allogeneic blood transfusion on the immune system of the recipient [15, 18]. There are no published data on the frequency of alloimmunization and related risk factors among Palestinian SCD patients. Thus, this study aimed to investigate the frequency of alloimmunization among these patients. The rate of alloimmunization observed in the present study was

7.76%, which is lower than that reported in many studies of RBC alloimmunization in SCD patients [10, 12–15, 19, 23–25]. Other studies present lower rates of RBC alloimmunization [16, 26–28]. These differences in the rate of RBC alloimmunization among SCD patients support the importance of ethnic/genetic differences between patients and donors. The low rate of alloimmunization in the present study (7.76%) may be due to the high phenotypic compatibility between SCD patients and blood donors although donors were not related to the patients, but they were all Palestinians. Although the cost of antigen matching is high, further studies are needed to investigate the influence of this factor on the rate of alloimmunization. Another factor that could contribute to the relatively low rate is that SCD patients are not checked for RBC alloantibodies after each transfusion which may lead to missing the detection of transitory alloantibodies. In the healthcare centers included in this study, antibody screening is performed at the pretransfusion stage and is not retested routinely unless a new transfusion is ordered. Our results showed that the majority of SCD patients had a single alloantibody rather than multiple alloantibodies. Of all alloantibodies detected, anti-K (33.3%) was the most frequent alloantibody followed by anti-E (22.2%), anti-D (11.1%), anti-C (11.1%), and anti-c (11.1%), respectively. Given that both Rh and Kell systems have highly immunogenic antigens and phenotype-matched RBC was not performed for these antigens except D, the prevalence of alloantibodies of both systems among our study subjects was similar to previous reports [9, 10, 13–16, 19]. Donor RBC phenotyping for Rh (D, C, E, c, and e) and K_1 (partial phenotype matching) is necessary to avoid alloimmunization and stop unwanted clinical consequences in SCD patients [25]. Castro et al. reported a drop in the rate of alloimmunization from 3% to 0.5% when SCD patients were transfused only with phenotype-matched RBC [29]. Anti-D was found in two SCD patients (22.2%) where in one case it was a single alloantibody and in the second case it was in combination with anti-C, a frequency higher than that reported in most studies [14–16, 19]. The two patients with anti-D were males, the first patient was 8 years old and the other patient with the anti-D and anti-C aged 54 years. The two patients had been typed as RhD+ by serology, and thus further molecular [30] and serological studies must be conducted in these patients to unequivocally establish their RhD status. Indeed, Natukunda et al. who performed genotyping for RhD in SCD patient's alloimmunized with anti-D found that such patients had either partial D or D pseudogenes [16]. These findings are encouraging to improve the standards of blood bank services in our centers. The current study showed that there was no association between gender and the rate of alloimmunization with 4 (6.3%) male patients and 5 (9.4%) female patients having alloantibodies, respectively (p=0.73) (Table 1). Only a few reports showed that gender was not a significant factor for RBC alloimmunization [13, 14]. Other studies reported a significant association between gender and RBC alloimmunization [25, 31]. Since none of the female subjects in our study get married and the majority of patients were predominantly in the pediatric age, gender was not a risk factor. Alloimmunization rate was not significantly depending on the type of sickle cell disease since HbSS and S/β-thal subjects showed alloimmunization rate with frequencies of 6.45% and 9.26%, respectively (P=0.73). Age has been associated with the risk of RBC alloimmunization in SCD [14, 15]. By analysis of the frequency of alloimmunization in different age groups, our data revealed that the highest rate (55.6%) was among patients with older age (> 20 years). These patients received multiple blood units for several years and thus were more exposed to allogeneic RBC in their life [14, 32]. The starting time of blood transfusion in our study population was difficult to identify because of the poor filing system. Rosse et al. reported that SCD children who were first transfused at age of 10 years and older had a higher rate of alloantibodies compared to those who were transfused before that age [14]. Other authors had reported similar results [32, 33]. Factors that modify the low rate of alloimmunization in SCD children include immune tolerance, absence of pregnancy, and lower frequency of blood transfusions [18]. Thus, starting transfusion at early age in pediatric SCD patients may provide protection against RBC alloantibodies because of immune tolerance induction. This study shows that the risk of alloimmunization increases with the number of blood units transfused. This finding is in agreement with previous reports that RBC allosensitization is more likely in patients with increased frequency of blood transfusion [34–36]. The alloimmunized SCD patients in Palestine received a high rate of transfusion (53.3 ± 22.2; range 20-98 RBC units). In the current study, twenty-five SCD patients underwent splenectomy of whom 7 (28%) had alloantibodies. Our findings revealed a significant association between splenectomy and rate of alloimmunization (P=0.009), since spleen plays an important role in red cell turnover. Additionally, our findings revealed that splenectomy is a risk factor for RBC alloimmunization and this is consistent with the findings of earlier reports [37, 38], while other studies revealed no significant association [39]. In the present study, one patient (0.86%) in the nonalloimmunized group developed an autoantibody. The pathogenesis of autoantibodies following transfusion in SCD patients is not well understood. Aygun et al. reported an association between IgG autoantibodies and clinically significant hemolysis in 8% of pediatrics and 9.7% of adults [40], while others found no clinical association with hemolysis [41].

5. Conclusion

This was the first report of the frequency of RBC alloimmunization and the related risk factors among SCD patients in Palestine. All alloantibodies identified among our study population were clinically significant and are mostly against Rh and Kell blood group systems. Thus we recommend that donors of RBC, as well as recipients' of RBC, should be phenotyped for Rh (D, C, E, c, and e) and K_1 (partial phenotype matching) before the first transfusion to avoid alloimmunization in SCD patients. Older age of patients, increase in number of blood units transfused, and splenectomy were the common risk factors for alloimmunization among our study population.

Disclosure

This study was presented at the 10th International Palestinian Conference of Laboratory Medicine and the 15th Arab Conference of Clinical Biology that took place on April 18 to 21, 2018, in Ramallah, Palestine, and the abstract of this study was also published in the abstract book of the conference.

Conflicts of Interest

The authors declare that they have no conflicts of interest.

Authors' Contributions

Fekri Samarah conducted experimental design, data interpretation, and manuscript writing. Mahmoud A. Srour conducted experimental design and interpretation of data and made a major contribution to writing the manuscript. Dirgham Yaseen conducted sample collection and analysis. Kamal Dumaidi contributed to data interpretation, statistical analysis, and manuscript writing. All authors read and approved the final manuscript.

Acknowledgments

The authors are grateful to the staff of the Thalassemia and Hematology Departments at Nablus, Jenin, and Tulkarem and the Palestinian Ministry of Health for their help in patient's recruitment and sample collection.

References

[1] D. J. Weatherall and J. B. Clegg, "Inherited haemoglobin disorders: an increasing global health problem," *Bulletin of the World Health Organization*, vol. 79, no. 8, pp. 704–712, 2001.

[2] Thalassemia Patients' Friends Society, *Thalassemia: Treatment Guidelines for Patients. Al-Bireh, Palestine*, 2014.

[3] Palestinian Central Bureau of Statistics, http://www.pcbs.gov .ps/site/lang_en/881/default.aspx?lang=en.

[4] H. Darwish, F. El-Khatib, and S. Ayesh, "Spectrum of β-globin gene mutations among thalassemia patients in the west bank region of palestine," *Hemoglobin*, vol. 29, no. 2, pp. 119–132, 2005.

[5] F. Samarah, S. Ayesh, M. Athanasiou, J. Christakis, and N. Vavatsi, "βs-globin gene cluster haplotypes in the west bank of palestine," *Hemoglobin*, vol. 33, no. 2, pp. 143–149, 2009.

[6] R. P. Rother, L. Bell, P. Hillmen, and M. T. Gladwin, "The clinical sequelae of intravascular hemolysis and extracellular plasma hemoglobin: a novel mechanism of human disease," *The Journal of the American Medical Association*, vol. 293, no. 13, pp. 1653–1662, 2005.

[7] M. J. Stuart and R. L. Nagel, "Sickle-cell disease," *The Lancet*, vol. 364, no. 9442, pp. 1343–1360, 2004.

[8] O. S. Platt, D. J. Brambilla, W. F. Rosse et al., "Mortality in sickle cell disease. Life expectancy and risk factors for early death," *The New England Journal of Medicine*, vol. 330, no. 23, pp. 1639–1644, 1994.

[9] C. D. Josephson, L. L. Su, K. L. Hillyer, and C. D. Hillyer, "Transfusion in the patient with sickle cell disease: a critical review of the literature and transfusion guidelines," *Transfusion Medicine Reviews*, vol. 21, no. 2, pp. 118–133, 2007.

[10] P. C. Desai, A. M. Deal, E. R. Pfaff et al., "Alloimmunization is associated with older age of transfused red blood cells in sickle cell disease," *American Journal of Hematology*, vol. 90, no. 8, pp. 691–695, 2015.

[11] S. O. Wanko and M. J. Telen, "Transfusion management in sickle cell disease," *Hematology/Oncology Clinics of North America*, vol. 19, no. 5, pp. 803–826, 2005.

[12] S. T. Chou, T. Jackson, S. Vege, K. Smith-Whitley, D. F. Friedman, and C. M. Westhoff, "High prevalence of red blood cell alloimmunization in sickle cell disease despite transfusion from Rh-matched minority donors," *Blood*, vol. 122, no. 6, pp. 1062–1071, 2013.

[13] U. Kangiwa, O. Ibegbulam, S. Ocheni, A. Madu, and N. Mohammed, "Pattern and prevelence of alloimmunization in multiply transfused patients with sickle cell disease in Nigeria," *Biomarker Research*, vol. 3, article 26, 2015.

[14] W. F. Rosse, D. Gallagher, T. R. Kinney et al., "Transfusion and alloimmunization in sickle cell disease. The cooperative study of sickle cell disease," *Blood*, vol. 76, no. 7, pp. 1431–1437, 1990.

[15] E. P. Vichinsky, A. Earles, R. A. Johnson, M. S. Hoag, A. Williams, and B. Lubin, "Alloimmunization in sickle cell anemia and transfusion of racially unmatched blood," *The New England Journal of Medicine*, vol. 322, no. 23, pp. 1617–1621, 1990.

[16] B. Natukunda, H. Schonewille, C. Ndugwa, and A. Brand, "Red blood cell alloimmunization in sickle cell disease patients in Uganda," *Transfusion*, vol. 50, no. 1, pp. 20–25, 2010.

[17] H. Schonewille, L. M. G. Van De Watering, D. S. E. Loomans, and A. Brand, "Red blood cell alloantibodies after transfusion: Factors influencing incidence and specificity," *Transfusion*, vol. 46, no. 2, pp. 250–256, 2006.

[18] J. M. Higgins and S. R. Sloan, "Stochastic modeling of human RBC alloimmunization: evidence for a distinct population of immunologic responders," *Blood*, vol. 112, no. 6, pp. 2546–2553, 2008.

[19] A. Pathare and S. Alkindi, "Alloimmunization in patients with sickle cell disease and thalassaemia: experience of single centre from oman," *Mediterranean Journal of Hematology and Infectious Diseases*, vol. 9, no. 1, 2017.

[20] R. G. Schneider, "Differentiation of electrophoretically similar hemoglobins— such as S, D, G and P; or A2, C, E, and O by electrophoresis of the globin chains," *Clinical Chemistry*, vol. 20, pp. 1111–1115, 1974.

[21] A. E. Kulozik, J. Lyons, E. Kohne, C. R. Bartram, and E. Kleihauer, "Rapid and non-radioactive prenatal diagnosis of β thalassaemia and sickle cell disease: application of the polymerase chain reaction (PCR)," *British Journal of Haematology*, vol. 70, no. 4, pp. 455–458, 1988.

[22] S. Asma, I. Kozanoglu, E. Tarım et al., "Prophylactic red blood cell exchange may be beneficial in the management of sickle cell disease in pregnancy," *Transfusion*, vol. 55, no. 1, pp. 36–44, 2015.

[23] L. Bashawri, "Red cell alloimmunization in sickle-cell anaemia patients," *Eastern Mediterranean Health Journal*, vol. 13, no. 5, pp. 1181–1189, 2007.

[24] R. Aly, M. R. El-sharnoby, and A. A. Hagag, "Frequency of red cell alloimmunization in patients with sickle cell anemia in an Egyptian referral hospital," *Transfusion and Apheresis Science*, vol. 47, no. 3, pp. 253–257, 2012.

[25] R. Ameen, S. Al Shemmari, and A. Al-Bashir, "Red blood cell alloimmunization among sickle cell Kuwaiti Arab patients who received red blood cell transfusion," *Transfusion*, vol. 49, no. 8, pp. 1649–1654, 2009.

[26] A. Olujohungbe, I. Hambleton, L. Stephens, B. Serjeant, and G. Serjeant, "Red cell antibodies in patients with homozygous sickle cell disease: A comparison of patients in Jamaica and the United Kingdom," *British Journal of Haematology*, vol. 113, no. 3, pp. 661–665, 2001.

[27] A. Mohammed, B. Ahmed, J. Nasreldin, and M. Adil, "Red blood cell alloimmunization among sudanese homozygous sickle cell disease patients," *American Journal of Medicine and Medical Sciences*, vol. 3, no. 4, pp. 61–67, 2013.

[28] E. Meda, P. M. Magesa, T. Marlow, C. Reid, D. J. Roberts, and J. Makani, "Red blood cell alloimmunization in sickle cell disease patients in Tanzania," *East African Journal of Public Health*, vol. 11, no. 2, pp. 775–780, 2014.

[29] O. Castro, S. G. Sandler, P. Houston-Yu, and S. Rana, "Predicting the effect of transfusing only phenotype-matched RBCs to patients with sickle cell disease: theoretical and practical implications.," *Transfusion*, vol. 42, no. 6, pp. 684–690, 2002.

[30] P. A. Maaskant-Van Wijk, B. H. W. Faas, J. A. M. De Ruijter et al., "Genotyping of RHD by multiplex polymerase chain reaction analysis of six RHD-specific exons," *Transfusion*, vol. 38, no. 11-12, pp. 1015–1021, 1998.

[31] A. M. Dias Zanette, M. de Souza Gonçalves, L. Vilasboas Schettini, and etal., "Alloimmunization and clinical profile of sickle cell disease patients from Salvador-Brazil," *Ethnicity & Disease*, vol. 20, no. 2, pp. 136–141, 2010.

[32] M. Murao and M. B. Viana, "Risk factors for alloimmunization by patients with sickle cell disease," *Brazilian Journal of Medical and Biological Research*, vol. 38, no. 5, pp. 675–682, 2005.

[33] S. Sarnaik, J. Schornack, and J. M. Lusher, "The incidence of development of irregular red cell antibodies in patients with sickle cell anemia," *Transfusion*, vol. 26, no. 3, pp. 249–252, 1986.

[34] S. A. Campbell-Lee, K. Gvozdjan, K. M. Choi et al., "Red blood cell alloimmunization in sickle cell disease: assessment of transfusion protocols during two time periods," *Transfusion*, 2018.

[35] M. E. M. Yee, C. D. Josephson, A. M. Winkler et al., "Red blood cell minor antigen mismatches during chronic transfusion therapy for sickle cell anemia," *Transfusion*, vol. 57, no. 11, pp. 2738–2746, 2017.

[36] S. Allali, T. Peyrard, D. Amiranoff et al., "Prevalence and risk factors for red blood cell alloimmunization in 175 children with sickle cell disease in a French university hospital reference centre," *British Journal of Haematology*, vol. 177, no. 4, pp. 641–647, 2017.

[37] S. T. Singer, V. Wu, R. Mignacca, F. A. Kuypers, P. Morel, and E. P. Vichinsky, "Alloimmunization and erythrocyte autoimmunization in transfusion-dependent thalassemia patients of predominantly Asian descent," *Blood*, vol. 96, no. 10, pp. 3369–3373, 2000.

[38] B. Keikhaei, A. Hirad Far, H. Abolghasemi et al., "Red blood cell alloimmunization in patients with thalassemia major and intermediate in southwest Iran," *Iranian Journal of Blood & Cancer*, vol. 6, no. 1, pp. 41–46, 2013.

[39] M. Amin, "Prevalence of alloimmunization against RBC antigens in thalassemia major patients in South East Of Iran," *Journal of Blood Disorders & Transfusion*, vol. 04, no. 04, 2013.

[40] B. Aygun, S. Padmanabhan, C. Paley, and V. Chandrasekaran, "Clinical significance of RBC alloantibodies and autoantibodies in sickle cell patients who received transfusions," *Transfusion*, vol. 42, no. 1, pp. 37–43, 2002.

[41] S. M. Castellino, M. R. Combs, S. A. Zimmerman, P. D. Issitt, and R. E. Ware, "Erythrocyte autoantibodies in paediatric patients with sickle cell disease receiving transfusion therapy: frequency, characteristics and significance," *British Journal of Haematology*, vol. 104, no. 1, pp. 189–194, 1999.

6

Haploidentical Transplantation in Children with Acute Leukemia: The Unresolved Issues

Sarita Rani Jaiswal[1,2] and Suparno Chakrabarti[1,2]

[1]*Department of Blood and Marrow Transplantation, Dharamshila Hospital and Research Centre, Vasundhara Enclave, New Delhi 110096, India*
[2]*Manashi Chakrabarti Foundation, Kolkata, India*

Correspondence should be addressed to Sarita Rani Jaiswal; drsaritaranij@gmail.com

Academic Editor: Nelson J. Chao

Allogeneic hematopoietic stem cell transplantation (HSCT) remains a curative option for children with high risk and advanced acute leukemia. Yet availability of matched family donor limits its use and although matched unrelated donor or mismatched umbilical cord blood (UCB) are viable options, they fail to meet the global need. Haploidentical family donor is almost universally available and is emerging as the alternate donor of choice in adult patients. However, the same is not true in the case of children. The studies of haploidentical HSCT in children are largely limited to T cell depleted grafts with not so encouraging results in advanced leukemia. At the same time, emerging data from UCBT are challenging the existing paradigm of less stringent HLA match requirements as perceived in the past. The use of posttransplantation cyclophosphamide (PTCY) has yielded encouraging results in adults, but data in children is sorely lacking. Our experience of using PTCY based haploidentical HSCT in children shows inadequacy of this approach in younger children compared to excellent outcome in older children. In this context, we discuss the current status of haploidentical HSCT in children with acute leukemia in a global perspective and dwell on its future prospects.

1. Introduction

Despite marked improvement in the outcome of children with acute leukemia with first-line chemotherapy, a significant proportion of patients require allogeneic hematopoietic stem cell transplantation (HSCT) either in first remission (CR1) or beyond. In the BFM 95, about 12% of children diagnosed with acute lymphoblastic leukemia (ALL) went on to receive an allogeneic HSCT and the number increased in subsequent studies with introduction of MRD based risk stratification [1]. Likewise in the trials involving children with acute myeloid leukemia (AML), up to 30% of patients underwent an allogeneic transplantation [2]. In addition, allogeneic HSCT is the preferred modality of intervention beyond CR1. Thus, a conservative estimation would be that 25% of children with ALL and 40% of those with AML might require an allogeneic HSCT either in CR1 or beyond.

HLA matched family donor (MFD) remains the donor of choice in any indication for allogeneic HSCT. But with restricted family sizes, the chances of obtaining a MFD for a child are substantially reduced. Thus, alternate donor HSCT would be needed for the majority when an allogeneic HSCT is indicated and the focus of the transplant community in the past two decades has been on development of alternate donor sources.

2. The Dilemma of HLA Matching: Time for Cord Blood As Well

Developments in unrelated donor registries for both marrow and cord blood repositories have enabled progress in the field of allogeneic HSCT. Initial registry based studies had established equivalence between a mismatched unrelated cord blood transplantation (UCBT) and matched unrelated donor (MUD) transplantation [3]. HLA matching based on high resolution typing has improved the outcome of MUD transplants over the last two decades [4]. The limitations of

North American and European registries in providing 8/8 HLA matched donors beyond the White Europeans have been largely addressed by the availability of ≥4/6 HLA matched UCB units from the existing public cord blood banks [5]. Whilst low resolution typing for HLA-A and HLA-B and high resolution typing for DRB1 were deemed optimal for UCBT aiming for 4–6/6 HLA matched units, recent studies have challenged this notion [6–9]. A retrospective analysis on 803 patients, mostly children, showed the importance of HLA-C matching to reduce transplant related mortality (TRM), which was hitherto considered redundant [6]. At the same time, high resolution allele level matching for both single and double cord units was shown to reduce TRM [7, 9]. The impact of allele level or extended HLA-C matching was shown to be independent of the cell dose. These findings, if taken to cognizance, would restrict the availability of suitably matched UCB such as ≤2 allele level mismatches including HLA-C. Thus, the attempts at optimizing the outcome of UCBT have pushed the quest for the third alternative that is HLA-haploidentical family donor (HFD) to the fore [7, 8].

3. Haploidentical Family Donor: Always Present but Barely Noticed until Now

The success of HSCT depends on establishment of bidirectional tolerance and compatibility of major HLA antigens is a prerequisite for the same. It has been aptly documented in the setting of unrelated donor HSCT that with each additional mismatch in HLA-A, HLA-B, HLA-C, or DRB1 the survival decreases by 10–20% [10–12]. Recent studies have highlighted the same regarding UCBT [8]. Early attempts at introducing haploidentical family donor as an alternate donor had failed miserably. Not unexpectedly, severe alloreactivity or graft rejection dominated the outcome and the concept of allograft from a HFD was not thought to be feasible [13].

4. Megadoses of Purified CD34+ Cell Infusion: The Door Opened but Questions Remained

The breakthrough came from murine experiments demonstrating the ability of megadoses of CD34+ cells to engraft across major HLA barriers [14–16]. This was translated to clinical reality by the group from Perugia when they reported 95% engraftment with virtually no serious graft-versus-host disease (GVHD) without employment of GVHD prophylaxis, in patients with advanced leukemia [17]. This was possible due to advent of growth factor mobilized peripheral blood stem cell (PBSC) collection which enabled collection of large amounts of CD34 cells which was not hitherto possible from marrow grafts. The other advancement of technology provided the ability to purify CD34 cells via immunomagnetic techniques drastically reducing the T and B cell content of the graft. This approach was based on infusing CD34 cells in excess of 10×10^6/kg with a CD3 cell inoculum of $<1 \times 10^5$/kg. In a pilot study on haploidentical HSCT with CD34 selected PBSC graft following myeloablative and immunoablative conditioning, Aversa et al. documented sustained engraftment in 41/43 patients with advanced leukemia without acute

or chronic GVHD and 28% long term disease-free survival (DFS) [17]. Importantly, no pharmacological GVHD prophylaxis was employed. The study population included both adults and children with an age range of 4 to 53 years. However, the major drawback of this approach was delayed immune reconstitution resulting in mortality from opportunistic infections in about 40% of the patients. The reconstitution of CD4 T cells was delayed beyond 12 months in the surviving patients. In a study on 39 children employing a similar approach, 36 patients engrafted promptly with little or no GVHD [18]. The DFS was 28% and TRM was 34%. Interestingly, immune reconstitution (IR) was noted to be better in those receiving $>20 \times 10^9$/kg CD34 cells. Subsequent studies by the Perugia group showed further improvement in outcome over the next decade, but TRM remained a major concern which was attributable to delayed IR [19–21]. Two studies from the UK highlighted similar findings with better results in patients in CR than those who were not in remission [22, 23]. The outcome with this approach was remarkably better in patients with AML as compared to those with ALL [19].

An EBMT Pediatric Disease Working Party survey on 127 children with ALL transplanted between 1995 and 2004 revealed some interesting facts [24]. They found that transplants carried out by centres performing more than 231 allografts in the specified period with a median of 8 HFD yielded a DFS of 39% compared to only 15% in those performing less than 231 allografts with a median of one HFD transplant. There was a trend towards lower relapse incidence (RI) and DFS amongst those receiving a higher dose of CD34 cells. These findings highlighted the fact that T cell depleted (TCD) HFD transplantation was a technically demanding procedure requiring experience and the results heavily depended on the CD34 cell content of the graft. The other major hindrance for its universal application was the high TRM associated with delayed IR. Whilst the major centres performing such procedures develop protocols and expertise in managing these complications, the ones performing TCD HFD transplants only occasionally were unlikely to achieve similar results.

5. Natural Killer (NK) Cell Alloreactivity: A New Kid in the Block

The focus of GVHD and GVL had remained on T cells until Ruggeri et al. highlighted the impact of natural killer (NK) cells in reduction of relapse in AML following CD34 selected PBSC grafts from haploidentical donors [25]. Since then, several groups have reported on the impact of NK cells in shaping the outcome of both haploidentical family donor and unrelated donor transplantation. The opinion has often been divided on this issue [26–28]. The last decade has witnessed an enormous effort in the understanding of NK cell biology within the context of allogeneic hematopoietic cell transplantation (HCT).

NK cells kill their target through direct cytotoxicity by engaging one or more activating receptors. However, the activating receptors are believed to be under the negative feedback control from inhibitory killer immunoglobulin-like receptors (KIRs). Cytotoxicity of NK cells in the steady state is under the constant negative feedback from inhibitory KIRs through binding to Self-Class 1 MHC molecules. Several key KIR genes have been identified along with their putative ligands, whilst others remain unidentified. Biallelic polymorphism in HLA-C (positions 77 and 80 of heavy chain) denoted as C_1 or C_2 and restricted polymorphism in HLA-B (positions 77–83 in heavy chain) denoted as BW4 have been identified as ligands for KIR 2DL2/3, 2DL1, and 3DL1, respectively [29].

When NK cells from biallelic donor (C_1 and C_2), for example, fail to find one of the alleles (C_1 or C_2) in the recipient, a subset of donor NK cells tend to lose the inhibitory feedback and target the host hematopoietic cells vis-a-vis the leukemia cells in cytotoxic killing. This phenomenon (missing self-theory) was described by the Perugia group as the key event responsible for the cure of high risk leukemia following CD34 selected haploidentical graft [29, 30]. Several other models of NK alloreactivity have been postulated, yet none have been proven beyond surrogacy in the clinical setting [29–32].

In recent years, the focus has shifted to the repertoire of activating genes in the donor NK cells. Sivori et al. reported on the beneficial outcome of donor KIR2DS1 expression in conjunction with C2 allele in the recipient [33]. Furthermore Cooley et al. showed that KIR haplotypes and the specific genes related to B haplotype in the donor at centromeric or telomeric positions might have a favourable impact on the outcome of both unrelated and haploidentical HCT [34].

6. Manipulating the Graft Further: Positive versus Negative Selection

The seminal findings on NK alloreactivity along with development of immunomagnetic cell selection gave researchers in the field the options to rid the graft of CD3 and CD19 cells, leaving behind CD34, CD56, and other cell types [35]. The Tuebingen group reported on 46 children undergoing HFD HSCT with CD3+/CD19+ depleted graft in 2014 [36]. The engraftment was 88% with 20% TRM at 5 years. However, the incidences of both acute and chronic GVHD were higher with this approach, unlike that witnessed with CD34 selected grafts. The same group studied NK cell reconstitution in 59 patients undergoing CD3/19 depletion as compared to 42 patients undergoing CD34 selection [37]. They observed superior NK cell recovery and cytotoxicity with the former approach.

However, despite achieving a DFS of 45% to 80% when children were in CR, both TCD approaches were associated with dismal outcomes in more advanced diseases [18, 22, 36–38]. Employment of other TCD approaches in HFD transplantation for children with advanced leukemia did not result in improved outcome [39].

Further refinement of this approach took place with a new TCD method that removes $\alpha\beta$+ T lymphocytes via a biotinylated anti-TCR$\alpha\beta$ antibody followed by an anti-biotin antibody conjugated to magnetic microbeads while retaining TCR $\gamma\delta$+ T lymphocytes, natural killer (NK) cells, and other

cells in the graft [40]. This approach was based on the fact that the TCR$\alpha\beta$ T cells were primarily responsible for GVHD and that TCR $\gamma\delta$ T cells had potent antileukemia and anti-pathogen activity which, coupled with NK cells in the graft, would boost both antitumor and anti-infective potency of the graft. This approach has yielded excellent results in children with nonmalignant diseases and in those with acute leukemia in CR [41–44]. The IR was accelerated with this approach compared to the previous ones. The incidence of both acute and chronic GVHD remained low more akin to the CD3/CD19 depletion approach. However, the outcome of children not in CR remained dismal [43].

Another innovative approach from the Perugia group has taken graft manipulation a level further [45]. In accordance with the animal studies, they infused CD4+ CD25+ FoxP3+ regulatory T cell subpopulation (Tregs) on day −4 at 2×10^6/kg following myeloablative conditioning [46]. This was followed by infusion of $>10 \times 10^6$/kg CD34 cells on day 0 along with 1×10^6/kg conventional T cells. This study was exclusively in adults and resulted in a DFS of 53% in patients with high risk leukemia, primarily in remission [46]. The authors claimed that this approach might reduce GVHD and yet augment the GVL effect. This approach is exciting but expensive and labor intensive.

Despite the encouraging results of TCD based approaches, two major caveats remain. Firstly, the approaches are technically demanding and expensive limiting its global application. Second, TCD based HSCT has uniformly yielded abysmal results in more advanced leukemia, particularly if not in remission [47].

7. Unmanipulated Haploidentical HSCT: Changing the Paradigm in Adults, but What about Children?

Two major approaches to HFD HSCT without graft manipulation in adults have changed the approach and outlook towards haploidentical transplantation in the last 5 years. The first approach pioneered by the Peking University group employed myeloablative conditioning with combined G-CSF stimulated marrow and PBSC grafts along with multiagent GVHD prophylaxis [48, 49]. Outcome data on 1210 transplants were reported in both adults and children with mostly ALL and AML with an impressive DFS of 67% and a NRM of 17% [50]. The incidences of acute and chronic GVHD were 40% and 50%, respectively. The RI was only 17%. The same group reported on the outcome of 212 children with a median age of 15 years with both AML and ALL [51]. They reported 100% engraftment with a NRM of 15% in those transplanted in CR1/CR2, but 25–40% in those beyond CR2. The incidences of both acute and chronic GVHD were similar to those reported in the combined population, but grades 3-4 GVHD which occurred in 15% of patients was identified as a risk factor for NRM. The RI was 7.2% and 19% in CR1 for AML and ALL, respectively, but was 2-4-fold higher beyond CR1. The overall DFS was 73% for AML and 57% for ALL. In those beyond CR2, the DFS was 42% for AML and 22% for ALL. These results compare favourably with TCD approaches reported thus far. Not surprisingly, the incidences of both acute and chronic GVHD were much higher with this approach.

The other approach which was pioneered by the Johns Hopkins group involved use of posttransplantation cyclophosphamide (PTCY) [52]. This simple but unique concept is based on the fact that activated T cells are susceptible to high dose cyclophosphamide if administered in the window of 72 hours after graft infusion. The hematopoietic stem cells as well as quiescent T cells are spared of the cytotoxic effects of PTCY due to higher amount of aldehyde dehydrogenase [53, 54]. It was shown in preclinical as well as the subsequent clinical studies that this approach resulted in 90% engraftment with very low incidences of both acute and chronic GVHD [55]. These studies were carried out in adults and the conditioning was nonmyeloablative (NMA) with marrow as the source of graft. The GVHD prophylaxis consisted of mycophenolate mofetil (MMF) for 35 days and tacrolimus for 180 days. In those grafted in CR1, the results were encouraging, but the ones with more advanced disease experienced very high incidences of relapse [56]. Subsequent studies on PTCY based HFD HSCT employing myeloablative conditioning reported better DFS with no significant increase in GVHD or NRM [57, 58]. At the same time, several groups have used PBSC graft instead of BM and the outcomes have been similar in terms of engraftment and NRM with some increase in acute GVHD [59–61]. Thus, these studies have established PTCY based haploidentical HSCT as a frontrunner when it comes to alternate donor HSCT, to the extent that many argue in favour of PTCY based HFD HSCT ahead of MUD or UCBT [62–64].

Despite the impressive results in adults, the literature has been largely silent on the use of PTCY in children. One study from Japan employed a modified PTCY based approach on day +3 alone and GVHD prophylaxis with steroids and tacrolimus in 15 children, 9 of whom had advanced leukemia [65]. They reported a higher incidence of graft failure with lower conditioning intensity. Although 46% of the patients achieved a CR, the long term outcome remained dismal.

We had carried out a pilot study with PTCY based haploidentical PBSC transplantation on 20 children with advanced leukemia, 13 with refractory or relapsed AML and 7 with high risk ALL in CR1 [66]. A myeloablative conditioning with Fludarabine, Busulfan, and Melphalan was employed and GVHD prophylaxis consisted of MMF for 14–21 days and cyclosporine for 60 days with further 2 weeks of tapering. All engrafted promptly with 35% experiencing grade 2–4 GVHD and 5% having mild chronic GVHD. NRM was 20% at 1 year and this was associated with grade 3-4 GVHD, similar to that reported by the Chinese group [51]. However, it was of note that grade 3-4 GVHD occurred exclusively in those below the age of 10 years in our study. The above-mentioned study from Japan also documented GVHD in 6/8 evaluable patients below the age of 10 years [65]. In addition, we also experienced a higher incidence of early alloreactivity in the form of hemophagocytic syndrome (HPS) in children below 10 years of age [67].

8. Why Are Younger Children at a Higher Risk of Early Alloreactivity following PTCY Based Haploidentical HSCT?

This finding is indeed intriguing and counterintuitive on the face of it. The high incidence of early alloreactivity in the younger children undermines the basic principle of the PTCY approach and contradicts the prevailing concept that GVHD occurs with increasing age rather than the other way around. The relative contents of CD34+ cells and CD3+ T cells in our study were similar in both younger and older children and hence the higher T lymphocyte content of PBSC graft is unlikely to be solely responsible for the disparate outcome in the younger children [66]. Based on these findings, we hypothesised that the possible reason for early alloreactivity could be related to the failure of elimination of the alloreactive T cells by PTCY in younger children. To support this hypothesis, the pharmacokinetic (PK) studies on CY metabolism in children have been shown to be extremely variable [68]. In a study on 38 children between the ages of 2 and 15 years, there was significant interpatient variability as well as variable activation of CY to its active metabolites [69, 70]. A pharmacokinetic study of high dose CY in children above the age of 10 years undergoing myeloablative conditioning for solid tumours did not reveal any impact of age on clearance or the volume of distribution of CY [71]. Extrapolating from the pharmacokinetic studies, this phenomenon might be explained by the reduced efficacy of PTCY in clearing alloreactive T cells in younger children, due to the variable metabolism of the drug in younger age group. Whether the alloreactivity would be less with marrow grafts is unclear due to the lack of data on the same. These findings once again serve as a reminder not to consider children as mere smaller adults and a regimen deemed successful in adults might not necessarily yield similar results in children.

9. Choice of Graft for Children in CR1 Lacking a Matched Donor?

In those in whom an allograft is recommended in CR1, traditionally, a MUD or UCBT from a cord unit with high cell dose and ≤2 allele mismatches would generally be preferred for both AML and ALL. In conventional algorithm, a TCD graft from a HFD would be considered appropriate if none of the above is available. The relevant studies on HFD HSCT in children have been summarised in Tables 1 and 2. Whilst this approach is feasible and can produce impressive results in experienced hands, the procedure remains challenging to most of the world due to financial and technical demands associated with it. However, the cost of procuring a cord or a MUD graft is even more and the absence of GVHD and its prophylaxis or treatment following TCD HFD graft largely balances out the upfront financial burden in the long term along with an improved quality of life due to lack of immunosuppression and chronic GVHD. The best results with this approach are obtained in patients in complete remission, CR1 or CR2, rather than those not in CR or beyond CR2 [18, 20, 36, 39, 43]. The newer approaches to TCD such as TCRαβ

TABLE 1: Outcome of T cell depleted haploidentical transplantation for children with acute leukemia.

Ref.	Patients with AL (total)	Age range (years)	Disease status	Conditioning	Graft manipulation	Graft composition CD34 (×10^6)	CD3 (×10^7)	Engraftment (%)	Acute GVHD (%)	Chronic GVHD (%)	NRM (%)	Relapse (%)	Overall survival (%)
Aversa et al. (1998) [17]	43	4–53	Advanced	FLU/TT/ATG/TBI	CD34 selection	14	2.7	95.3%	None	None	40%	AML: 13% ALL: 63%	AML: 36% ALL: 17%
Handgretinger et al. (2001) [18]	21 (39)	(0.5–18)	NR = 9 CR = 12	MA	CD34 selection	20.7	1.5	92.3%	5%	None	28%	33%	NR: 14% CR: 39%
Goldman et al. (2000) [39]	52	1–19	AML Rel./Ref.	TBI: 40 Non-TBI: 12	Bone marrow CD2 depletion	MNC×10^8	3.04	71%	44%	None	71%	26%	2%
Ortin et al. (2002) [23]	16 (21)	2–16	CR	CY/TBI	CD34 selection	8.5	5.6	100%	43%	25%	4.8%	18.7%	81.3%
Marks et al. (2006) [22]	34	1–16	CR 18 NR 16	CY/TBI/Campath/ATG	CD34 selection	13.8	0.3–5.2	91.7%	29%	12%	29.4%	CR: 13% NR: 100%	26% AML CR: 28% ALL CR: 38%
Klingebiel et al. (2010) [24]	127	0.6–16	ALL NR 25 CR 102	MA	CD34 selection	12.3	5.0	91%	37%	16.7%	37%	36%	CR: 22–39% NR: 0%
Leung et al. (2011) [38]	38	<16	NR 5 CR 30	TBI: 20 Non-TBI: 15	CD34 selection: 13 CD3 depletion: 17 Others: 5	NA	9–44	NA	25.7%	NA	23.9%	14.7%	<2002: 19% >2002: 88%
Lang et al. (2014) [36]	46	1.1–23.7	NR 20 CR 26	FLU/TT/MEL +ATG/OKT3	CD3/19 depletion	14.5	0.59	81.6%	26%	21%	10.8%	38%	CR: 31% NR: 20%
Lang et al. (2015) [43]	29 (41)	<16	NR 9 CR 20	NA	TCRα/β and CD3 depletion	14.9	1.69	88%	24%	18%	NA%	47.2%	CR1–CR3: 100% NR: 0%

AL: acute leukemia; ALL: acute lymphoblastic leukemia; AML: acute myeloid leukemia; ATG: antithymocyte globulin; CR: complete remission; CY: cyclophosphamide; GVHD: graft-versus-host disease; FLU: Fludarabine; MA: myeloablative conditioning; Mel.: Melphalan; NR: not in remission; NRM: nonrelapse mortality; Ref.: refractory; Rel.: relapsed; TBI: total body irradiation; TT: thiotepa.

TABLE 2: Outcome of haploidentical transplantation for children with acute leukemia without T cell depletion.

Ref.	Number of patients with AL (total)	Age range (years)	Disease status	Conditioning	Graft composition		GVHD prophylaxis	Engraftment (%)	Acute GVHD (%)	Chronic GVHD (%)	NRM (%)	Relapse (%)	Overall survival (%)
					CD34 (×10^6)	CD3 (×10^7)							
Liu et al. (2013) [51]	212	3–18	NR = 24 CR = 188	AraC/BU/CY Semustin/ATG	2.5	1.88	Multiagent	100%	48.8%	40.1%	<2008: 16.8% >2008: 12.2%	<2008: 28.3% >2008: 17.5%	<2008: 61.1% >2008: 71.5%
Sawada et al. (2014) [65]	9 (15)	2–17	Ref./Rel.: 7 CR = 2	FLU/MEL	NA	NA	PTCY based	80%	55.6%	NA	28.5%	57.1%	Ref./Rel.: 14.2% CR = 100%
Jaiswal et al. (2016) [66, 67]	20	2–20	AML Rel./Ref.: 13 ALL CR: 7	FLU/BU/MEL	7.5	6.85	PTCY based	100%	35%	5%	20%	25.7%	64.3%

AL: acute leukemia; ALL: acute lymphoblastic leukemia; AML: acute myeloid leukemia; ATG: antithymocyte globulin; BU: Busulfan; CR: complete remission; CY: cyclophosphamide; GVHD: graft-versus-host disease; FLU: Fludarabine; MA: myeloablative conditioning; Mel.: Melphalan; NR: not in remission; NRM: nonrelapse mortality; Ref.: refractory; Rel.: relapsed; TBI: total body irradiation; TT: thiotepa.

depletion might be more appropriate than CD34 selection due to the poor immune reconstitution associated with the latter resulting in significant infection associated mortality [20, 39, 43, 72]. However, the data on the former is scanty and follow-ups are short to allow any definitive verdict in favour of either. Furthermore, NK cell alloreactivity plays an important role in reducing relapses for myeloid malignancies following TCD grafts in the HFD setting [32, 73]. The same is not established unequivocally in the context of ALL [73]. Some studies have suggested that NK cell alloreactivity might be effective in T cell ALL as well, whilst another study suggested an improved outcome in childhood ALL with a donor NK cell KIR B haplotype with higher B score [74].

The preferred modality of graft manipulation would be subject to the experience of individual centres with the main thrust on administering high number of CD34 cells, preferably in the range of $15-20 \times 10^6$/kg. An NK alloreactive donor would be preferred as would be a maternal donor, if the graft is T cell depleted [75]. The issue of donor NK haplotype and B score might be relevant but remains uncertain pending further studies. However, if more than one NK alloreactive HFD is available, choosing one with a B haplotype and/or higher B score might be preferred. Although the data on NK cell alloreactivity is more robust in HFD transplants for AML, the limited data should not preclude the choice of the same in ALL.

If TCD is not feasible due to technical or financial reasons, should one opt for an unmanipulated graft and if so, what should dictate the choice of the donor? Given the limited data on non-TCD approaches, the recommendations would be more tailored to the individual situation. The study by the Chinese group has yielded impressive results in both AML and ALL in CR1. However, data is not available from other centres employing a similar approach and it remains unclear if the results would be similar in other ethnic groups. This is exemplified by a much higher incidence of HPS following both UCBT and HFD HSCT from Asia as compared to Europe and Northern America [67, 76]. The data on PTCY based approach is limited, but early data indicates that this approach is best limited to children above the age of 10 years due to a higher risk of early alloreactivity [66].

The next issue that needs to be addressed is related to the choice of the haploidentical family donor. If the former approach is chosen, the choice of donor might be more definitive as donor issues have been extensively studied by the researchers from Peking University [50]. Interestingly, in direct contradiction to the data from TCD HFD [75], maternal donors were found to be associated with poorer outcomes. Three factors stood out in this analysis, donor gender, donor age, and noninherited maternal antigen (NIMA) mismatch. Thus, a NIMA mismatched younger male sibling would be a preferred donor followed by the father over mother or a sister. The same group had shown a detrimental effect of NK cell alloreactivity on the outcome, which was again contrary to the findings from TCD approach [77]. The same, however, cannot be extrapolated to other forms of unmanipulated HFD grafts and, pending further studies, a NIMA mismatched sibling donor might be a reasonable option. However, given

the increased number of single child nuclear families, one might be left to choose between the parents. The Johns Hopkins group had shown that there might not be an impact of NK cell alloreactivity in the context of NMA PTCY based haploidentical transplantation [78]. Rather, a HFD with NK B haplotype might yield better results. This again remains unproven in the pediatric setting following myeloablative conditioning.

The current excellent results of TCD haploidentical HSCT could challenge the current hierarchical algorithm of alternate donor choice of MUD and UCBT in preference to HFD grafts, especially when the financial implications of the latter are more favourably balanced in the long term. It would not be unwise to assume that continued advances in the field of HFD HSCT might make this form of alternate donor HSCT the preferred option in the near future.

10. The Choice of Graft beyond CR1/CR2

The results of TCD approaches have been uniformly dismal even with newer methods of graft manipulation in these patients [43, 47] and a non-TCD approach might be preferred. Given the high risk of treatment failure, higher incidence of both acute and chronic GVHD following an unmanipulated graft might be more acceptable. Similar to TCD approaches, the choice would be centre specific with the main aim of the regimen directed at reducing both relapse and NRM. However, if a TCD approach is employed, this needs to be combined with immunotherapy. Whether infusion of NK cells or even $\gamma\delta$T cells can improve the outcome remains to be seen but poses an exciting area of research [41, 79, 80]. The other approach being studied is the use of suicide gene modified T cells [81, 82]. Thus, it might be prudent to enroll such patients in one of the trials employing any of these approaches. At our centre, we continue with Flu-Bu-Mel conditioning and PBSC graft with PTCY and attenuated courses of both MMF and CSA in those above 10 years old. In those under the age of 10 years, we are currently enrolling patients with relapsed refractory leukemia in a study exploring inhibitors of T cell activation with PTCY to prevent early alloreactivity or TCD grafts with active immunotherapy.

11. Optimizing NK Cell Mediated GVL Effect in Unmanipulated Haploidentical HSCT

NK cell alloreactivity is unequivocally demonstrable following TCD haploidentical HSCT and yet has not been discernable with an unmanipulated graft. This paradox has never been addressed but undoubtedly deserves a closer look. There could be several explanations for this phenomenon. Ligand mismatches are not the only prerequisite for realising the antileukemia effect of alloreactive NK cells. Studies on HFD transplantation with unmanipulated graft have employed MMF as GVHD prophylaxis and have routinely employed G-CSF after transplant. Both of these interventions compromise NK cell cytotoxicity [83, 84] and so does sirolimus [85]. On the other hand, CSA probably does not impair NK cell activity and might even augment it [85, 86].

High dose CY has also been shown to enhance NK cell activation. Administration of high doses of CY improved the antitumor effect of IL-2 activated NK cells in animal models [87]. The cytotoxic activity of NK cells was increased by over 300% when they were incubated with CY. This effect was demonstrable after 2 hours and maximised after 8 hours of incubation [88]. In a clinical study on adoptive immunotherapy with haploidentical NK cells in patients with refractory AML, the use of high dose CY was associated with increased expansion of donor NK cells [89]. This was attributed to a marked rise in endogenous IL-15, a phenomenon not witnessed with low dose CY.

Thus, the combination of PTCY and CSA might provide the ideal platform to exploit the antileukemic potential of alloreactive NK cells, if the use of MMF or G-CSF could be limited. Furthermore, the use of PBSC graft rather than marrow might contribute to this phenomenon.

12. Conclusion

Haploidentical HSCT has come a long way since the initial failures in the 1980s [90]. The concepts of both the veto effect of CD34 cells when infused alone in large amounts and the utilisation of metabolic principles of cyclophosphamide in eradicating activated T cells immediately after transplantation have ushered a new era in alternate donor transplantation. Newer methods of graft manipulation with adoptive immunotherapy might pave the way for greater successes in the field of HFD transplantation for children with acute leukemia. At the same time, improving on the approaches to unmanipulated haploidentical HSCT is essential to realise the global potential of this procedure.

Competing Interests

The authors declare that there is no conflict of interests regarding the publication of this paper.

References

[1] A. Möricke, A. Reiter, M. Zimmermann et al., "Risk-adjusted therapy of acute lymphoblastic leukemia can decrease treatment burden and improve survival: treatment results of 2169 unselected pediatric and adolescent patients enrolled in the trial ALL-BFM 95," *Blood*, vol. 111, no. 9, pp. 4477–4489, 2008.

[2] H. Hasle, "A critical review of which children with acute myeloid leukaemia need stem cell procedures," *British Journal of Haematology*, vol. 166, no. 1, pp. 23–33, 2014.

[3] V. Rocha, J. Cornish, E. L. Sievers et al., "Comparison of outcomes of unrelated bone marrow and umbilical cord blood transplants in children with acute leukemia," *Blood*, vol. 97, no. 10, pp. 2962–2971, 2001.

[4] S. J. Lee, J. Klein, M. Haagenson et al., "High-resolution donor-recipient HLA matching contributes to the success of unrelated donor marrow transplantation," *Blood*, vol. 110, no. 13, pp. 4576–4583, 2007.

[5] L. Gragert, M. Eapen, E. Williams et al., "HLA match likelihoods for hematopoietic stem-cell grafts in the U.S. registry,"

The New England Journal of Medicine, vol. 371, no. 4, pp. 339–348, 2014.

[6] M. Eapen, J. P. Klein, G. F. Sanz et al., "Effect of donor-recipient HLA matching at HLA A, B, C, and DRB1 on outcomes after umbilical-cord blood transplantation for leukaemia and myelodysplastic syndrome: a retrospective analysis," *The Lancet Oncology*, vol. 12, no. 13, pp. 1214–1221, 2011.

[7] M. Eapen, J. P. Klein, A. Ruggeri et al., "Impact of allele-level HLA matching on outcomes after myeloablative single unit umbilical cord blood transplantation for hematologic malignancy," *Blood*, vol. 123, no. 1, pp. 133–140, 2014.

[8] B. Oran and E. J. Shpall, "Allele-Level HLA cord blood matching matters," *Blood*, vol. 123, no. 1, pp. 8–9, 2014.

[9] B. Oran, K. Cao, R. M. Saliba et al., "Better allele-level matching improves transplant-related mortality after double cord blood transplantation," *Haematologica*, vol. 100, no. 10, pp. 1361–1370, 2015.

[10] B. E. Shaw, "The clinical implications of HLA mismatches in unrelated donor haematopoietic cell transplantation," *International Journal of Immunogenetics*, vol. 35, no. 4-5, pp. 367–374, 2008.

[11] M. R. Verneris, S. J. Lee, K. W. Ahn et al., "HLA mismatch is associated with worse outcomes after unrelated donor reduced-intensity conditioning hematopoietic cell transplantation: an analysis from the center for international blood and marrow transplant research," *Biology of Blood and Marrow Transplantation*, vol. 21, no. 10, pp. 1783–1789, 2015.

[12] D. Weisdorf, S. Spellman, M. Haagenson et al., "Classification of HLA-matching for retrospective analysis of unrelated donor transplantation: revised definitions to predict survival," *Biology of Blood and Marrow Transplantation*, vol. 14, no. 7, pp. 748–758, 2008.

[13] R. L. Powles, H. E. M. Kay, H. M. Clink et al., "Mismatched family donors for bone-marrow transplantation as treatment for acute leukaemia," *The Lancet*, vol. 321, no. 8325, pp. 612–615, 1983.

[14] N. Or-Geva and Y. Reisner, "Megadose stem cell administration as a route to mixed chimerism," *Current Opinion in Organ Transplantation*, vol. 19, no. 4, pp. 334–341, 2014.

[15] N. Or-Geva and Y. Reisner, "Exercising 'veto' power to make haploidentical hematopoietic stem cell transplantation a safe modality for induction of immune tolerance," *Regenerative Medicine*, vol. 10, no. 3, pp. 239–242, 2015.

[16] Y. Reisner and M. F. Martelli, "Transplantation tolerance induced by 'mega dose' CD34$^+$ cell transplants," *Experimental Hematology*, vol. 28, no. 2, pp. 119–127, 2000.

[17] F. Aversa, A. Tabilio, A. Velardi et al., "Treatment of high-risk acute leukemia with T-cell-depleted stem cells from related donors with one fully mismatched hla haplotype," *The New England Journal of Medicine*, vol. 339, no. 17, pp. 1186–1193, 1998.

[18] R. Handgretinger, T. Klingebiel, P. Lang et al., "Megadose transplantation of purified peripheral blood CD34$^+$ progenitor cells from HLA-mismatched parental donors in children," *Bone Marrow Transplantation*, vol. 27, no. 8, pp. 777–783, 2001.

[19] F. Aversa, A. Terenzi, R. Felicini et al., "Haploidentical stem cell transplantation for acute leukemia," *International Journal of Hematology*, vol. 76, supplement 1, pp. 165–168, 2002.

[20] F. Aversa, Y. Reisner, and M. F. Martelli, "The haploidentical option for high-risk haematological malignancies," *Blood Cells, Molecules, and Diseases*, vol. 40, no. 1, pp. 8–12, 2008.

[21] F. Aversa, "T cell depleted haploidentical transplantation: positive selection," *Pediatric Reports*, vol. 3, supplement 2, article e14, 2011.

[22] D. I. Marks, N. Khattry, M. Cummins et al., "Haploidentical stem cell transplantation for children with acute leukaemia," *British Journal of Haematology*, vol. 134, no. 2, pp. 196–201, 2006.

[23] M. Ortín, R. Raj, E. Kinning, M. Williams, and P. J. Darbyshire, "Partially matched related donor peripheral blood progenitor cell transplantation in paediatric patients adding fludarabine and antilymphocyte gamma-globulin," *Bone Marrow Transplantation*, vol. 30, no. 6, pp. 359–366, 2002.

[24] T. Klingebiel, J. Cornish, M. Labopin et al., "Results and factors influencing outcome after fully haploidentical hematopoietic stem cell transplantation in children with very high-risk acute lymphoblastic leukemia: Impact of center size: an analysis on behalf of the Acute Leukemia and Pediatric Disease Working Parties of the European Blood and Marrow Transplant group," *Blood*, vol. 115, no. 17, pp. 3437–3446, 2010.

[25] L. Ruggeri, M. Capanni, E. Urbani et al., "Effectiveness of donor natural killer cell alloreactivity in mismatched hematopoietic transplants," *Science*, vol. 295, no. 5562, pp. 2097–2100, 2002.

[26] E. J. Lowe, V. Turner, R. Handgretinger et al., "T-cell alloreactivity dominates natural killer cell alloreactivity in minimally T-cell-depleted HLA-non-identical paediatric bone marrow transplantation," *British Journal of Haematology*, vol. 123, no. 2, pp. 323–326, 2003.

[27] S. M. Davies, L. Ruggeri, T. DeFor et al., "Evaluation of KIR ligand incompatibility in mismatched unrelated donor hematopoietic transplants," *Blood*, vol. 100, no. 10, pp. 3825–3827, 2002.

[28] A. Bishara, D. De Santis, C. C. Witt et al., "The beneficial role of inhibitory *KIR* genes of HLA class I NK epitopes in haploidentically mismatched stem cell allografts may be masked by residual donor-alloreactive T cells causing GVHD," *Tissue Antigens*, vol. 63, no. 3, pp. 204–211, 2004.

[29] A. Moretta, C. Bottino, D. Pende et al., "Identification of four subsets of human CD3-CD16+ Natural Killer (NK) cells by the expression of clonally distributed functional surface molecules: correlation between subset assignment of NK clones and ability to mediate specific alloantigen recognition," *Journal of Experimental Medicine*, vol. 172, no. 6, pp. 1589–1598, 1990.

[30] L. Ruggeri, M. Capanni, M. Casucci et al., "Role of natural killer cell alloreactivity in HLA-mismatched hematopoietic stem cell transplantation," *Blood*, vol. 94, no. 1, pp. 333–339, 1999.

[31] K. C. Hsu, T. Gooley, M. Malkki et al., "KIR ligands and prediction of relapse after unrelated donor hematopoietic cell transplantation for hematologic malignancy," *Biology of Blood and Marrow Transplantation*, vol. 12, no. 8, pp. 828–836, 2006.

[32] L. Ruggeri, A. Mancusi, M. Capanni et al., "Donor natural killer cell allorecognition of missing self in haploidentical hematopoietic transplantation for acute myeloid leukemia: challenging its predictive value," *Blood*, vol. 110, no. 1, pp. 433–440, 2007.

[33] S. Sivori, S. Carlomagno, M. Falco, E. Romeo, L. Moretta, and A. Moretta, "Natural killer cells expressing the KIR2DS1-activating receptor efficiently kill T-cell blasts and dendritic cells: implications in haploidentical HSCT," *Blood*, vol. 117, no. 16, pp. 4284–4292, 2011.

[34] S. Cooley, D. J. Weisdorf, L. A. Guethlein et al., "Donor selection for natural killer cell receptor genes leads to superior survival after unrelated transplantation for acute myelogenous leukemia," *Blood*, vol. 116, no. 14, pp. 2411–2419, 2010.

[35] R. C. Barfield, M. Otto, J. Houston et al., "A one-step large-scale method for T- and B-cell depletion of mobilized PBSC for allogeneic transplantation," *Cytotherapy*, vol. 6, no. 1, pp. 1–6, 2004.

[36] P. Lang, H.-M. Teltschik, T. Feuchtinger et al., "Transplantation of CD3/CD19 depleted allografts from haploidentical family donors in paediatric leukaemia," *British Journal of Haematology*, vol. 165, no. 5, pp. 688–698, 2014.

[37] M. M. Pfeiffer, T. Feuchtinger, H.-M. Teltschik et al., "Reconstitution of natural killer cell receptors influences natural killer activity and relapse rate after haploidentical transplantation of T- and B-cell depleted grafts in children," *Haematologica*, vol. 95, no. 8, pp. 1381–1388, 2010.

[38] W. Leung, D. Campana, J. Yang et al., "High success rate of hematopoietic cell transplantation regardless of donor source in children with very high-risk leukemia," *Blood*, vol. 118, no. 2, pp. 223–230, 2011.

[39] F. D. Goldman, S. L. Rumelhart, P. DeAlacron et al., "Poor outcome in children with refractory/relapsed leukemia undergoing bone marrow transplantation with mismatched family member donors," *Bone Marrow Transplantation*, vol. 25, no. 9, pp. 943–948, 2000.

[40] M. Schumm, P. Lang, W. Bethge et al., "Depletion of T-cell receptor α/β and CD19 positive cells from apheresis products with the CliniMACS device," *Cytotherapy*, vol. 15, no. 10, pp. 1253–1258, 2013.

[41] I. Airoldi, A. Bertaina, I. Prigione et al., "$\gamma\delta$ T-cell reconstitution after HLA-haploidentical hematopoietic transplantation depleted of TCR-$\alpha\beta^+$/CD19$^+$ lymphocytes," *Blood*, vol. 125, no. 15, pp. 2349–2358, 2015.

[42] A. Bertaina, P. Merli, S. Rutella et al., "HLA-haploidentical stem cell transplantation after removal of $\alpha\beta+$ T and B cells in children with nonmalignant disorders," *Blood*, vol. 124, no. 5, pp. 822–826, 2014.

[43] P. Lang, T. Feuchtinger, H. M. Teltschik et al., "Improved immune recovery after transplantation of TCR$\alpha\beta$/CD19-depleted allografts from haploidentical donors in pediatric patients," *Bone Marrow Transplantation*, vol. 50, supplement 2, pp. S6–S10, 2015.

[44] F. Locatelli, A. Bauquet, G. Palumbo, F. Moretta, and A. Bertaina, "Negative depletion of α/β^+ T cells and of CD19+ B lymphocytes: a novel frontier to optimize the effect of innate immunity in HLA-mismatched hematopoietic stem cell transplantation," *Immunology Letters*, vol. 155, no. 1-2, pp. 21–23, 2013.

[45] M. F. Martelli, M. D. Ianni, L. Ruggeri et al., "Next generation HLA-haploidentical HSCT," *Bone Marrow Transplantation*, vol. 5, supplement 2, pp. S63–S66, 2015.

[46] M. F. Martelli, M. D. Ianni, L. Ruggeri et al., "HLA-haploidentical transplantation with regulatory and conventional T-cell adoptive immunotherapy prevents acute leukemia relapse," *Blood*, vol. 124, no. 4, pp. 638–644, 2014.

[47] F. Aversa, "T-cell depletion: from positive selection to negative depletion in adult patients," *Bone Marrow Transplantation*, vol. 50, pp. S11–S13, 2015.

[48] Y.-Q. Sun, J. Wang, Q. Jiang et al., "Haploidentical hematopoietic SCT may be superior to conventional consolidation/maintenance chemotherapy as post-remission therapy for high-risk adult ALL," *Bone Marrow Transplantation*, vol. 50, no. 1, pp. 20–25, 2015.

[49] C.-H. Yan, Q. Jiang, J. Wang et al., "Superior survival of unmanipulated haploidentical hematopoietic stem cell transplantation compared with chemotherapy alone used as post-remission

therapy in adults with standard-risk acute lymphoblastic leukemia in first complete remission," *Biology of Blood and Marrow Transplantation*, vol. 20, no. 9, pp. 1314–1321, 2014.

[50] Y. Wang, Y.-J. Chang, L.-P. Xu et al., "Who is the best donor for a related HLA haplotype-mismatched transplant?" *Blood*, vol. 124, no. 6, pp. 843–850, 2014.

[51] D.-H. Liu, L.-P. Xu, K.-Y. Liu et al., "Long-term outcomes of unmanipulated haploidentical HSCT for paediatric patients with acute leukaemia," *Bone Marrow Transplantation*, vol. 48, no. 12, pp. 1519–1524, 2013.

[52] P. V. O'Donnell, L. Luznik, R. J. Jones et al., "Nonmyeloablative bone marrow transplantation from partially HLA-mismatched related donors using posttransplantation cyclophosphamide," *Biology of Blood and Marrow Transplantation*, vol. 8, no. 7, pp. 377–386, 2002.

[53] C. G. Kanakry, S. Ganguly, M. Zahurak et al., "Aldehyde dehydrogenase expression drives human regulatory T cell resistance to posttransplantation cyclophosphamide," *Science Translational Medicine*, vol. 5, no. 211, Article ID 211ra157, 2013.

[54] L. Luznik, S. Jalla, L. W. Engstrom, R. Iannone, and E. J. Fuchs, "Durable engraftment of major histocompatibility complex-incompatible cells after nonmyeloablative conditioning with fludarabine, low-dose total body irradiation, and posttransplantation cyclophosphamide," *Blood*, vol. 98, no. 12, pp. 3456–3464, 2001.

[55] L. Luznik, P. V. O'Donnell, H. J. Symons et al., "HLA-haploidentical bone marrow transplantation for hematologic malignancies using nonmyeloablative conditioning and high-dose, posttransplantation cyclophosphamide," *Biology of Blood and Marrow Transplantation*, vol. 14, no. 6, pp. 641–650, 2008.

[56] S. R. McCurdy, J. A. Kanakry, M. M. Showel et al., "Risk-stratified outcomes of nonmyeloablative HLA-haploidentical BMT with high-dose posttransplantation cyclophosphamide," *Blood*, vol. 125, no. 19, pp. 3024–3031, 2015.

[57] A. M. Raiola, A. Dominietto, A. Ghiso et al., "Unmanipulated haploidentical bone marrow transplantation and posttransplantation cyclophosphamide for hematologic malignancies after myeloablative conditioning," *Biology of Blood and Marrow Transplantation*, vol. 19, no. 1, pp. 117–122, 2013.

[58] S. R. Solomon, C. A. Sizemore, M. Sanacore et al., "TBI-based myeloablative haploidentical stem cell transplantation is a safe and effective alternative to unrelated donor transplantation in patients without matched sibling donors," *Biology of Blood and Marrow Transplantation*, vol. 124, no. 21, p. 426, 2015.

[59] L. Castagna, R. Crocchiolo, S. Furst et al., "Bone marrow compared with peripheral blood stem cells for haploidentical transplantation with a nonmyeloablative conditioning regimen and post-transplantation cyclophosphamide," *Biology of Blood and Marrow Transplantation*, vol. 20, no. 5, pp. 724–729, 2014.

[60] K. Raj, A. Pagliuca, K. Bradstock et al., "Peripheral blood hematopoietic stem cells for transplantation of hematological diseases from related, haploidentical donors after reduced-intensity conditioning," *Biology of Blood and Marrow Transplantation*, vol. 20, no. 6, pp. 890–895, 2014.

[61] S. R. Solomon, C. A. Sizemore, M. Sanacore et al., "Haploidentical transplantation using T cell replete peripheral blood stem cells and myeloablative conditioning in patients with high-risk hematologic malignancies who lack conventional donors is well tolerated and produces excellent relapse-free survival: results of a prospective phase II trial," *Biology of Blood and Marrow Transplantation*, vol. 18, no. 12, pp. 1859–1866, 2012.

[62] A. Bashey, X. Zhang, C. A. Sizemore et al., "T-cell-replete HLA-haploidentical hematopoietic transplantation for hematologic malignancies using post-transplantation cyclophosphamide results in outcomes equivalent to those of contemporaneous HLA-matched related and unrelated donor transplantation," *Journal of Clinical Oncology*, vol. 31, no. 10, pp. 1310–1316, 2013.

[63] S. O. Ciurea, M.-J. Zhang, A. A. Bacigalupo et al., "Haploidentical transplant with posttransplant cyclophosphamide vs matched unrelated donor transplant for acute myeloid leukemia," *Blood*, vol. 126, no. 8, pp. 1033–1040, 2015.

[64] A. M. Raiola, A. Dominietto, C. di Grazia et al., "Unmanipulated haploidentical transplants compared with other alternative donors and matched sibling grafts," *Biology of Blood and Marrow Transplantation*, vol. 20, no. 10, pp. 1573–1579, 2014.

[65] A. Sawada, M. Shimizu, K. Isaka et al., "Feasibility of HLA-haploidentical hematopoietic stem cell transplantation with post-transplantation cyclophosphamide for advanced pediatric malignancies," *Pediatric Hematology and Oncology*, vol. 31, no. 8, pp. 754–764, 2014.

[66] S. R. Jaiswal, A. Chakrabarti, S. Chatterjee et al., "Haploidentical peripheral blood stem cell transplantation with posttransplantation cyclophosphamide in children with advanced acute leukemia with fludarabine-, busulfan-, and melphalan-based conditioning," *Biology of Blood and Marrow Transplantation*, vol. 22, no. 3, pp. 499–504, 2016.

[67] S. R. Jaiswal, A. Chakrabarti, S. Chatterjee, S. Bhargava, K. Ray, and S. Chakrabarti, "Hemophagocytic syndrome following haploidentical peripheral blood stem cell transplantation with post-transplant cyclophosphamide," *International Journal of Hematology*, vol. 103, no. 2, pp. 234–242, 2016.

[68] S. M. Yule, A. V. Boddy, M. Cole et al., "Cyclophosphamide metabolism in children," *Cancer Research*, vol. 55, no. 4, pp. 803–809, 1995.

[69] S. M. Yule, A. V. Boddy, M. Cole et al., "Cyclophosphamide pharmacokinetics in children," *British Journal of Clinical Pharmacology*, vol. 41, no. 1, pp. 13–19, 1996.

[70] S. M. Yule, L. Price, M. Cole, A. D. J. Pearson, and A. V. Boddy, "Cyclophosphamide metabolism in children following a 1-h and a 24-h infusion," *Cancer Chemotherapy and Pharmacology*, vol. 47, no. 3, pp. 222–228, 2001.

[71] G. Chinnaswamy, J. Errington, A. Foot, A. V. Boddy, G. J. Veal, and M. Cole, "Pharmacokinetics of cyclophosphamide and its metabolites in paediatric patients receiving high-dose myeloablative therapy," *European Journal of Cancer*, vol. 47, no. 10, pp. 1556–1563, 2011.

[72] R. Handgretinger, X. Chen, M. Pfeiffer et al., "Cellular immune reconstitution after haploidentical transplantation in children," *Biology of Blood and Marrow Transplantation*, vol. 14, no. 1, pp. 59–65, 2008.

[73] F. Locatelli, D. Pende, M. C. Mingari et al., "Cellular and molecular basis of haploidentical hematopoietic stem cell transplantation in the successful treatment of high-risk leukemias: role of alloreactive NK cells," *Frontiers in Immunology*, vol. 4, article 15, 2013.

[74] L. Oevermann, S. U. Michaelis, M. Mezger et al., "KIR B haplotype donors confer a reduced risk for relapse after haploidentical transplantation in children with ALL," *Blood*, vol. 124, no. 17, pp. 2744–2747, 2014.

[75] M. Stern, L. Ruggeri, A. Mancusi et al., "Survival after T cell-depleted haploidentical stem cell transplantation is improved using the mother as donor," *Blood*, vol. 112, no. 7, pp. 2990–2995, 2008.

[76] S. Takagi, K. Masuoka, N. Uchida et al., "High incidence of hae-mophagocytic syndrome following umbilical cord blood transplantation for adults," *British Journal of Haematology*, vol. 147, no. 4, pp. 543–553, 2009.

[77] X.-J. Huang, X.-Y. Zhao, D.-H. Liu, K.-Y. Liu, and L.-P. Xu, "Deleterious effects of KIR ligand incompatibility on clinical outcomes in haploidentical hematopoietic stem cell transplantation without in vitro T-cell depletion," *Leukemia*, vol. 21, no. 4, pp. 848–851, 2007.

[78] Y. L. Kasamon, L. Luznik, M. S. Leffell et al., "Nonmyeloablative HLA-haploidentical bone marrow transplantation with high-dose posttransplantation cyclophosphamide: effect of HLA disparity on outcome," *Biology of Blood and Marrow Transplantation*, vol. 16, no. 4, pp. 482–489, 2010.

[79] F. Locatelli, P. Merli, and S. Rutella, "At the bedside: innate immunity as an immunotherapy tool for hematological malignancies," *Journal of Leukocyte Biology*, vol. 94, no. 6, pp. 1141–1157, 2013.

[80] H. Norell, A. Moretta, B. Silva-Santos, and L. Moretta, "At the bench: preclinical rationale for exploiting NK cells and $\gamma\delta$ T lymphocytes for the treatment of high-risk leukemias," *Journal of Leukocyte Biology*, vol. 94, no. 6, pp. 1123–1139, 2013.

[81] R. Greco, G. Oliveira, M. T. Stanghellini et al., "Improving the safety of cell therapy with the TK-suicide gene," *Frontiers in Pharmacology*, vol. 6, article 95, 2015.

[82] G. Oliveira, E. Ruggiero, M. T. L. Stanghellini et al., "Tracking genetically engineered lymphocytes long-term reveals the dynamics of T cell immunological memory," *Science Translational Medicine*, vol. 7, no. 317, Article ID 317ra198, 2015.

[83] K. Ohata, J. L. Espinoza, X. Lu, Y. Kondo, and S. Nakao, "Mycophenolic acid inhibits natural killer cell proliferation and cytotoxic function: a possible disadvantage of including mycophenolate mofetil in the graft-versus-host disease prophylaxis regimen," *Biology of Blood and Marrow Transplantation*, vol. 17, no. 2, pp. 205–213, 2011.

[84] L. Schlahsa, Y. Jaimes, R. Blasczyk, and C. Figueiredo, "Granulocyte-colony-stimulatory factor: a strong inhibitor of natural killer cell function," *Transfusion*, vol. 51, no. 2, pp. 293–305, 2011.

[85] L.-E. Wai, M. Fujiki, S. Takeda, O. M. Martinez, and S. M. Krams, "Rapamycin, but not cyclosporine or FK506, alters natural killer cell function," *Transplantation*, vol. 85, no. 1, pp. 145–149, 2008.

[86] M. T. Kasaian and C. A. Biron, "Cyclosporin A inhibition of interleukin 2 gene expression, but not natural killer cell proliferation, after interferon induction in vivo," *Journal of Experimental Medicine*, vol. 171, no. 3, pp. 745–762, 1990.

[87] R. H. Goldfarb, M. Ohashi, K. W. Brunson et al., "Augmentation of IL-2 activated natural killer cell adoptive immunotherapy with cyclophosphamide," *Anticancer Research*, vol. 18, no. 3, pp. 1441–1446, 1998.

[88] B. Sharma and N. D. Vaziri, "Augmentation of human natural killer cell activity by cyclophosphamide in vitro," *Cancer Research*, vol. 44, no. 8, pp. 3258–3261, 1984.

[89] J. S. Miller, Y. Soignier, A. Panoskaltsis-Mortari et al., "Successful adoptive transfer and in vivo expansion of human haploidentical NK cells in patients with cancer," *Blood*, vol. 105, no. 8, pp. 3051–3057, 2005.

[90] Y. Reisner, F. Aversa, and M. F. Martelli, "Haploidentical hematopoietic stem cell transplantation: state of art," *Bone Marrow Transplantation*, vol. 50, supplement 2, pp. S1–S5, 2015.

7

Outcomes of Six-Dose High-Dose Cytarabine as a Salvage Regimen for Patients with Relapsed/Refractory Acute Myeloid Leukemia

Brandi Anders,[1] Lauren Veltri,[2] Abraham S. Kanate,[3] Alexandra Shillingburg,[1,3] Nilay Shah,[3] Michael Craig,[3] and Aaron Cumpston[1,3]

[1]Department of Pharmacy, West Virginia University Medicine, Morgantown, WV, USA
[2]Section of Hematology/Oncology, Department of Internal Medicine, West Virginia University, Morgantown, WV, USA
[3]Osborn Hematopoietic Malignancy and Transplantation Program, MBRCC, West Virginia University, Morgantown, WV, USA

Correspondence should be addressed to Aaron Cumpston; cumpstona@wvumedicine.org

Academic Editor: Meral Beksac

Relapsed/refractory acute myeloid leukemia (RR-AML) is associated with poor prognosis and long-term disease-free survival requires allogeneic hematopoietic cell transplantation (allo-HCT). Limited data exists, regarding the optimal regimen to obtain remission prior to allo-HCT. Single agent high-dose cytarabine (10–12 doses administered every 12 hours) has been previously used as induction therapy. Six-dose high-dose cytarabine (HiDAC-6), commonly used as a consolidation regimen, has never been evaluated as induction therapy. We present a retrospective review of 26 consecutive patients with RR-AML receiving single agent cytarabine 3 g/m^2 intravenously every 12 hours on days 1, 3, and 5 for a total of six doses (HiDAC-6). Median follow-up for surviving patients was 10.4 months (range 1.6–112.2 months). Complete remission was obtained in 62% (54% CR and 8% CRi) of the patients. The median relapse-free survival (RFS) was 22.3 months (range 0.7–112 months), event-free survival (EFS) was 4.7 months (range 0.5–112 months), and the overall survival (OS) was 9.6 months (range 1–112 months). Thirty-five percent of patients were able to subsequently proceed to allo-HCT. Treatment-related toxicities included neutropenic fever (38%), infection (35%), neurotoxicity (8%), and skin toxicity (8%). This is the first study to demonstrate HiDAC-6 as an active treatment option for younger patients with RR-AML which can effectively serve as a bridge to allo-HCT without significant toxicity.

1. Introduction

Acute myeloid leukemia (AML) remains the most common form of acute leukemia among adults and is responsible for the largest number of deaths from leukemia in the United States [1]. Standard front-line induction therapy achieves complete response (CR) rates of 60–80%; however these remissions are often transient and the majority of patients recur within one to three years after diagnosis [2–4]. Patients who do not enter remission or relapse within 6 months of achieving CR have relatively low response rates to reinduction therapy [5–7]. There are several salvage regimens that can be considered for patients with relapsed/refractory AML (RR-AML), with limited data to guide selection of the optimal regimen. Single agent high-dose cytarabine is established for

consolidation of AML [8, 9] and has also been studied in the relapsed/refractory setting either as monotherapy or in combination with another agent, frequently an anthracycline [10, 11]. The maximum tolerated dose was found to be 3 g/m^2 every 12 hours for six days for a total of 12 doses (HiDAC-12) with toxicities associated with higher dose and extended duration including conjunctivitis and liver, dermatologic, and CNS toxicity [10]. HiDAC-12 demonstrated improved response rates with the higher dose and complete remission rate of 63% in patients with RR-AML [10]. The HiDAC regimen utilized in the consolidation phase of treatment has been reduced to 6 doses (HiDAC-6) to reduce cerebellar toxicities. The current era HiDAC-6 regimen has never been evaluated as a salvage regimen for RR-AML. We conducted a retrospective evaluation of response rates and toxicities of

HiDAC-6 at our institution in the RR-AML patient population.

2. Methods

This retrospective study was conducted at West Virginia University Hospitals. Patients included were admitted to the inpatient adult hematologic malignancy service between June 2001 and July 2015 for RR-AML. All patients received induction chemotherapy with single agent cytarabine $3\,g/m^2$ intravenously (IV) every 12 hours on days 1, 3, and 5 for a total of 6 doses (HiDAC-6). This study was approved by the Protocol Review and Monitoring Committee and the Institutional Review Board.

The primary outcome was complete remission [CR + CR with incomplete remission (CRi)] after reinduction with HiDAC-6. The secondary outcomes included overall survival (OS), event-free survival (EFS), and relapse-free survival (RFS), evaluating CR rates stratified by cytogenetic abnormalities, ability to undergo allogeneic transplant, and regimen-related toxicities. Disease responses (CR, CRi, OS, EFS, and RFS) and genetic risk groups were defined according to recommendations published by Döhner et al. [3]. Toxicity assessments were defined according to common terminology criteria of adverse events (CTCAE) version 4.03 [12]. Platelet and neutrophil recovery were defined as platelet count greater than 100×10^9/L and absolute neutrophil count (ANC) > 1.0 $\times 10^9$, respectively. All primary and secondary outcomes were reported with the use of descriptive statistics.

2.1. Supportive Care. All patients received antibacterial (levofloxacin), antifungal (fluconazole/posaconazole), and antiviral (acyclovir) prophylaxis from the start of chemotherapy until resolution of neutropenia. Other supportive care received by each patient included standard antiemetic prophylaxis with 5HT3 receptor antagonists, dexamethasone eye drops to prevent conjunctivitis, and white blood cell growth factor support. Cerebellar assessments were performed prior to each dose of cytarabine. Routine transfusion support included red blood cell and platelet infusions administered for hemoglobin <8 g/dL and platelet count <10 × 10^9/L, respectively.

3. Results

Baseline characteristics of the patients are presented in Table 1. A total of 26 patients with a median age of 46 (range 20–58) were included in the study. The majority of patients had a diagnosis of de novo AML and had received a median of one (range 1–4) prior therapy. Eighty-eight percent of patients had previously received 7 + 3 (cytarabine + anthracycline) and 31% had prior HiDAC. At the time of treatment with HiDAC-6 reinduction, 69% (n = 18) had refractory disease and 31% (n = 8) of patients had relapsed from prior treatment. Two patients had undergone prior allogeneic hematopoietic cell transplant (allo-HCT).

Median follow-up for surviving patients was 10.4 months (range 1.6–112.2 months). The complete response rate for the

TABLE 1: Patient characteristics.

Characteristics	$N = 26$
Median age, years (range)	46 (20–58)
Male gender, n (%)	16 (62%)
Median BMI (range)	28.2 (18.4–39.6)
AML diagnosis, n (%)	
(i) De novo	23 (88%)
(ii) Treatment-related	3 (12%)
Prior MDS, n (%)	3 (12%)
ECOG performance status, median (range)	1 (0–2)
Disease status, n (%)	
(i) Refractory	18 (69%)
(ii) Relapsed	8 (31%)
Prior therapies, median (range)	1 (1–4)
Prior treatments	
7 + 3	23 (88%)
HiDAC	8 (31%)
Etoposide/mitoxantrone	2 (8%)
Prior allo-HCT, n (%)	2 (8%)
Genetic risk group [3], n (%)	
Favorable	5 (19%)
Intermediate I	10 (39%)
Intermediate II	6 (23%)
Poor risk	5 (19%)

BMI: body mass index, AML: acute myeloid leukemia, MDS: myelodysplastic syndromes, ECOG: Eastern Cooperative Oncology Group, 7 + 3: cytarabine + anthracycline chemotherapy, HiDAC: high-dose cytarabine, and HCT: hematopoietic cell transplant.

TABLE 2: Response stratified by genetic risk group.

Risk group	CR + CRi N (%)
Favorable ($N = 5$)	4 (80)
Intermediate I ($N = 10$)	7 (70)
Intermediate II ($N = 6$)	3 (50)
Poor ($N = 5$)	2 (40)

CR: complete response; CRi: complete response with incomplete count recovery.

26 patients included in the study was 62% (n = 16) and included CR in 54% (n = 14) and CRi in 8% (n = 2). The median RFS, EFS, and OS were 22.3 months (range 0.7–112 months), 4.7 months (range 0.5–112 months), and 9.6 months (range 1–112 months), respectively. Stratified according to the genetic risk groups, 73% (n = 11) of patients in the favorable/intermediate I risk group achieved CR, whereas 45% (n = 5) in the intermediate II/poor risk group achieved CR (Table 2). Thirty-five percent (n = 9) of patients were able to subsequently proceed to allo-HCT.

All patients in the study experienced grade 4 thrombocytopenia and neutropenia. Median time to neutrophil and platelet recovery was 23 days (range 15–53 days) and

TABLE 3: Nonhematological adverse events.

Toxicity	Number of patients (%)
Liver toxicity (Grade 2)	1 (4)
Mucositis	
(i) Grade 1 (mild)	1 (4)
(ii) Grade ≥ 2 (moderate-severe)	2 (8)
Cerebellar toxicity	2 (8)
Neutropenic fever	10 (38)
Infection	
(i) Fungal pneumonia	4 (15)
(ii) Pneumonia, unknown pathogen	1 (4)
(iii) Bacteremia	4 (15)
(iv) Cellulitis	1 (4)
Skin toxicity	2 (8)
Other toxicities: nausea (1) and pericardial effusion ($n = 1$)	

23 days (range 13–53 days), respectively. The most common nonhematological adverse event associated with HiDAC-6 was neutropenic fever (38%). Nine patients (35%) had confirmed infection, most commonly fungal pneumonia (15%) or bacteremia (15%). Additional nonhematological toxicities and associated frequencies are listed in Table 3.

4. Discussion

To the best of our knowledge, this is the only report evaluating HiDAC-6 as a salvage reinduction regimen for RR-AML. With a CR rate of 62%, HiDAC-6 may be considered an effective salvage regimen and demonstrates similar CR rates compared to previously reported data evaluating more intense HiDAC-12 regimen (CR = 63%) and combination chemotherapy with cytarabine (CR = 30–60%) [7, 13–15].

Clinical impact of cytogenetic abnormalities and gene mutations on AML outcomes was not well described at the time of most prior single agent HiDAC salvage regimens. We had cytogenetic data on all patients and molecular mutations on 58% ($n = 15$). Although limited by a small sample size, reasonable CR rates were noted across all risk-categories of AML. However, as expected, better responses were noted in those in "better-risk" groups. While only 40% of those with poor risk cytogenetics achieved CR, 80% of patients in favorable risk group entered CR with HiDAC-6. These response rates are especially noteworthy considering the majority of the patients had refractory disease (69%, $n = 18$), which is uniformly associated with poor outcomes [3, 16]. With HiDAC-6, 67% ($n = 12$) of these patients were able to proceed to allo-HCT. Among those with relapsed AML 31% ($n = 8$), CR was noted in 50% ($n = 4$) and 2 proceeded to allo-HCT. Salvage therapy with HiDAC-6 appears to be a feasible bridge to allo-HCT in patients with RR-AML.

HiDAC-6 was well tolerated, with primary nonhematologic complications being neutropenic fever and fungal pneumonia. Infectious complications are anticipated due to prolonged neutropenia associated with AML induction

regimens and prophylactic antimicrobials and supportive care are vital components of therapy. Specifically, the high rate of fungal pneumonia ($n = 4$) highlights the need for mold prophylaxis in these patients. All 4 patients with fungal pneumonia were prior to the availability of posaconazole, which has been shown to reduce fungal infections in this patient population [17]. In the Cancer and Leukemia Group B (CALGB) study evaluating HiDAC-6 consolidation, 71% of patients required hospitalization for neutropenic fever or other complications [8]. The CNS toxicity in the CALGB study was 12% with a higher rate (32%) among those older than 60 years of age [8]. Two patients (8%) in our study developed cerebellar toxicity with prompt resolution of symptoms with discontinuation of therapy.

5. Conclusions

Albeit limited by a small sample size and retrospective design, HiDAC-6 may be considered an effective salvage reinduction regimen for younger patients with RR-AML and can be utilized as a bridge to allo-HCT.

Disclosure

This work was presented in part at the Annual Meeting of the Hematology/Oncology Pharmacy Association (HOPA), Austin, TX, March 25–28, 2015, and further updated at the American Society of Clinical Oncology (ASCO) Annual Meeting, Chicago, IL, June 3–7, 2016.

Conflicts of Interest

The authors declare that there are no conflicts of interest regarding the publication of this article.

Authors' Contributions

Brandi Anders and Lauren Veltri contributed equally to this work.

References

[1] R. Siegel, J. Ma, Z. Zou, and A. Jemal, "Cancer statistics, 2014," *CA: A Cancer Journal for Clinicians*, vol. 64, no. 1, pp. 9–29, 2014.

[2] F. Thol, R. F. Schlenk, M. Heuser, and A. Ganser, "How i treat refractory and early relapsed acute myeloid leukemia," *Blood*, vol. 126, no. 3, pp. 319–327, 2015.

[3] H. Döhner, E. H. Estey, S. Amadori et al., "Diagnosis and management of acute myeloid leukemia in adults: recommendations from an international expert panel, on behalf of the European LeukemiaNet," *Blood*, vol. 115, no. 3, pp. 453–474, 2010.

[4] D. Pulte, A. Gondos, and H. Brenner, "Expected long-term survival of patients diagnosed with acute myeloblastic leukemia during 2006–2010," *Annals of Oncology*, vol. 21, no. 2, pp. 335–341, 2010.

[5] D. A. Breems, W. L. J. Van Putten, P. C. Huijgens et al., "Prognostic index for adult patients with acute myeloid leukemia in first relapse," *Journal of Clinical Oncology*, vol. 23, no. 9, pp. 1969–1978, 2005.

[6] E. Estey, S. Kornblau, S. Pierce, H. Kantarjian, M. Beran, and M. Keating, "A stratification system for evaluating and selecting therapies in patients with relapsed or primary refractory acute myelogenous leukemia," *Blood*, no. article 756, 1996.

[7] L. H. Leopold and R. Willemze, "The treatment of acute myeloid leukemia in first relapse: A comprehensive review of the literature," *Leukemia and Lymphoma*, vol. 43, no. 9, pp. 1715–1727, 2002.

[8] R. J. Mayer, R. B. Davis, C. A. Schiffer et al., "Intensive postremission chemotherapy in adults with acute myeloid leukemia," *New England Journal of Medicine*, vol. 331, pp. 896–903, 1994.

[9] G. L. Phillips, D. E. Reece, J. D. Shepherd et al., "High-dose cytarabine and daunorubicin induction and postremission chemotherapy for the treatment of acute myelogenous leukemia in adults," *Blood*, vol. 77, no. 7, pp. 1429–1435, 1991.

[10] R. H. Herzig, H. M. Lazarus, S. N. Wolff, and G. P. Herzig, "High-dose cytosine arabinoside therapy with and without anthracycline antibiotics for remission reinduction of acute nonlymphoblastic leukemia," *Journal of Clinical Oncology*, vol. 3, no. 7, pp. 992–997, 1985.

[11] C. Karanes, K. J. Kopecky, D. R. Head et al., "A phase III comparison of high dose ARA-C (HIDAC) versus HIDAC plus mitoxantrone in the treatment of first relapsed or refractory acute myeloid leukemia. Southwest oncology group Study," *Leukemia Research*, vol. 23, no. 9, pp. 787–794, 1999.

[12] A. C. Dueck, T. R. Mendoza, S. A. Mitchell et al., "Validity and reliability of the US National cancer institute's patient-reported outcomes version of the common terminology criteria for adverse events (PRO-CTCAE)," *JAMA Oncology*, vol. 1, no. 8, pp. 1051–1059, 2015.

[13] P. Raanani, O. Shpilberg, S. Gillis et al., "Salvage therapy of refractory and relapsed acute leukemia with high dose mitoxantrone and high dose cytarabine," *Leukemia Research*, vol. 23, no. 8, pp. 695–700, 1999.

[14] T. Dang, P. Hilden, S. M. Devlin et al., "High-dose cytarabine monotherapy versus intermediate or high-dose cytarabine in combination with other agents as second-line salvage therapy in patients with acute myeloid leukemia who did not respond to initial induction therapy," *Blood*, vol. 122, no. article 2695, p. 122, 2013.

[15] Y.-G. Lee, J.-H. Kwon, I. Kim, S. S. Yoon, J.-S. Lee, and S. Park, "Effective salvage therapy for high-risk relapsed or refractory acute myeloid leukaemia with cisplatin in combination with high-dose cytarabine and etoposide," *European Journal of Haematology*, vol. 92, no. 6, pp. 478–484, 2014.

[16] W. Kern, T. Haferlach, C. Schoch et al., "Early blast clearance by remission induction therapy is a major independent prognostic factor for both achievement of complete remission and long-term outcome in acute myeloid leukemia: data from the German AML cooperative group (AMLCG) 1992 trial," *Blood*, vol. 101, no. 1, pp. 64–70, 2003.

[17] O. A. Cornely, J. Maertens, D. J. Winston et al., "Posaconazole vs. fluconazole or itraconazole prophylaxis in patients with neutropenia," *The New England Journal of Medicine*, vol. 356, pp. 348–359, 2007.

8

The Evolution of Prognostic Factors in Multiple Myeloma

Amr Hanbali, Mona Hassanein, Walid Rasheed, Mahmoud Aljurf, and Fahad Alsharif

King Faisal Specialist Hospital and Research Center, Riyadh, Saudi Arabia

Correspondence should be addressed to Amr Hanbali; ahanbali@kfshrc.edu.sa

Academic Editor: David H. Vesole

Multiple myeloma (MM) is a heterogeneous hematologic malignancy involving the proliferation of plasma cells derived by different genetic events contributing to the development, progression, and prognosis of this disease. Despite improvement in treatment strategies of MM over the last decade, the disease remains incurable. All efforts are currently focused on understanding the prognostic markers of the disease hoping to incorporate the new therapeutic modalities to convert the disease into curable one. We present this comprehensive review to summarize the current standard prognostic markers used in MM along with novel techniques that are still in development and highlight their implications in current clinical practice.

1. Introduction

Multiple myeloma (MM) is a heterogeneous hematologic malignancy involving the proliferation of plasma cells derived by different genetic events contributing to the development, progression, and prognosis of this disease. Despite improvement in treatment strategies of MM over the last decade, the disease remains incurable in most cases, although in recent years overall survival of patients has been significantly increased. All current efforts are focused on the development of novel diagnostic and therapeutic modalities hoping to convert the disease into a curable one. Over the last 15 years, new techniques in prognostic markers and novel imaging modalities became available.

Risk stratification of MM is essential for understanding the prognosis and modifications of therapeutic modalities. Patients with MM who are stratified as high risk, such as those with 17p13 deletion, generally have poor outcome with current treatment strategies and all efforts currently are focused on establishing alternative strategies for management of such patients. For the low-risk patients, they have at least 50% chance of surviving more than 10 years.

Our aim of this review is to summarize the current standard prognostic markers used in MM along with novel techniques that are still in development and highlight their implications in current clinical practice.

The prognostic factors of MM will be divided into 4 major sections:

(1) Risk Stratification, which includes Staging of MM, Plasma Cell Labeling index (PCLI), Cytogenetics and Gene Expression Profiling (GEP)

(2) Monitoring of Response Tools, which includes Serum-Free Light Chain Assay, serum Heavy/Light Chain (HLC) Assay (Hevylite™), and Advanced Imaging Modalities.

(3) Minimal Residual Disease (MRD) Monitoring Methods, which includes Circulating Plasma Cells, MRD Monitoring in General, and the Value of Depth of Response

(4) Novel Prognostic Markers

2. Risk Stratification

2.1. Staging of MM. Determining the prognosis in MM requires the knowledge of tumor and host factors. Work on stratifying MM into different stages started in the 1960s and early 1970s when a number of clinical and laboratory parameters were identified, including hemoglobin level, serum calcium, serum creatinine, and severity of bone lesions [1, 2]. In 1975, Durie and Salmon [3] developed a Durie-Salmon Staging (DS) system as a prognostic model using the following parameters that predicted myeloma cell tumor burden: hemoglobin level, serum calcium level, the number of bone lesions on bone X-ray, and the level and type of monoclonal protein.

Durie-Salmon staging system for multiple myeloma (see [3, 4]) is as follows.

Stage I. Low cell mass is $<0.6 \times 10^{12}$ cells/m^2 plus all of the following:

(i) Hgb > 10 g/dL

(ii) Serum IgG < 5 g/dL

(iii) Serum IgA < 3 g/dL

(iv) Normal serum calcium

(v) Urine monoclonal protein excretion < 4 g/day

(vi) No generalized lytic bone lesions.

Stage II. Intermediate cell mass is neither stage I nor stage III.

Stage III. High cell mass is $>1.2 \times 10^{12}$ cells/m^2 plus one or more of the following:

(i) Hgb < 8.5 g/dL

(ii) Serum IgG > 7 g/dL

(iii) Serum IgA > 5 g/dL

(iv) Serum calcium > 12 mg/dL (3 μmol/L)

(v) Urine monoclonal protein excretion > 12 g/day

(vi) Advanced lytic bone lesions

Stage III is subclassified as IIIA or IIIB based on serum creatinine:

(A) Serum creatinine < 2 mg/dL (177 μmol/L)

(B) Serum creatinine ≥ 2 mg/dL

DS system was adopted as a standard method for MM staging for many years and it became the most commonly used prognostic scheme in patients with newly diagnosed MM. The drawbacks of this system included the following: it focuses on variables correlate with myeloma mass and it does not take into account the biologic variability of the disease. Also, one of the important elements of DS system is the number of lytic lesions seen on skeletal survey, which is operator dependent. Since then, several other staging systems have been proposed using other known prognostic factors, including C-reactive protein albumin and plasma cell labeling index [5–8], but the one that gained wide acceptance was the international staging system (ISS) that was published in 2005 [4]. ISS is a simple staging system that is based on the serum beta-2 microglobulin (Sβ2M) and albumin.

International staging system for myeloma (see [4]) is as follows:

Stage 1: β2M < 3.5 and ALB ≥ 3.5

Stage 2: ALB < 3.5 and β2M < 3.5; ALB < 3.5; or β2M 3.5–<5.5

Stage 3: β2M ≥ 5.5

where β2M is serum β2 microglobulin in mg/dL and ALB is serum albumin in g/dL.

The ISS evolved from a statistical model focusing on survival duration [4]. The ISS is a major improvement over the DSS in that it separates patients into cohorts using easily measurable, objective, and reproducible parameters [9]. The major criticism of ISS was the lack of the use of known other prognostic markers in MM including cytogenetics abnormalities (CA) and LDH. In 2015, Palumbo et al. [10] published revised international staging system (ISS-R) which combined ISS with CA and LDH as follows.

Revised international staging system (see [10]) is as follows:

Stage I: ISS I, standard risk by FISH and normal LDH

Stage II: not R-ISS I or III

Stage III: ISS III, either high risk by FISH or high LDH

where (i) high risk by FISH is presence of del(17p) and/or translocation t(4;14) and/or t(14;16), (ii) standard risk by FISH is no high-risk chromosomal abnormalities, (iii) normal LDH is serum LDH < the upper limit of normal, and (iv) high LDH is serum LDH > the upper limit of normal.

ISS-R is proving to be a powerful prognostic staging system, but currently its use in practical practice is limited and it is used primarily for risk stratification of patients in clinical trials.

2.2. Plasma Cell Labeling Index. MM is characterized by proliferation of monoclonal plasma cells (PCs) in the bone marrow. There are certain characteristics of this proliferation that correlate with prognosis of MM, including plasma cell labeling index (PCLI), circulating plasma cells, and plasmablastic morphology.

PCLI is a measure of marrow plasma cells in S phase of the cell cycle, which provides a good estimate of the proliferative capacity of the malignant clonal plasma cells [11]. In 1993, Greipp et al. demonstrated that PCLI and B2M measured at diagnosis are independent prognostic factors in MM [12]. This was confirmed in other studies, including the study by Steensma et al., which demonstrated that high PCLI in patients with apparently stable, plateau phase MM is an adverse parameter that may predict a short time to disease progression and death [13]. Another study by Li et al. showed that PCLI was higher among patients with del (13q14), and patients with a high PCLI had a short time to disease progression [14]. Currently PCLI is rarely used because of the availability of more practical prognostic methods.

2.3. Cytogenetics. MM is a malignancy of plasma cells which develops through genetic aberrations, epigenetic changes, and the bone marrow microenvironment interaction. In the past decade, nonrandom chromosomal aberrations such as t(4;14), t(14;16), t(14;20), amp1q21, and del 17p have been shown to be associated with poor prognosis, and moreover, recent progress in genome-wide deep sequencing studies revealed mutations and intratumor subclonal heterogeneity which may explain the clinical phenotype and therapeutic resistance.

2.3.1. t(4;14). The prognostic significance of t(4;14) as detected by RT-PCR on BM and PB samples of 208 patients with MM and 52 patients with monoclonal gammopathy of undetermined significance (MGUS) was assessed. The results showed that the presence of this translocation is associated with poor survival ($P = 0.006$) and poor response to first-line chemotherapy ($P = 0.05$) [15]. At Mayo Clinic, in a series of 238 patients studied between 1990 and 2001, t(4;14) was determined in 153 patients, suggesting that high-dose therapy, as used to be in their practice, has minimal benefit for these patients with a median time to progression of only 8.2 months after stem cell therapy [16]. In another study, 19 patients with t(4;14) showed a good response to vincristine, doxorubicin, and dexamethasone (VAD) induction chemotherapy or pulsed dexamethasone alone, but early progression was common before HDT, with evident resistance to alkylating agents [17]. The results after a long term follow-up of 100 cases of MM with t(4;14), treated in IFM99 trials with tandem transplantation, revealed a heterogeneity in patients expressing t(4;14). They usually have similar overall response rates after both induction and HDT, to those achieved in patients without t(4;14). However, achievement of CR or VGPR after HDT in patients with t(4;14) was a powerful independent prognostic factor of outcome, with high risk of early relapse and dismal outcome in patients achieving only PR or less. In this study, the heterogeneity was not only related to response; the authors found that patients, who had b2-microglobulin of <4 mg/L and Hb level of ≥10 g/dL at diagnosis (45%), experienced improved survival after tandem transplant and benefited from HDT [18]. A clear separation of two groups of t(4;14) patients was reported by the Arkansas group using a 70-gene expression model [19]. The results of the 260 myeloma patients, enrolled in the GEM-2000 Spanish transplant protocol, reinforced the previous results from other series and confirmed that the presence of t(4;14) was sufficient for shortening MM patient survival [20]. The poor prognosis of patients with t(4; 14) may be in part due to its association with upregulation of the fibroblast growth factor receptor 3 (FGFR3). Data from the preclinical studies suggest that patients with increased expression of FGFR3 may benefit from the use of FGFR3 inhibitors [21]. Another interesting study showed that t(4;14) can be gained at time of relapse, which was observed in 14 out of 268 patients who did not express t(4;14) at diagnosis. Hypotheses that explain the acquisition of the t(4;14) at relapse include evolution of already present subclones or its acquisition during evolution [22].

2.3.2. t(11;14). A different translocation involving immunoglobulin heavy chain gene on chromosome 14, which is commonly associated with lymphomas, especially mantle cell lymphoma, was identified in 24 cases of multiple myeloma, by standard cytogenetic analysis; in most of these cases

t(11;14)(q13;q32) was part of a complex karyotype and strong cyclin D1 overexpression by immunohistochemical stain [23]. In a large cohort including more than 350 myeloma patients, who participated in the Eastern Cooperative Oncology Group phase III clinical trial E9486, t(11;14)(q13;q32) was detected in approximately one-sixth of patients, and it was associated with a low serum monoclonal protein and plasma cell labeling index and is less likely to be hyperdiploid by DNA content analysis, which appeared to correlate with a better survival and prognosis in those patients [24]. The previous study, in addition to other studies, reported that the presence of t(11;14)(q13;q32) was always associated with small mature lymphoplasmacytoid morphology [24–26], and in more than 60% of the cases with CD20 expression [27]. Moreau et al. reported markedly improved long term survival in 26 patients with t(11;14)(q13;q32) after HDT [28], whereas patients with this translocation, who were treated within the Eastern Cooperative Oncology Group protocol with HDT, showed borderline improvement [24]. However, no effect on survival or time to progression was seen in patients with t(11;14)(q13;q32), treated with HDT at Mayo Clinic between 1990 and 2001 [16]. On the other hand, patients with t(11;14)(q13;q32) showed higher risk of extramedullary plasmacytoma- (EMP-) specific relapse compared to other cytogenetic abnormalities [29, 30] and a lower response rate, if they have EMP at presentation [31], which is supposed to be due to downregulation of CD56, which facilitate disease dissemination and malignant plasma cells extramedullary spread [32, 33]. In a further analysis of three hundred and four patients with newly diagnosed MM treated at Mayo Clinic between January 2004 and December 2012, who underwent serial cytogenetic evaluations, patients with t(11;14) showed an increased cytogenetic stability during the follow-up, with decreased odds of cytogenetic evolution (odds ratio (OR) = 0.22, 95% confidence interval (CI) = 0.09–0.56, $P = 0.001$) [34]. In contrast, Kaufman and colleagues reported inferior overall survival of patients with t(11;14) when compared with the classical standard risk patients in their cohort, which included 409 patients treated with HDT following doublet or triplet novel agent induction [35].

2.3.3. t(14;16). The data about t(14;16) are conflicting; on a retrospective analysis of over 1000 myeloma patients, the 32 patients with t(14;16) did not show any survival difference from patients lacking this translocation, and it was not proved to be an independent prognostic factor on multivariate analysis [50], while some studies reported that t(14;16) have a negative impact on prognosis [51, 52].

2.3.4. Chromosome 13 Deletions. Chromosome 13 deletions either partial or complete detected by metaphase cytogenetics (CG) proved to have poor prognostic impact on patients with MM [53]. In subsequent studies, the rate of del(13q) detection was increased 2 to 3 times using interphase fluorescence in situ hybridization (FISH), but it remains an independent adverse prognostic [54–57]. In a further study that included 238 patients treated with HDT patients who expressed 13q del alone by FISH did not have a significantly shorter overall survival, but the presence of both 13q del and t(4;14) together had a significant adverse effect on outcome [58]. In addition, the presence or absence of del(13q14) did not seem to affect overall response to single agent bortezomib in 62 patients with relapsed/refractory MM [59].

2.3.5. 17p13 Deletion. TP53 gene is located at 17p13; deletion of 17p13 is expressed in up to 11% of newly diagnosed myeloma patients. TP53 mutation, a well-known poor prognostic factor in many cancers, has also a strong correlation with poor outcome and resistance to therapy in patients with MM, less frequently expressed at diagnosis, but it becomes more detected at relapse or with advanced disease [60–62]. The work done by Lodè and colleagues showed that TP53 mutations are exclusively associated with del(17p); by sequencing for TP53 gene in 92 newly diagnosed myeloma patients, 37% of 54 patients with del(17p) have mutations of the TP53 gene (63% are homozygous), while none of the patients without del(17p) expressed TP53 mutation [60]. It is evident that the negative prognostic impact of del(17p) is demonstrated when at least 60% of plasma cells have it [63].

2.3.6. Chromosome 1 Abnormalities. Chromosome 1 abnormalities are frequently detected in MM [31]; del 1p lead to loss of tumor suppressor genes and emerged as a poor prognostic factor in myeloma [64, 65]. The adverse prognostic role was confirmed in a study, which included 15 patients with del 1p; associated 13 q del was detected in 10 out of the 15 patients. Del 1p did not affect PFS in these patients after HDT and Autotransplant [66]. In addition, the role of chromosome 1 abnormalities was investigated in elderly patients (>65 years) enrolled in a phase III randomized clinical trial comparing VMP versus VMPT-VT; the abnormalities are when thalidomide appears to have a detrimental effect in elderly patients with newly diagnosed MM and abnormal chr1, while bortezomib can overcome its negative prognostic impact [67].

2.3.7. Gene Expression Profile (GEP). Several studies tried to identify molecular subgroups of multiple myeloma, using gene expression profiling on purified by CD138+ plasma cells. A study done in the University of Arkansas for Medical Science (UAMS), using plasma cells (PCs) from 74 newly diagnosed myeloma patients, 5 with monoclonal gammopathy of undetermined significance (MGUS), and 31 healthy volunteers (normal PCs), identified 4 distinct subgroups of MM (MM1, MM2, MM3, and MM4), ranging from MM1 that is more like normal PCs and MGUS, whereas MM4 showed more poor prognostic features as abnormal karyotype and high serum b2-microglobulin levels [68]. In a later study from (UAMS), they defined 7 subgroups rather than 4, using samples from over 400 newly diagnosed myeloma patients and more specific genes such as c-MAF and MAFB, CCND1, CCND3, ASS, IL6R, MMSET, FGFR3, CCNB2, FRZB, and DKK1. They described the UAMS classification 7 clusters, CD-1, CD-2, MS, MF, HY, PR, and LB [69]. Three novel subsets of multiple myeloma were identified, using data of the 320 newly diagnosed myeloma patients included in the Dutch-Belgian/German HOVON-65/GMMG-HD4 trial,

in addition to 7 subgroups described in the 2006 UAMS classification, which were NFκB, CTA, and PRL3 clusters [70].

Myeloma can be roughly divided into two equal disease entities: hyperdiploid multiple myeloma (H-MM) and Non-hyperdiploid multiple myeloma (NH-MM). A gene expression profiling study was conducted at Mayo Clinic trying to characterize the molecular profile of H-MM. Four nonoverlapping clusters were identified, each with distinct clinical and biological features, including a subgroup with a poor prognosis and a subgroup that responds fairly well to bortezomib [71].

The 15 most stable genes associated with survival from the 7,508-gene set used in the IFM 99 trials were used to stratify myeloma patients included in the trials into low-risk and high-risk groups; the authors concluded that high-risk patients have a 6.8-fold increased risk of death compared with low-risk patients (95% CI, 3.92 to 11.73; $P < 0.001$), with more than 90% survival rates for low-risk group and less than 50% for high-risk group at 3 years [72].

Another gene signature called EMC-92-gene signature was generated from gene expression profile used in the HOVON65/GMMG-HD4 trial. The performance of the EMC-92-gene signature was validated in newly diagnosed and relapsed myeloma patients, and it was proved to be independent of other prognostic factors on multivariate analysis. In addition, it was reported to be the best compared to other used signatures [73]. In another study done by Kuiper et al., they evaluated twenty risk markers, including t(4;14) and deletion of 17p (FISH), EMC92, and UAMS70 (GEP classifiers), and ISS. Their results showed that the EMC92-ISS combination is the strongest predictor for overall survival, resulting in a 4-group risk classification. The median survival was 24 months for the highest risk group and 47 and 61 months for the intermediate risk groups, and the median was not reached after 96 months for the lowest risk group [74].

2.4. Risk Stratification Models. Several risk stratification models have been developed for prognostication of MM patients. The most widely used are shown in Table 1.

3. Monitoring of Response Tools

3.1. Serum Light Chain Assay. Standard work-up of newly diagnosed MM includes assessment of both serum and urine for monoclonal protein. These biological markers have also proven to be essential in the disease progression detection and monitoring. A panel of members of the 2009 International Myeloma Workshop developed guidelines for standard investigative work-up of patients with suspected multiple myeloma. Both serum and urine should be assessed for monoclonal protein. Measurement of monoclonal protein both by the densitometer tracing and/by nephelometric quantitation is recommended, and immunofixation is required for confirmation. The serum-free light chain (sFLC) assay is recommended in all newly diagnosed patients with plasma cell dyscrasias [75]. Multiple studies have showed sFLCR to be a superior prognostic marker for plasma cell dyscrasias in contrast to M-spike. As an example, Dimopoulos et al.

TABLE 1: Various risk stratification models.

Risk stratification model	Prognostic markers	OS	Reference
mSMART	(i) Cytogenetics (ii) GEP (iii) PCLI	(i) Low risk: 10 years (ii) Intermediate risk: 4.5 years (iii) High risk: 3 years	[36]
IMWG	(i) ISS (ii) Cytogenetics	(i) Low risk: >10 years (ii) Standard risk: 7 years (iii) High risk: 2 years	[37]
IFM	(i) LDH (ii) ISS (iii) Cytogenetics	Score 0–3. Score 3 had very poor prognosis	[38]

showed that, in patients with monoclonal gammopathy of undetermined significance (MGUS), the risk of progression in patients with an abnormal sFLC ratio (sFLCR) was significantly higher compared with patients with a normal ratio (hazard ratio, 3.5; 95% confidence interval [CI], 2.3–5.5; $P < 0.001$) and was independent of the size and type of the serum monoclonal (M) protein [75]. For patients with smoldering MM (SMM), Rajkumar et al. demonstrated that a high sFLCR > 100 is a predictor of imminent progression, and such patients may be considered candidates for early treatment intervention [76]. The prognostic value of sFLC was also seen in patients with solitary plasmacytoma of bone with significant higher progression to MM in patients with abnormal sFLCR [77]. In MM, abnormal sFLCR was shown to be an independent prognostic factor, with one study showing 5-year disease-specific survival of 82% in patients with sFLCR ≤ than the median compared to 30% in patients with sFLCR > the median ($P = 0.0001$) [78]. Because the half-life of FLC is <6 hours, FLC measurements at short sampling intervals allow real-time measurement of treatment-induced tumor kill and provide prompt indications of chemosensitivity [79].

3.2. Serum Heavy/Light Chain (HLC) Assay (Hevylite). Immunofixation (IFE) is a standard method for detecting monoclonal immunoglobulins and characterizing its isotype. Recently clonality can also be determined by using immunoglobulin (Ig) heavy chain/light chain immunoassays (HLC), Hevylite. HLC separately measures in pairs light chain types of each intact Ig class generating ratio of monoclonal Ig/uninvolved polyclonal Ig concentrations [80]. Studies have shown that the HLC ratio (HLCR) is of prognostic significance in MM. According to results from a study by Koulieris et al. [81], high HLCR was associated with anemia, high serum FLCR, extensive bone marrow infiltration, and increased β2-microglobulin. In addition, increased HLCR and the presence of immunoparesis correlated with time to treatment initiation. Patients with high HLCR had a significantly shorter survival ($P = 0.022$). At the moment, HLC is considered novel immunoassays with multiple studies showing its utility in disease monitoring and outcome prediction in plasma cell dyscrasias. Its use is currently being cleared by the US Food and Drug Agency (FDA).

3.2.1. Advanced Imaging Modalities. Imaging studies in MM include metastatic skeletal survey (MSS), computed tomography (CT), magnetic resonant imaging (MRI), and, more recently, positron emission tomography (PET) with fluorodeoxyglucose (FDG). MSS continues to be the standard diagnostic study in MM. Unfortunately, for MSS to detect bone destruction, the damage has to reach approximately 50% [82]. The national cancer center network (NCCN) MM panel recommends additional tests that may be useful under some circumstances. These include MRI and PET/CT [83]. Both MRI and PET scan are proven to give important information in patients with MM including detection of bone lesions, bone marrow infiltration, and disease monitoring posttherapy. A study by Baur-Melnyk et al. showed that patients without bone marrow infiltration have a significantly longer survival than patients with bone marrow infiltration in MRI at the time of diagnosis. However, even in stage I disease (Durie and Salmon) and negative X-ray films bone marrow infiltration in MRI may be detected in 29–50% of patients. Those patients typically show an earlier disease progression [84]. IMWG consensus considered MRI to be the gold-standard imaging technique for detection of bone marrow involvement [85]. The panel also discussed the prognostic value of MRI explaining that focal pattern on MRI gives prognostic information in symptomatic MM, and diffuse pattern also correlates with worse prognosis. Another study by Bredella et al. evaluated the value of FDG PET in the assessment of patient with MM and showed that FDG PET has sensitivity in detecting myelomatous involvement of 85% and specificity of 92%. FDG PET is able to detect bone marrow involvement in patients with MM and it is useful in assessing extent of disease at time of initial diagnosis, contributing to staging that is more accurate [86].

Despite numerous potential advantages of both MRI and PET-CT in MM, they are not yet the established gold standard for disease evaluation at diagnosis or at completion of therapy. Concerns with the serial use of these techniques exist due to the heterogeneity of visual criteria and the lack of consistency in the interpretation of results. Standardization of disease definitions for MRI and PET-CT imaging is needed to improve the specificity and positive predictive value of these tools [87].

Novel techniques can detect more lytic lesions compared to conventional radiography. Whole body, multidetector, low-dose computed tomography (WBLD-CT) is more sensitive for the detection of lytic lesions in myeloma compared to conventional radiography; it is very easy to perform (the examination is performed in 2 min or less), has a more accurate evaluation of areas with instability or at risk of fracture, and is superior regarding the planning for radiotherapy or surgical interventions [88].

For initial diagnosis of patients with multiple myeloma bone disease, use of an imaging test with a superior detection rate such as WBLDCT would find more lesions and presumably upstage patients, but definitive studies have yet to be completed defining the prognostic value of WBLDCT. WBLDCT can reliably exclude bone disease to confirm MGUS and complement laboratory monitoring. It remains unproven whether clinical benefit could be obtained by treating patients earlier or more aggressively based on WBLDCT findings. Nevertheless, recent data showing that early treatment of smoldering multiple myeloma leads to improved overall survival suggest that a more sensitive imaging method might help to detect lytic lesions and provide earlier treatment and thus improve survival [89]. Currently WBLDCT is considered a diagnostic tool, not a prognostic one.

4. Minimal Residual Disease (MRD) Monitoring Methods

4.1. Circulating Plasma Cells. Circulating PC detected by flow cytometry also is considered one of predictors of survival in patients with newly diagnosed MM. Nowakowski et al. studied the relationship between the number of circulating PCs in patients with newly diagnosed MM and survival and they concluded that it is an independent predictor of survival [90]. The increase in PC may be accompanied by morphological differences, like plasmablastic features, and can distinguish patients with a poor prognosis. Greipp et al. studied the prognostic significance of plasmablastic (PB) MM and the authors concluded that PB MM is a discrete entity associated with more aggressive disease and shortened survival [91]. However, since the prognostic values of these factors are not easily reproducible, they are not widely adopted [92].

4.2. Minimal Residual Disease (MRD). It is currently well established that there is a direct relationship between depth of response and prolonged survival in MM [93, 94]. Still, the vast majority of patients who achieve complete response (CR) per the current definition criteria will eventually relapse. Because of that, the international Myeloma Working Group (IMWG), working on refining the criteria of CR in an effort to improve the outcome of the patients and in 2006, introduced normalization of sFLCs and absence of clonal PCs in BM biopsies by immunohistochemistry and/or immunofluorescence as additional requirements to define more stringent CR criteria [95]. Another CR definition that had emerged is molecular complete response (mCR), which is defined as absence of detectable disease by polymerase chain reaction

(PCR) for Ig gene rearrangement [96]. Currently, the most sensitive approaches to detect MRD in MM include Multiparameter Flow Cytometry (MFC) and Ig allele-specific oligonucleotide-based quantitative PCR (ASO-PCR) [29]. The role of next generation sequencing (NGS) of Ig genes is emerging as a future sensitive tool to assess MRD. The sensitivity of these methods is comparable (MFC: 10^{-5} to 10^{-6}, ASO-PCR: 10^{-5} to 10^{-6}, NGS: 10^{-6}) [97].

The prognostic value of MRD in MM has been explored in multiple studies. San Miguel et al. [98] studied the prognostic value of multiparametric immunophenotyping of PC compartment in patients with MM and found that ASCT provided a significantly greater reduction in the level of residual tumor PCs and with better recovery of normal PCs. The authors also found that patients in whom at least 30% of gated PCs had a normal phenotype after treatment had a significantly longer progression-free survival (60 months versus 34 months; $P = 0.02$). Paiva et al. on behalf of the GEM/PETHEMA cooperative study group [99] showed in MM patients who were treated with ASCT that median PFS (71 versus 37 months, $P < 0.001$) and median OS (not reached versus 89 months, $P < .002$) were longer in patients who were MRD negative versus MRD positive by multiparameter flow at day 100 after ASCT. Puig et al. compared ASO RQ-PCR with multiparameter FCM in patients with MM and found a significant correlation in MRD quantitation by both techniques ($r = 0.881$, $P < 0.001$), being reflective of treatment intensity. Patients with $<10^{-4}$ residual tumor cells showed PFS compared with the rest (not reached (NR) versus 31 months, $P = 0.002$), with similar results observed with MFC. Among complete responders ($n = 62$), PCR discriminated two risk groups with different PFS (49 versus 26 months, $P = 0.001$) and overall survival (NR versus 60 months, $P = 0.008$) [100]. Martinez-Lopez et al. assessed the prognostic value of MRD detection in MM patients using a NGS tool and showed that the applicability of deep sequencing was 91%. Concordance between sequencing and MFC and ASO-PCR was 83% and 85%, respectively. Patients who were MRD– by sequencing had a significantly longer time to tumor progression (TTP) (median 80 versus 31 months; $P < 0.0001$) and overall survival (median not reached versus 81 months; $P = 0.02$), compared with patients who were MRD+ [101]. The conclusion from the above-mentioned studies and many other studies is that MRD assessment in MM using different methods is associated with improvement in PFS and OS which supports the rationale for implementing MRD assessment to redefine and improve current CR criteria in MM [97].

Another way of detecting MRD is by the use of MRI and PET/CT through the detection of possible patchy BM infiltration or extramedullary involvement with an MRD-negative BM [97]. MRI is very sensitive in detecting bone marrow involvement in the spine. PET/CT is able to detect extramedullary disease which has an adverse prognostic impact [102].

A study that compared PET/CT and whole body MRI in transplant-candidate patients showed that, against conventional response criteria, PET/CT had the same sensitivity but higher specificity than whole body MRI [103].

TABLE 2: Summary of some of the novel prognostic markers that were published recently.

Authors	Novel prognostic marker	Conclusion
Li et al. 2015 [39]	The expression patterns of miR-15a/16-1	miR-15a seems to be linked with disease progression and prognosis while miR-16-1 acts as a valuable diagnostic marker
Wang et al. 2015 [40]	Immune checkpoint signaling	The overall response rate to treatment was higher in low sPD-L1 patients than in high sPD-L1 patients
Jung et al. 2016 [41]	Inverse platelet to lymphocyte ratio (iPLR)	Staging by iPLR group had predictive value for PFS and OS
Zhou et al. 2015 [42]	Dysregulated long noncoding RNAs (lncRNAs)	Four lncRNAs were identified to be significantly associated with OS
Lee et al. 2015 [43]	Bone marrow (BM) microvessel density (MVD)	PFS was significantly lower in the high MVD group than in the low MVD group
Ma et al. 2015 [44]	N-Cadherin	OS is worse with high expression of N-Cadherin which may be related to 1q21 amplification.
Lullo et al. 2015 [45]	Th22 cells	Increased frequency of IL-22(+)IL-17(−)IL-13(+) T cells correlates with poor prognosis
Li et al. 2015 [46]	Downregulated miR-33b	miR-33b low expression had significantly shortened PFS and OS
Bolomsky et al. 2015 [47]	Insulin-like growth factor binding protein 7 (IGFBP7) expression	IGFBP7 expression is linked to translocation t(4;14) showing clinical features of adverse prognosis
Jung et al. 2015 [48]	Autophagic markers beclin 1 and LC3	Higher immunoreactivity for autophagic markers in MM is associated with superior patient survival
Trotter et al. 2015 [49]	Myeloma cell-derived Runx2	Runx2 expression is a major regulator of MM progression in bone and myeloma bone disease

Many studies have shown the value of MRD diagnostics for evaluation of the efficacy of specific treatment stages. Both the Spanish [104] and UK [105] study groups showed the importance of MRD in identifying chemosensitivity before and after ASCT. Failure to eradicate MRD levels before ASCT will show significantly superior PFS if MRD negativity is achieved after ASCT. Another example is a study by Rawstron et al. that showed that patients who achieved MRD negativity with maintenance therapy experienced significantly prolonged PFS [105].

Depth of response was evaluated in different studies. An early study of 126 consecutive patients, of whom 33% achieved CR with SCT, CR did not influence outcome, on either high or low-risk group [99]. Another study at Mayo Clinic showed no significant difference in time to progression (TTP) between the small group of patients who achieved CR before HDT-ASCT (BCR) and those who achieved CR after HDT-ASCT (ACR), at more than 6 years follow-up, and the median OS was not reached at time of analysis [100]. With the advent of novel agents, more CR rates are achieved and its prognostic impact is studied in both relapsed and newly diagnosed MM. Multiple prospective studies of newly diagnosed myeloma patients demonstrated either a longer EFS and/or a better OS in patients who achieved CR or at least VGPR, after a single [101, 102] or tandem ASCT [103–106]. In a large series, including 1000 patients treated with MEL-based tandem high-dose therapy (HDT) trials with autologous hematopoietic stem cell (AHSC) support, superior overall survival was seen in relapsed patients, who achieved a complete remission [107]. However, in a retrospective study which analyzed the outcome of over 500 patients who did not achieve at least

a PR after initial induction, there was no difference in median OS between patients who received salvage chemotherapy and those who did not receive any additional therapy to augment response prior to transplant [108]. At this time, we believe that new tools of disease burden are needed to define CR in a more precise way in the era of newer treatments and to study the impact of deeper CR on overall survival.

5. Novel Prognostic Markers in MM

Over the past year, there were multiple publications on novel prognostic markers in MM. These include markers in immunophenotyping, genetics, immune signaling, biomarkers, bone marrow environment, and imaging techniques. We selected some of these novel markers. Table 2 provides summary of some of these promising markers.

6. Conclusion and Future Directions

Understanding the prognostic factors in MM is important for optimal care of MM patients.

Our comprehension of the prognostic markers in MM has developed significantly over the last 10 years. Incorporation of different prognostic markers of MM in risk stratification of the disease is evolving with the presence of multiple models in the literature. The ultimate goal of establishing prognostic models in MM is to develop risk-adaptive therapeutic strategies. Our aim of this review is to summarize the current standard prognostic markers used in MM along with novel techniques that are still in development and highlight their implications in current clinical practice. Currently, the most powerful prognostic markers in MM that has clinical implication are genetics abnormalities. The classification of MM into high risk, intermediate risk, and standard risk is based primarily on the impact of genetic aberrations. Selection of therapies nowadays is also directed by this risk stratification. Development of novel prognostic markers is evolving and soon will be part of the standard risk classification in MM and these include GEP and next generation sequencing (NGS).

We believe that refinement of the prognostic models in MM will eventually lead to enhancement of the efficacy of the therapeutic approaches and ultimately will improve the outcome of the disease.

Competing Interests

All authors do not have financial disclosure.

References

[1] P. P. Carbone, L. E. Kellerhouse, and E. A. Gehan, "Plasmacytic myeloma. A study of the relationship of survival to various clinical manifestations and anomalous protein type in 112 patients," *The American Journal of Medicine*, vol. 42, no. 6, pp. 937–948, 1967.

[2] G. Costa, R. L. Engle, A. Schilling et al., "Melphalan and prednisone: an effective combination for the treatment of multiple myeloma," *The American Journal of Medicine*, vol. 54, no. 5, pp. 589–599, 1973.

[3] B. G. M. Durie and S. E. Salmon, "A clinical staging system for multiple myeloma," *Cancer*, vol. 36, pp. 842–854, 1975.

[4] P. R. Greipp, J. S. Miguel, B. G. M. Dune et al., "International staging system for multiple myeloma," *Journal of Clinical Oncology*, vol. 23, no. 15, pp. 3412–3420, 2005.

[5] G. Merlini, J. G. Waldenstrom, and S. D. Jayakar, "A new improved clinical staging system for multiple myeloma based on analysis of 123 treated patients," *Blood*, vol. 55, no. 6, pp. 1011–1019, 1980.

[6] R. Bataille, B. G. M. Durie, J. Grenier, and J. Sany, "Prognostic factors and staging in multiple myeloma: a reappraisal," *Journal of Clinical Oncology*, vol. 4, no. 1, pp. 80–87, 1986.

[7] J. Blade, C. Rozman, F. Cervantes, J.-C. Reverter, and E. Montserrat, "A new prognostic system for multiple myeloma based on easily available parameters," *British Journal of Haematology*, vol. 72, no. 4, pp. 507–511, 1989.

[8] Medical Research Council's Working Party on Leukemia in Adults, "Prognostic features in the third MRC myelomatosis trial," *British Journal of Cancer*, vol. 42, no. 6, pp. 831–840, 1980.

[9] P. N. Hari, M.-J. Zhang, V. Roy et al., "Is the international staging system superior to the Durie-Salmon staging system? A comparison in multiple myeloma patients undergoing autologous transplant," *Leukemia*, vol. 23, no. 8, pp. 1528–1534, 2009.

[10] A. Palumbo, H. Avet-Loiseau, S. Oliva et al., "Revised international staging system for multiple myeloma: a report from international myeloma working group," *Journal of Clinical Oncology*, vol. 33, no. 26, pp. 2863–2869, 2015.

[11] S. Kumar, S. V. Rajkumar, P. R. Greipp, and T. E. Witzig, "Cell proliferation of myeloma plasma cells: comparison of the blood and marrow compartments," *American Journal of Hematology*, vol. 77, no. 1, pp. 7–11, 2004.

[12] P. R. Greipp, J. A. Lust, W. M. O'Fallon, J. A. Katzmann, T. E. Witzig, and R. A. Kyle, "Plasma cell labeling index and β2-microglobulin predict survival independent of thymidine kinase and C-reactive protein in multiple myeloma," *Blood*, vol. 81, no. 12, pp. 3382–3387, 1993.

[13] D. P. Steensma, M. A. Gertz, P. R. Greipp et al., "A high bone marrow plasma cell labeling index in stable plateau-phase multiple myeloma is a marker for early disease progression and death," *Blood*, vol. 97, no. 8, pp. 2522–2523, 2001.

[14] C. Li, L. Chen, X. Gao et al., "Plasma cell labeling index correlates with deletion of 13q14 in multiple myeloma," *Leukemia and Lymphoma*, vol. 52, no. 2, pp. 260–264, 2011.

[15] J. J. Keats, T. Reiman, C. A. Maxwell et al., "In multiple myeloma, t(4;14)(p16;q32) is an adverse prognostic factor irrespective of FGFR3 expression," *Blood*, vol. 101, no. 4, pp. 1520–1529, 2003.

[16] M. A. Gertz, M. Q. Lacy, A. Dispenzieri et al., "Clinical implications of t(11;14)(q13;q32), t(4;14)(p16.3;q32), and -17p13 in myeloma patients treated with high-dose therapy," *Blood*, vol. 106, no. 8, pp. 2837–2840, 2005.

[17] W. Jaksic, S. Trudel, H. Chang et al., "Clinical outcomes in t(4;14) multiple myeloma: a chemotherapy-sensitive disease characterized by rapid relapse and alkylating agent resistance," *Journal of Clinical Oncology*, vol. 23, no. 28, pp. 7069–7073, 2005.

[18] P. Moreau, M. Attal, F. Garban et al., "Heterogeneity of t(4;14) in multiple myeloma. Long-term follow-up of 100 cases treated with tandem transplantation in IFM99 trials," *Leukemia*, vol. 21, no. 9, pp. 2020–2024, 2007.

[19] J. D. Shaughnessy Jr., F. Zhan, B. E. Burington et al., "A validated gene expression model of high-risk multiple myeloma is defined by deregulated expression of genes mapping to chromosome 1," *Blood*, vol. 109, no. 6, pp. 2276–2284, 2007.

[20] N. C. Gutiérrez, M. V. Castellanos, M. L. Martín et al., "Prognostic and biological implications of genetic abnormalities in multiple myeloma undergoing autologous stem cell transplantation: t(4;14) is the most relevant adverse prognostic factor, whereas RB deletion as a unique abnormality is not associated with adverse prognosis," *Leukemia*, vol. 21, no. 1, pp. 143–150, 2007.

[21] A. Kalff and A. Spencer, "The t(4;14) translocation and FGFR3 overexpression in multiple myeloma: prognostic implications and current clinical strategies," *Blood Cancer Journal*, vol. 2, article no. 37, 2012.

[22] B. Hébraud, D. Caillot, J. Corre et al., "The translocation t(4;14) can be present only in minor subclones in multiple myeloma," *Clinical Cancer Research*, vol. 19, no. 17, 2013.

[23] J. D. Hoyer, C. A. Hanson, R. Fonseca, P. R. Greipp, G. W. Dewald, and P. J. Kurtin, "The (11;14)(q13;q32) translocation in multiple myeloma: A Morphologic and Immunohistochemical Study," *American Journal of Clinical Pathology*, vol. 113, no. 6, pp. 831–837, 2000.

[24] R. Fonseca, E. A. Blood, M. M. Oken et al., "Myeloma and the t(11;14)(q13;q32); evidence for a biologically defined unique subset of patients," *Blood*, vol. 99, no. 10, pp. 3735–3741, 2002.

[25] R. Garand, H. Avet-Loiseau, F. Accard, P. Moreau, J. L. Harousseau, and R. Bataille, "t(11;14) and t(4;14) translocations correlated with mature lymphoplasmacytoid and immature morphology, respectively, in multiple myeloma," *Leukemia*, vol. 17, no. 10, pp. 2032–2035, 2003.

[26] H. Avet-Loiseau, R. Garand, L. Lodé, J.-L. Harousseau, and R. Bataille, "Translocation t(11;14)(q13;q32) is the hallmark of IgM, IgE, and nonsecretory multiple myeloma variants," *Blood*, vol. 101, no. 4, pp. 1570–1571, 2003.

[27] N. Robillard, H. Avet-Loiseau, R. Garand et al., "CD20 is associated with a small mature plasma cell morphology and t(11;14) in multiple myeloma," *Blood*, vol. 102, no. 3, pp. 1070–1071, 2003.

[28] P. Moreau, T. Facon, X. Leleu et al., "Recurrent 14q32 translocations determine the prognosis of multiple myeloma, especially in patients receiving intensive chemotherapy," *Blood*, vol. 100, no. 5, pp. 1579–1583, 2002.

[29] R. Fonseca, T. E. Witzig, M. A. Gertz et al., "Multiple myeloma and the translocation t(11;14)(q13;q32): a report on 13 cases," *British Journal of Haematology*, vol. 101, no. 2, pp. 296–301, 1998.

[30] E. Parkins, M. Boll, S. J. M. O'Connor, A. C. Rawstron, and R. G. Owen, "Extramedullary plasmacytoma with a t(11;14)(q13;q32) and aggressive clinical course," *Leukemia and Lymphoma*, vol. 51, no. 7, pp. 1360–1362, 2010.

[31] J. D. Shaughnessy, F. Zhan, B. E. Burington et al., "A validated gene expression model of high-risk multiple myeloma is defined by deregulated expression of genes mapping to chromosome 1," *Blood*, vol. 109, no. 6, pp. 2276–2284, 2007.

[32] H.-J. Shin, K. Kim, J.-J. Lee et al., "The t(11;14)(q13;q32) translocation as a poor prognostic parameter for autologous stem cell transplantation in myeloma patients with extramedullary plasmacytoma," *Clinical Lymphoma, Myeloma and Leukemia*, vol. 15, no. 4, pp. 227–235, 2015.

[33] G. An, Y. Xu, L. Shi et al., "T(11;14) multiple myeloma: a subtype associated with distinct immunological features, immunophenotypic characteristics but divergent outcome," *Leukemia Research*, vol. 37, no. 10, pp. 1251–1257, 2013.

[34] M. Binder, S. V. Rajkumar, R. P. Ketterling et al., "Occurrence and prognostic significance of cytogenetic evolution in patients with multiple myeloma," *Blood Cancer Journal*, vol. 6, 2016.

[35] G. P. Kaufman, M. A. Gertz, A. Dispenzieri et al., "Impact of cytogenetic classification on outcomes following early high-dose therapy in multiple myeloma," *Leukemia*, vol. 30, no. 3, pp. 633–639, 2015.

[36] J. R. Mikhael, D. Dingli, V. Roy et al., "Management of newly diagnosed symptomatic multiple myeloma: updated mayo stratification of myeloma and risk-adapted therapy (mSMART) consensus guidelines 2013," *Mayo Clinic Proceedings*, vol. 88, no. 4, pp. 360–376, 2013.

[37] H. Iriuchishima, T. Saitoh, H. Handa et al., "A new staging system to predict prognosis of patients with multiple myeloma in an era of novel therapeutic agents," *European Journal of Haematology*, vol. 94, no. 2, pp. 145–151, 2015.

[38] P. Moreau, M. Cavo, P. Sonneveld et al., "Combination of International Scoring System 3, highlactate dehydrogenase, and t(4;14) and/or del(17p) identifies patients with multiple myeloma (MM) treated with front-line autologous stem-cell transplantation at high risk of early MM progression-related death," *Journal of Clinical Oncology*, vol. 32, no. 20, pp. 2173–2180, 2014.

[39] F. Li, Y. Xu, S. Deng et al., "MicroRNA-15a/16-1 cluster located at chromosome 13q14 is down-regulated but displays different expression pattern and prognostic significance in multiple myeloma," *Oncotarget*, vol. 6, no. 35, pp. 38270–38282, 2015.

[40] L. Wang, H. Wang, H. Chen et al., "Serum levels of soluble programmed death ligand 1 predict treatment response and progression free survival in multiple myeloma," *Oncotarget*, vol. 6, no. 38, pp. 41228–41236, 2015.

[41] S.-H. Jung, J. S. Kim, W. S. Lee et al., "Prognostic value of the inverse platelet to lymphocyte ratio (iPLR) in patients with multiple myeloma who were treated up front with a novel agent-containing regimen," *Annals of Hematology*, vol. 95, no. 1, pp. 55–61, 2016.

[42] M. Zhou, H. Zhao, Z. Wang et al., "Identification and validation of potential prognostic lncRNA biomarkers for predicting survival in patients with multiple myeloma," *Journal of Experimental and Clinical Cancer Research*, vol. 34, article 102, 2015.

[43] N. Lee, H. Lee, S. Y. Moon et al., "Adverse prognostic impact of bone marrow microvessel density in multiple myeloma," *Annals of Laboratory Medicine*, vol. 35, no. 6, pp. 563–569, 2015.

[44] J. Ma, Q.-F. Yu, X.-Y. Liu et al., "Expression of N-cadherin in patients with multiple myeloma and its clinical significance," *Zhongguo Shi Yan Xue Ye Xue Za Zhi*, vol. 23, no. 4, pp. 1044–1048, 2015.

[45] G. D. Lullo, M. Marcatti, S. Heltai et al., "Th22 cells increase in poor prognosis multiple myeloma and promote tumor cell growth and survival," *OncoImmunology*, vol. 4, no. 5, 2015.

[46] F. Li, M. Hao, X. Feng et al., "Downregulated miR-33b is a novel predictor associated with disease progression and poor prognosis in multiple myeloma," *Leukemia Research*, vol. 39, no. 7, pp. 793–799, 2015.

[47] A. Bolomsky, D. Hose, M. Schreder et al., "Insulin like growth factor binding protein 7 (IGFBP7) expression is linked to poor prognosis but may protect from bone disease in multiple myeloma," *Journal of Hematology and Oncology*, vol. 8, article 10, Article ID 13045, 2015.

[48] G. Jung, J. Roh, H. Lee et al., "Autophagic markers BECLIN 1 and LC3 are associated with prognosis of multiple myeloma," *Acta Haematologica*, vol. 134, no. 1, pp. 17–24, 2015.

[49] T. N. Trotter, M. Li, Q. Pan et al., "Myeloma cell-derived Runx2 promotes myeloma progression in bone," *Blood*, vol. 125, no. 23, pp. 3598–3608, 2015.

[50] I. Vande Broek, K. Vanderkerken, B. Van Camp, and I. Van Riet, "Extravasation and homing mechanisms in multiple myeloma," *Clinical and Experimental Metastasis*, vol. 25, no. 4, pp. 325–334, 2008.

[51] H. Avet-Loiseau, F. Malard, L. Campion et al., "Translocation t(14;16) and multiple myeloma: is it really an independent prognostic factor?" *Blood*, vol. 117, no. 6, pp. 2009–2011, 2011.

[52] B. Nair, F. Van Rhee, J. D. Shaughnessy Jr. et al., "Superior results of total therapy 3 (2003-33) in gene expression profiling-defined low-risk multiple myeloma confirmed in subsequent trial 2006-66 with VRD maintenance," *Blood*, vol. 115, no. 21, pp. 4168–4173, 2010.

[53] R. Fonseca, "Clinical and biologic implications of recurrent genomic aberrations in myeloma," *Blood*, vol. 101, no. 11, pp. 4569–4575, 2003.

[54] G. Tricot, B. Barlogie, S. Jagannath et al., "Poor prognosis in multiple myeloma is associated only with partial or complete deletions of chromosome 13 or abnormalities involving 11q and not with other karyotype abnormalities," *Blood*, vol. 86, no. 11, pp. 4250–4256, 1995.

[55] N. Zojer, R. Königsberg, J. Ackermann et al., "Deletion of 13q14 remains an independent adverse prognostic variable in multiple myeloma despite its frequent detection by interphase fluorescence in situ hybridization," *Blood*, vol. 95, no. 6, pp. 1925–1930, 2000.

[56] N. Worel, H. Greinix, J. Ackermann et al., "Deletion of chromosome 13q14 detected by FISH has prognostic impact on survival after high-dose therapy in patients with multiple myeloma," *Annals of Hematology*, vol. 80, pp. 345–348, 2001.

[57] R. Fonseca, D. Harrington, M. M. Oken et al., "Biological and prognostic significance of interphase fluorescence *in situ* hybridization detection of chromosome 13 abnormalities (Δ13) in

multiple myeloma: An Eastern Cooperative Oncology Group Study," *Cancer Research*, vol. 62, no. 3, pp. 715–720, 2002.

[58] H. Kaufmann, E. Krömer, T. Nösslinger et al., "Both chromosome 13 abnormalities by metaphase cytogenetics and deletion of 13q by interphase FISH only are prognostically relevant in multiple myeloma," *European Journal of Haematology*, vol. 71, no. 3, pp. 179–183, 2003.

[59] V. Sagaster, H. Ludwig, H. Kaufmann et al., "Bortezomib in relapsed multiple myeloma: response rates and duration of response are independent of a chromosome 13q-deletion," *Leukemia*, vol. 21, no. 1, pp. 164–168, 2007.

[60] L. Lodé, M. Eveillard, V. Trichet et al., "Mutations in TP53 are exclusively associated with del(17p) in multiple myeloma," *Haematologica*, vol. 95, no. 11, pp. 1973–1976, 2010.

[61] W. Xiong, X. Wu, S. Starnes et al., "An analysis of the clinical and biologic significance of TP53 loss and the identification of potential novel transcriptional targets of TP53 in multiple myeloma," *Blood*, vol. 112, no. 10, pp. 4235–4246, 2008.

[62] J. Drach, J. Ackermann, E. Fritz et al., "Presence of a p53 gene deletion in patients with multiple myeloma predicts for short survival after conventional-dose chemotherapy," *Blood*, vol. 92, no. 3, pp. 802–809, 1998.

[63] B. Lucani, G. Papini, M. Bocchia, and A. Gozzetti, "P53 and molecular genetics of multiple myeloma," *Journal of Blood Disorders*, vol. 1, no. 1, p. 3, 2014.

[64] A. D. Panani, A. D. Ferti, C. Papaxoinis, S. A. Raptis, and C. Roussos, "Cytogenetic data as a prognostic factor in multiple myeloma patients: involvement of 1p12 region an adverse prognostic factor," *Anticancer Research*, vol. 24, no. 6, pp. 4141–4146, 2004.

[65] Y. Marzin, D. Jamet, N. Douet-Guilbert et al., "Chromosome 1 abnormalities in multiple myeloma," *Anticancer Research*, vol. 26, no. 2, pp. 953–959, 2006.

[66] M. H. Qazilbash, R. M. Saliba, B. Ahmed et al., "Deletion of the short arm of chromosome 1 (del 1p) is a strong predictor of poor outcome in myeloma patients undergoing an autotransplant," *Biology of Blood and Marrow Transplantation*, vol. 13, no. 9, pp. 1066–1072, 2007.

[67] S. Caltagirone, M. Ruggeri, S. Aschero et al., "Chromosome 1 abnormalities in elderly patients with newly diagnosed multiple myeloma treated with novel therapies," *Haematologica*, vol. 99, no. 10, pp. 1611–1617, 2014.

[68] F. Zhan, J. Hardin, B. Kordsmeier et al., "Global gene expression profiling of multiple myeloma, monoclonal gammopathy of undetermined significance, and normal bone marrow plasma cells," *Blood*, vol. 99, no. 5, pp. 1745–1757, 2002.

[69] F. Zhan, Y. Huang, S. Colla et al., "The molecular classification of multiple myeloma," *Blood*, vol. 108, no. 6, pp. 2020–2028, 2006.

[70] A. Broyl, D. Hose, H. Lokhorst et al., "Gene expression profiling for molecular classification of multiple myeloma in newly diagnosed patients," *Blood*, vol. 116, no. 14, pp. 2543–2553, 2010.

[71] W. J. Chng, S. Kumar, S. VanWier et al., "Molecular dissection of hyperdiploid multiple myeloma by gene expression profiling," *Cancer Research*, vol. 67, no. 7, pp. 2982–2989, 2007.

[72] O. Decaux, L. Lodé, F. Magrangeas et al., "Prediction of survival in multiple myeloma based on gene expression profiles reveals cell cycle and chromosomal instability signatures in high-risk patients and hyperdiploid signatures in low-risk patients: a study of the Intergroupe Francophone du Myélome," *Journal of Clinical Oncology*, vol. 26, no. 29, pp. 4798–4805, 2008.

[73] R. Kuiper, A. Broyl, Y. De Knegt et al., "A gene expression signature for high-risk multiple myeloma," *Leukemia*, vol. 26, no. 11, pp. 2406–2413, 2012.

[74] R. Kuiper, M. Van Duin, M. H. Van Vliet et al., "Prediction of high- and low-risk multiple myeloma based on gene expression and the international staging system," *Blood*, vol. 126, no. 17, pp. 1996–2004, 2015.

[75] M. Dimopoulos, R. Kyle, J. P. Fermand et al., "Consensus recommendations for standard investigative workup: report of the International Myeloma Workshop Consensus Panel 3," *Blood*, vol. 117, no. 18, pp. 4701–4705, 2011.

[76] S. V. Rajkumar, R. A. Kyle, T. M. Therneau et al., "Serum free light chain ratio is an independent risk factor for progression in monoclonal gammopathy of undetermined significance," *Blood*, vol. 106, no. 3, pp. 812–817, 2005.

[77] J. T. Larsen, S. K. Kumar, A. Dispenzieri, R. A. Kyle, J. A. Katzmann, and S. V. Rajkumar, "Serum free light chain ratio as a biomarker for high-risk smoldering multiple myeloma," *Leukemia*, vol. 27, no. 4, pp. 941–946, 2013.

[78] D. Dingli, R. A. Kyle, S. V. Rajkumar et al., "Immunoglobulin free light chains and solitary plasmacytoma of bone," *Blood*, vol. 108, no. 6, pp. 1979–1983, 2006.

[79] S. Jagannath, "Value of serum free light chain testing for the diagnosis and monitoring of monoclonal gammopathies in hematology," *Clinical Lymphoma and Myeloma*, vol. 7, no. 8, pp. 518–523, 2007.

[80] M. Kraj, "Immunoglobulin heavy chain/light chain pairs (Hlc, Hevylite™) assays for diagnosing and monitoring monoclonal gammopathies," *Advances in Clinical and Experimental Medicine*, vol. 23, no. 1, pp. 127–133, 2014.

[81] E. Koulieris, P. Panayiotidis, S. J. Harding et al., "Ratio of involved/uninvolved immunoglobulin quantification by Hevylite™ assay: clinical and prognostic impact in multiple myeloma," *Experimental Hematology & Oncology*, vol. 1, no. 9, 2012.

[82] F. E. Lecouvet, B. C. Vande Berg, J. Malghem, and B. E. Maldague, "Magnetic resonance and computed tomography imaging in multiple myeloma," *Seminars in Musculoskeletal Radiology*, vol. 5, no. 1, pp. 43–56, 2001.

[83] National Comprehensive Cancer Network (NCCN), Clinical Practice Guidelines in Oncology, Multiple myeloma, V.1.2016.

[84] A. Baur-Melnyk, S. Buhmann, H. R. Dürr, and M. Reiser, "Role of MRI for the diagnosis and prognosis of multiple myeloma," *European Journal of Radiology*, vol. 55, no. 1, pp. 56–63, 2005.

[85] M. A. Dimopoulos, J. Hillengass, S. Usmani et al., "The role of magnetic resonance imaging in the management of patients with multiple myeloma: a consensus statement on behalf of the international myeloma working group," *Journal of Clinical Oncology*, vol. 33, no. 6, pp. 657–664, 2015.

[86] M. A. Bredella, L. Steinbach, G. Caputo, G. Segall, and R. Hawkins, "Value of FDG PET in the assessment of patients with multiple myeloma," *American Journal of Roentgenology*, vol. 184, no. 4, pp. 1199–1204, 2005.

[87] P. Moreau, "PET-CT in MM: a new definition of CR," *Blood*, vol. 118, no. 23, pp. 5984–5985, 2011.

[88] E. Terpos, M. Kleber, M. Engelhardt et al., "European myeloma network guidelines for the management of multiple myeloma-related complications," *Haematologica*, vol. 100, no. 10, pp. 1254–1266, 2015.

[89] M. J. Pianko, E. Terpos, G. D. Roodman et al., "Whole-body low-dose computed tomography and advanced imaging techniques for multiple myeloma bone disease," *Clinical Cancer Research*, vol. 20, no. 23, pp. 5888–5897, 2014.

[90] G. S. Nowakowski, T. E. Witzig, D. Dingli et al., "Circulating plasma cells detected by flow cytometry as a predictor of survival in 302 patients with newly diagnosed multiple myeloma," *Blood*, vol. 106, no. 7, pp. 2276–2279, 2005.

[91] P. R. Greipp, T. Leong, J. M. Bennett et al., "Plasmablastic morphology—an independent prognostic factor with clinical and laboratory correlates: eastern Cooperative Oncology Group (ECOG) myeloma trial E9486 report by the ECOG myeloma laboratory group," *Blood*, vol. 91, no. 7, pp. 2501–2507, 1998.

[92] W. J. Chng, A. Dispenzieri, C.-S. Chim et al., "IMWG consensus on risk stratification in multiple myeloma," *Leukemia*, vol. 28, no. 2, pp. 269–277, 2014.

[93] F. Gay, A. Larocca, P. Wijermans et al., "Complete response correlates with long-term progression-free and overall survival in elderly myeloma treated with novel agents: analysis of 1175 patients," *Blood*, vol. 117, no. 11, pp. 3025–3031, 2011.

[94] J. J. Lahuerta, M. V. Mateos, J. Martínez-López et al., "Influence of pre- and post-transplantation responses on outcome of patients with multiple myeloma: sequential improvement of response and achievement of complete response are associated with longer survival," *Journal of Clinical Oncology*, vol. 26, no. 35, pp. 5775–5782, 2008.

[95] B. G. Durie, J. L. Harousseau, J. S. Miguel et al., "International uniform response criteria for multiple myeloma," *Leukemia*, vol. 20, no. 9, pp. 1467–1473, 2006.

[96] S. Vincent Rajkumar, J.-L. Harousseau, B. Durie et al., "Consensus recommendations for the uniform reporting of clinical trials: report of the International Myeloma Workshop Consensus Panel 1," *Blood*, vol. 117, no. 18, pp. 4691–4695, 2011.

[97] B. Paiva, J. J. M. Van Dongen, and A. Orfao, "New criteria for response assessment: role of minimal residual disease in multiple myeloma," *Blood*, vol. 125, no. 20, pp. 3059–3068, 2015.

[98] J. F. S. San Miguel, J. Almeida, G. Mateo et al., "Immunophenotypic evaluation of the plasma cell compartment in multiple myeloma: a tool for comparing the efficacy of different treatment strategies and predicting outcome," *Blood*, vol. 99, no. 5, pp. 1853–1856, 2002.

[99] B. Paiva, M. B. Vidriales, J. Cerveró et al., "Multiparameter flow cytometric remission is the most relevant prognostic factor for multiple myeloma patients who undergo autologous stem cell transplantation," *Blood*, vol. 112, no. 10, pp. 4017–4023, 2008.

[100] N. Puig, M. E. Sarasquete, A. Balanzategui et al., "Critical evaluation of ASO RQ-PCR for minimal residual disease evaluation in multiple myeloma. A comparative analysis with flow cytometry," *Leukemia*, vol. 28, no. 2, pp. 391–397, 2014.

[101] J. Martinez-Lopez, J. J. Lahuerta, F. Pepin et al., "Prognostic value of deep sequencing method for minimal residual disease detection in multiple myeloma," *Blood*, vol. 123, no. 20, pp. 3073–3079, 2014.

[102] J. Bladé, C. Fernández de Larrea, L. Rosiñol, M. T. Cibeira, R. Jiménez, and R. Powles, "Soft-tissue plasmacytomas in multiple myeloma: incidence, mechanisms of extramedullary spread, and treatment approach," *Journal of Clinical Oncology*, vol. 29, no. 28, pp. 3805–3812, 2011.

[103] J. Hillengass, T. Bäuerle, R. Bartl et al., "Diffusion-weighted imaging for non-invasive and quantitative monitoring of bone marrow infiltration in patients with monoclonal plasma cell disease: a comparative study with histology," *British Journal of Haematology*, vol. 153, no. 6, pp. 721–728, 2011.

[104] B. Paiva, M. B. Vidriales, J. Cerveró et al., "Multiparameter flow cytometric remission is the most relevant prognostic factor for multiple myeloma patients who undergo autologous stem cell transplantation," *Blood*, vol. 112, no. 10, pp. 4017–4023, 2008.

[105] A. C. Rawstron, J. A. Child, R. M. de Tute et al., "Minimal residual disease assessed by multiparameter flow cytometry in multiple myeloma: impact on outcome in the Medical Research Council Myeloma IX Study," *Journal of Clinical Oncology*, vol. 31, no. 20, pp. 2540–2547, 2013.

[106] M. E. Gore, C. Viner, M. Meldrum et al., "Intensive treatment of multiple myeloma and criteria for complete remission," *The Lancet*, vol. 334, no. 8668, pp. 879–882, 1989.

[107] J. Bladé, D. Samson, D. Reece et al., "Criteria for evaluating disease response and progression in patients with multiple myeloma treated by high-dose therapy and haemopoietic stem cell transplantation," *British Journal of Haematology*, vol. 102, no. 5, pp. 1115–1123, 1998.

[108] B. G. Durie, J. L. Harousseau, J. S. San Miguel et al., "International uniform response criteria for multiple myeloma," *Leukemia*, vol. 20, no. 9, pp. 1467–1473, 2006.

9

Sp17 Protein Expression and Major Histocompatibility Class I and II Epitope Presentation in Diffuse Large B Cell Lymphoma Patients

Kamel Ait-Tahar,[1] **Amanda P. Anderson,**[1] **Martin Barnardo,**[2] **Graham P. Collins,**[3] **Chris S. R. Hatton,**[3] **Alison H. Banham,**[1] **and Karen Pulford**[1]

[1]*Nuffield Division of Clinical Laboratory Sciences, Radcliffe Department of Medicine, University of Oxford, Oxford, UK*
[2]*Transplant Immunology & Immunogenetics, Oxford Transplant Centre, Churchill Hospital, Oxford, UK*
[3]*Department of Clinical Haematology, Churchill Hospital, Oxford, UK*

Correspondence should be addressed to Karen Pulford; karen.pulford@ndcls.ox.ac.uk

Academic Editor: Shaji Kumar

Improved therapies are urgently needed for patients with diffuse large B cell lymphoma (DLBCL). Success using immune checkpoint inhibitors and chimeric antigen receptor T cell technology has fuelled demand for validated cancer epitopes. Immunogenic cancer testis antigens (CTAs), with their widespread expression in many tumours but highly restricted normal tissue distribution, represent attractive immunotherapeutic targets that may improve treatment options for DLBCL and other malignancies. Sperm protein 17 (Sp17), a CTA reported to be immunogenic in ovarian cancer and myeloma patients, is expressed in DLBCL. The aim of the present study was to investigate Sp17 epitope presentation via the presence of a cytotoxic T cell (CTL) and a CD4 T-helper (Th) response in DLBCL patients. A significant γ-interferon CTL response was detected in peripheral blood mononuclear cells of 13/31 DLBCL patients following short-term cell stimulation with two novel HLA-A*0201 peptides and one previously reported HLA-A*0101-restricted nine-mer Sp17 peptide. No significant responses were detected in the HLA-A*0201-negative DLBCL patients or four healthy subjects. A novel immunogenic 20-mer CD4 Th Sp17 peptide was detected in 8/17 DLBCL patients. This is the first report of a CTL and a CD4 Th response to Sp17 in DLBCL and supports Sp17 as a potential immunotherapeutic target for DLBCL.

1. Introduction

DLBCL is the most common form of mature B cell lymphoma and is heterogeneous with respect to morphology, clinical features, and immunophenotype [1]. A significant proportion of patients with DLBCL fail to achieve long-term remission despite advances in the definition of clinically relevant subtypes and treatment [2]. The development of improved immunotherapeutic options for the treatment of DLBCL thus remains urgent. The recent breakthroughs using immune checkpoint inhibitors and chimeric antigen receptor (CAR) T cell technology have opened up new avenues for achieving these objectives [3, 4]. However, the identification of relevant antigenic targets, particularly those presented on the cell surface of primary tumours and not just cancer cell lines, remains a priority.

Tumour-associated antigens (TAAs), recognized by the immune system of the patient, have been studied extensively in haematological malignancies. Evidence in support of their potential therapeutic benefit has been provided by autologous bone marrow transplantation and donor lymphocyte infusion studies, demonstrating that donor cells can recognize and respond to TAAs in a variety of malignancies, such as multiple myeloma and myeloid leukaemia [5, 6]. TAAs that are of current particular interest for improving treatment regimens are the family of cancer testis antigens (CTAs). Previous studies have reported expression of various CTAs in haematological malignancies, such as lymphomas [7, 8] and myeloid malignancies [9, 10], and in multiple myeloma [11–15]. These immunogenic molecules are highly tumour-specific and frequently expressed in various types of cancer, properties which make them promising candidate targets for cancer immunotherapy, including cancer vaccination and adoptive T cell transfer with chimeric T cell receptors [16–18].

One of the CTAs under intense investigation is the Sp17 protein. Its restricted expression in testis and its reported expression and immunogenicity in ovarian cancer [19–21], non-small cell lung cancer [22], and myeloma [23–25] patients make it an attractive candidate immunotherapeutic target in these malignancies. Moreover, Sp17 was found to be present on the surface of malignant lymphoid cells, including B- and T-lymphoid cell lines, and on the surface of primary cells isolated from two patients having B-lymphoid tumours [26]. We have also previously reported Sp17 protein expression in both primary DLBCL and DLBCL cell lines [27]. It has been suggested that Sp17 is an "oncofetal antigen" since it is expressed in embryonic as well as adult neoplastic cells, but not in normal tissues, and has been associated with the motility and migratory capacity of tumour cells [28]. As demonstrated with other CTAs, this functional role in tumour biology makes Sp17 a good immunotherapeutic target as it is unlikely to lose expression under therapeutic selection pressure. The current study was performed to explore the immunogenicity of the Sp17 protein and its expression in DLBCL patients.

2. Materials and Methods

2.1. Subjects and Samples. Peripheral blood was obtained from 31 patients with B cell lymphoma attending the Haematology Departments of the John Radcliffe Hospital, Oxford ($n = 25$), and Milton Keynes General Hospital ($n = 6$). The patient cohort (previously described in earlier studies on the PASD1 CTA [29, 30]) consisted of 22 patients with de novo DLBCL (two with relapsed DLBCL), seven patients with transformed DLBCL, and two patients with T cell rich B cell lymphoma. The patients presented with differing stages of disease and their clinical details and treatment protocols are summarized in Supplementary Table 1 in Supplementary Material available online at https://doi.org/10.1155/2017/6527306. Normal testis and tonsil tissues were obtained from the Department of Pathology, John Radcliffe Hospital, and used as positive and negative controls, respectively. Peripheral blood samples were also obtained from four healthy subjects. HLA typing was done by polymerase chain reaction (PCR) as previously described [31]. Ethical approval and written consent were obtained from the Oxfordshire Research Ethics Committee B (C02.356) for all blood samples collected and tissue sections used in the immunolabelling studies.

2.2. Peptides. CTL peptides: Two 9-amino-acid peptides, predicted with high binding affinity to the major histocompatibility complex (MHC) class I HLA-A*0201 allele, were identified using the web-based SYFPEITHI (http://www.syfpeithi.de) and the HLA peptide prediction site of the Bioinformatics and Molecular Analysis Section (BIMAS, National Institutes of Health, Bethesda, USA) programmes. The peptides identified were as follows: Sp17(1)$_{43-52}$ (SLLEKREKT); Sp17(2)$_{19-27}$ (LLEGLTREI). Sp17(3)$_{102-110}$ (ILDSSEEDK) previously identified as immunogenic in an HLA-A1 healthy

donor [24] was also investigated. A control irrelevant peptide from the HIV-1 reverse transcriptase (ILKEPVHGV) that binds to HLA-A*0201 was used in the CD8 T cell ELISPOT assays (Invitrogen, Paisley, UK). The Sp17 peptides were synthesized by standard chemistry on a multiple peptide synthesizer (Proimmune, Oxford, UK) and were >90% pure. Lyophilized peptides were dissolved in dimethyl sulfoxide and stored at −20°C.

CD4 T-Helper (Th) Peptides. The TEPITOPE prediction algorithm and SYPETHI (http://www.syfpeithi.de) programs were used to select three 20-mer Sp17 peptides predicted to be immunogenic in the context of HLA-DRB1 *0101, *0301, *0401, *0701, *1101, and *1501 (the most prevalent alleles among the Caucasian population) [31]. The peptides identified were as follows: Sp17(4)$_{9-28}$ (YRIPQGFGNLLEGLTREILR); Sp17(5)$_{67-86}$ (FYNNHAFEEQEPPEKSDPKQ); and Sp17(6)$_{118-139}$ (VKIQAAFRGHIAREEAKKMK). The irrelevant control peptide was HIV-1$_{121-140}$ (DESFRKYTAFTIPSMNNETP) (Invitrogen, Paisley, UK).

2.3. Antibodies. The anti-Sp17 monoclonal antibody was a kind gift from S. H. Lim (Texas). Antibodies to BCL6 (PG-B6p), CD10 (56C6), CD4 (T4-10, IgG1 isotype), and CD20 (DAKO-L26, IgG2a isotype) were purchased from DakoCytomation (Ely, Cambridgeshire, UK) while anti-CD8 (X-107, IgG1 isotype, used undiluted) was prepared in the authors' laboratory. Anti-MUM1 was a kind gift from Professor B. Fallini (Perugia, Italy). The anti-HLA-A*0201 (BB7.2) used in the CD8 T cell blocking experiments was purchased from BD BioSciences (Oxford, UK). Major histocompatibility complex (MHC) class II expression was studied using the monoclonal anti-HLA-DP, DQ, and DR antibody (CR3/43) (DakoCytomation, Glostrup, Denmark). Unless stated, all antibodies were used at dilutions recommended by the manufacturers. Rabbit anti-CD3 (DAKO-CD3, diluted 1:100) and the Envision-horseradish peroxidase (HRP) labelling system were obtained from DakoCytomation. The MACH 3™ HRP-polymer detection kit was purchased from Biocare Medical (Wokingham, Berkshire, UK). Goat anti-rabbit immunoglobulin (Ig) and anti-mouse Ig-isotype specific antibodies conjugated to either fluorescein isothiocyanate (FITC) or Texas Red™ (diluted 1:100) were obtained from Invitrogen Ltd. (Paisley, UK).

2.4. Immunolabelling. Paraffin-embedded tissue sections were dewaxed and heat-induced antigen retrieval was performed using 50 mM Tris: 2 mM EDTA at pH 9.0. Immunolabelling for anti-MHC-class II was carried out using the Envision-HRP labelling kit (DAKO, Ely, UK). The method of staining for Sp17 protein expression and the subtyping of the DLBCL cases (germinal or nongerminal center subtypes [32]) was performed as previously described [27].

2.5. Preparation and Culture of PBMCs. Peripheral blood mononuclear cells (PBMCs) were prepared in RPMI 1640 medium containing 10% fetal calf serum (FCS) (RPMI

1640/FCS, Invitrogen Ltd.) as described previously [33]. PBMCs (0.5×10^5) in 200 μl of RPMI 1640/FCS were added to each well of a 96-well round-bottomed plate and incubated for 8–10 days with 10 μmol of one of the following: Sp17(1), Sp17(2), Sp17(3), Sp17(4), Sp17(5), Sp17(6), or the control HIV peptides, 10 μg/ml phytohaemagglutinin (PHA; Sigma-Aldrich Co. Ltd., Dorset, UK), or tissue culture media only. Recombinant interleukin-2 (rIL-2: 20 iu/ml; Roche Diagnostics, Indianapolis, IN, USA) and rIL-7 (25 ng/ml; R&D Systems, Minneapolis, MN, USA) were added on days 2, 5, and 7.

2.6. Enzyme-Linked Immunospot Assay (ELISPOT). After 8–10 days of culture, the cells were washed and incubated for 18 h with RPMI 1640/FCS at 37°C in 5% CO_2 with one of the Sp17 peptides, HIV control peptide, PHA, or medium only. Peptides were used at 10 μmol and all cultures were carried out in triplicate. Gamma-interferon (γ-IFN) release assays were performed according to manufacturer's instructions (Mabtech, Stockholm, Sweden). Spots were counted using an automated ELISPOT reader (Autoimmun-Diagnostika, Strasberg, Germany). Results were considered positive if the number of spots in the test wells was at least twice those present in the control cultures (media only or containing the irrelevant HIV-1 peptide) and assays were excluded if there were more than 25 spots per well in the absence of peptides. All tests were performed in triplicate.

2.7. Generation of CD8 T Cell Lines, Depletion, and Blocking Experiments. PBMCs cultured at a density of 2×10^6 cells/ml were cultured in RPMI 1640/FCS containing 10 μmol of the appropriate Sp17 peptides. After 72 h, an equal volume of RPMI 1640/FCS containing 50 IU of rIL-2 per ml was added. Half of the medium was removed and replaced with fresh medium every 3 d. The cells were restimulated weekly for 6 weeks with the Sp17 peptides before being used in an ELISPOT assay. In some experiments, CD8-positive T cells were enriched from the CTL lines using magnetic beads coated with anti-human CD8 antibody according to the manufacturer's instructions (Dynabeads, Dynal, Oslo, Norway) before assay. In other experiments, the anti-HLA-A*0201 antibody (BB7.2) was added at a concentration of 10 μg/ml to block γ-IFN release.

2.8. Statistical Analysis. Student's t-test was used to analyse the results obtained in the ELISPOT assays and the immune response while Fisher's exact test was used to analyse the presence of a CTL response with Sp17 protein expression in patients who were HLA-A*0201 or HLA-A*0101 positive. P values < 0.05 were considered significant.

3. Results

3.1. Sp17 Protein Expression in DLBCL Patient Biopsies. Routinely fixed tissue sections from diagnostic biopsies were available for 20 of the 31 DLBCL patients to investigate Sp17 protein expression by immunohistochemistry (IHC). Clinicopathological characteristics of the DLBCL patients including their cell-of-origin classification, results of the

Sp17 immunolabelling of tumour biopsies, and MHC class I and II expression are summarized in Tables 1 and 2 and Supplementary Table 1. Labelling with the Sp17 antibody was detected in the tumour cells derived from nine patients. Both nuclear and cytoplasmic labelling of Sp17 were observed in five cases, while scattered nuclear labelling was observed in the remaining four cases. Sp17 protein was not detected in the remaining 11 patients. In normal testis sections, the anti-Sp17 antibody detected weak staining of protein in the cytoplasm of the spermatogonia and in the cytoplasm and nuclei of the primary spermatocytes and the spermatozoa (strong staining). Sp17 protein expression was absent in normal tonsil. These data are consistent with those illustrated in our initial pilot study of Sp17 expression in DLBCL [27].

3.2. CD8 T Cell Responses to Sp17. The results of the γ-IFN response ELISPOT assay are summarized in Table 1. Significant γ-IFN responses to Sp17 were observed in 14/31 DLBCL patients after short-term culture with the Sp17 peptides compared to those results obtained from the control cultures (cells stimulated with the irrelevant HIV peptide or medium only, $P < 0.05$) and eight patients showed a response to more than one peptide. The Sp17 γ-IFN responses correlated with Sp17 protein expression in eight patients expressing Sp17 (0.0497, $P < 0.05$). With the exception of patients (9 and 39) who had a response to Sp17(1) peptide, no significant γ-IFN responses were detected in the eight patients with tumours where Sp17 protein was not detected. This suggests that the responses are antigen-driven. Two of the five HLA-A*0101-positive patients (7 and 39) responded to the Sp17(3) peptide, previously identified as immunogenic in an HLA-A1 healthy donor [24]. Conversely, none of the HLA-A*0201-positive patients responded to the Sp17(3) peptide, possibly reflecting the HLA-restricted nature of the responses. Frequencies of Sp17-responding T cells varied between patients, ranging from 1 : 600 (0.2%) PBMCs in patient 8 to 1 : 2000 (0.05%) in patient 39. Sp17(1) was identified as the most immunogenic peptide since it induced significant responses in the majority of the responding patients (13/15). No significant responses to any of the Sp17 peptides were detected in the four healthy donors examined.

3.3. CD4 T Cell Responses to Sp17. CD4 Th responses were examined in PBMCs of 17 DLBCL patients, eight of which displayed Sp17 protein expression. A significant response to Sp17(4) was observed in 8/17 patients (Table 2). None of the patients displayed a significant response to either Sp17(5) or Sp17(6). Patients 8 and 12 displayed the highest CD4 Th responses. It is noteworthy that some of the patients who responded most vigorously to either of the CTL peptides Sp17(1) and Sp17(2) (Table 1) also displayed the highest responses to the Sp17(4) peptide (patients 1, 8, and 12 in Table 2). Seven patients with a CD4 Th response also exhibited a CTL response to Sp17.

3.4. Persistence and Specificity of the γ-IFN Response to Sp17. The CD8 T cell responses to Sp17(1) and Sp17(2) were investigated in samples from two HLA-A*0201-positive patients (1 and 2), who were both in remission one year

TABLE 1: Summary of the CD8 T cell responses to the Sp17 peptides by DLBCL patients.

Patients	Diagnosis	HLA status	Pattern of Sp17 staining	γ-IFN response to peptides per 50,000 cells					
				Sp17(1)	Sp17(2)	Sp17(3)	No peptide	HIV-1	PHA
Significant response									
1	DLBCL(dn)	A*0201+	Cytoplasm and <10% nuclei	**84 ± 12**	**46 ± 10**	24 ± 6	12 ± 2	18 ± 4	126 ± 28
2	DLBCL(dn)	A*0201+	Scattered nuclei	**58 ± 10**	**74 ± 14**	30 ± 8	18 ± 4	20 ± 4	94 ± 16
5	DLBCL(dn)	A*0201+	—	**48 ± 4**	34 ± 16	30 ± 8	16 ± 4	20 ± 4	104 ± 18
7	DLBCL(dn)	A*0101+	<10% nuclei	16 ± 4	14 ± 2	**48 ± 6**	12 ± 2	10 ± 2	124 ± 16
8	DLBCL(dn)	A*0201+	ND	**102 ± 16**	24 ± 4	32 ± 8	20 ± 4	16 ± 4	204 ± 24
9	DLBCL(dn)	A*0201+	—	**86 ± 12**	40 ± 8	38 ± 10	12 ± 4	20 ± 4	128 ± 18
12	DLBCL(dn)	A*0201+	Weak cytoplasm and < 5% nuclei	**98 ± 14**	**76 ± 14**	42 ± 6	22 ± 2	16 ± 4	154 ± 16
14	DLBCL(dn)	A*0201+	ND	**66 ± 6**	**44 ± 8**	26 ± 6	12 ± 6	14 ± 2	84 ± 14
18	DLBCL(dn)	A*0201+	Weak cytoplasm and <5% nuclei	**68 ± 12**	**54 ± 4**	30 ± 8	18 ± 4	20 ± 2	94 ± 16
19	DLBCL(t)	A*0201+	<10% nuclei	**56 ± 10**	**62 ± 14**	22 ± 4	20 ± 2	18 ± 4	86 ± 12
21	DLBCL(dn)	A*0201+	Cytoplasm + scattered < 5% nuclei	**46 ± 4**	14 ± 2	30 ± 8	12 ± 0	16 ± 2	110 ± 12
22	DLBCL(t)	A*0201+	ND	**86 ± 8**	**64 ± 14**	40 ± 8	20 ± 4	10 ± 1	88 ± 10
37	DLBCL(dn)	A*0101+	<5% nuclei	**38 ± 4**	24 ± 14	**32 ± 4**	12 ± 2	6 ± 1	178 ± 8
39	T cell rich	A*0201+	—	**28 ± 2**	12 ± 2	22 ± 4	10 ± 2	6 ± 1	108 ± 10
No significant response									
3	DLBCL(dn)	A*0201+	—	28 ± 8	42 ± 6	28 ± 4	16 ± 8	20 ± 4	88 ± 22
4	DLBCL(dn)	A*0201+	—	40 ± 6	38 ± 12	22 ± 4	20 ± 4	16 ± 6	132 ± 18
6	DLBCL(dn)	A*0201+	ND	10 ± 2	12 ± 4	20 ± 2	12 ± 6	6 ± 2	148 ± 10
10	DLBCL(dn)	A*0101+	ND	24 ± 4	26 ± 2	16 ± 2	18 ± 2	12 ± 6	106 ± 18
11	DLBCL(dn)	A*0201+	ND	36 ± 10	22 ± 4	20 ± 8	18 ± 6	22 ± 4	112 ± 10
13	DLBCL(dn)	A*0201+	—	32 ± 8	24 ± 4	18 ± 8	12 ± 6	16 ± 4	98 ± 12
15	DLBCL(dn)	A*0101+	ND	16 ± 2	20 ± 6	28 ± 8	10 ± 6	6 ± 2	86 ± 10
16	DLBCL(dn)	A*0201+	—	36 ± 6	32 ± 8	30 ± 8	12 ± 6	20 ± 10	94 ± 16
17	DLBCL(dn)	A*0201+	—	16 ± 1	14 ± 2	22 ± 2	16 ± 2	10 ± 4	114 ± 10
20	DLBCL(dn)	A*0101+	Cytoplasm + scattered < 5% nuclei	32 ± 1	28 ± 8	**36 ± 8**	18 ± 4	16 ± 1	134 ± 16
38	DLBCL(dn)	A*0201+	ND	26 ± 2	24 ± 4	32 ± 2	20 ± 6	16 ± 10	114 ± 18
40	DLBCL(dn)	A*0201-negative, A*0101-negative	ND	16 ± 4	14 ± 4	26 ± 4	14 ± 2	10 ± 2	64 ± 12
41	DLBCL(dn)	A*0201-negative, A*0101-negative	—	18 ± 6	20 ± 4	12 ± 4	10 ± 2	8 ± 2	66 ± 10
42	DLBCL(dn)	A*0201-negative, A*0101-negative	ND	26 ± 4	22 ± 6	18 ± 6	22 ± 4	20 ± 2	102 ± 16
43	DLBCL(dn)	A*0201-negative, A*0101-negative	—	24 ± 10	34 ± 14	20 ± 8	22 ± 4	16 ± 2	>500
48	DLBCL(dn)	A*0201-negative, A*0101-negative	—	16 ± 4	24 ± 14	28 ± 8	22 ± 6	20 ± 2	94 ± 16
49	DLBCL(dn)	A*0201-negative, A*0101-negative	ND	24 ± 2	18 ± 4	22 ± 6	14 ± 2	10 ± 4	144 ± 18
Healthy donors									
1		A*0201+	ND	16 ± 4	12 ± 4	16 ± 4	18 ± 4	8 ± 2	68 ± 12
2		A*0201+	ND	18 ± 2	20 ± 2	12 ± 4	8 ± 4	6 ± 2	76 ± 10
3		A*0201+	ND	32 ± 4	36 ± 4	24 ± 6	16 ± 4	20 ± 2	112 ± 18
4		A*0301+	ND	26 ± 10	28 ± 8	12 ± 2	10 ± 4	16 ± 2	88 ± 14

DLBCL(dn): de novo diffuse large B cell lymphoma; DLBCL(t): diffuse large B cell lymphoma transformed; TCR: T cell rich B cell lymphoma. The results +/− are from triplicate ELISPOT cultures. The SD was calculated using standard techniques. Significant γ-IFN responses are highlighted in bold. ND, not determined.

TABLE 2: Summary of the CD4 T cell responses to the Sp17 peptides by DLBCL patients.

Patients	MHC class II status	Sp17 protein	γ-IFN response to peptides per 50,000 cells					
			Sp17(4)	Sp17(5)	Sp17(6)	No peptide	HIV-1	PHA
Significant response								
1	DRB1*0102,*1104	+	**42 ± 4**	16 ± 2	14 ± 4	12 ± 2	10 ± 4	92 ± 4
2	DRB1*0101,*0701	+	**28 ± 2**	8 ± 2	18 ± 2	10 ± 2	6 ± 1	72 ± 12
5	DRB1*0301,*0401	−	**26 ± 4**	12 ± 2	14 ± 2	8 ± 2	4 ± 0	108 ± 10
8	DRB1*1501,*0803	ND	**52 ± 4**	12 ± 2	14 ± 4	10 ± 2	6 ± 2	78 ± 14
10	DRB1*0101	ND	**36 ± 4**	20 ± 2	10 ± 4	8 ± 2	4 ± 2	86 ± 6
12	DRB1*0401,*1401	+	**50 ± 2**	22 ± 4	28 ± 4	16 ± 2	12 ± 4	128 ± 16
14	DRB1*1403,*0401	ND	**38 ± 4**	14 ± 2	24 ± 6	8 ± 2	4 ± 2	78 ± 14
18	DRB1*0401,*0401	+	**32 ± 6**	18 ± 2	16 ± 4	6 ± 2	10 ± 2	66 ± 12
No significant response								
7	DRB1*0301,*0701	+	18 ± 6	22 ± 2	26 ± 4	14 ± 2	12 ± 2	58 ± 8
9	DRB1*0301,*1601	−	16 ± 8	32 ± 4	20 ± 4	18 ± 2	14 ± 4	108 ± 10
15	DRB1*1301,*1101	ND	10 ± 2	12 ± 2	20 ± 4	10 ± 2	14 ± 2	58 ± 8
19	DRB1*0401,*0901	+	14 ± 2	18 ± 2	6 ± 1	12 ± 2	8 ± 2	50 ± 8
20	DRB1*1104,*1501	+	24 ± 4	26 ± 2	14 ± 4	14 ± 2	12 ± 2	72 ± 10
21	DRB1*0301,*1303	+	10 ± 2	14 ± 2	18 ± 2	9 ± 2	8 ± 2	86 ± 6
39	DRB1*0701	−	32 ± 4	26 ± 2	14 ± 2	16 ± 2	14 ± 2	112 ± 16
43	DRB1*0101,*1101	−	24 ± 4	32 ± 2	28 ± 2	18 ± 4	20 ± 2	98 ± 12
48	DRB1*0101,*0405	−	28 ± 4	10 ± 2	18 ± 2	18 ± 4	14 ± 2	98 ± 8

DLBCL(dn): de novo diffuse large B cell lymphoma; DLBCL(t): diffuse large B cell lymphoma transformed; TCR: T cell rich B cell lymphoma. The results +/− are from triplicate ELISPOT cultures. The SD was calculated using standard techniques. Significant γ-IFN responses are highlighted in bold. ND, not determined.

after initial diagnosis. A significant γ-IFN response to both Sp17 peptides was still detectable in the two patients after one year (Figure 1(a)) suggesting the persistence of a pool of circulating memory CD8-positive T cells to the Sp17 protein.

PBMCs from the HLA-A*0201-positive patient 1 were maintained in culture to permit further analysis of their functional activity. PBMCs were restimulated weekly with rIL-2 and with one of the following: Sp17(1), Sp17(2), or the irrelevant HIV peptide. After 3 weeks, cells were tested for their γ-IFN secreting activity to the Sp17 and control peptides in an overnight ELISPOT assay. T cells were found to expand and respond specifically to both Sp17 peptides. After three rounds of expansion, Sp17(1)- and Sp17(2)-specific CD8+ T cells increased almost three- and twofold, respectively, compared to the nonexpanded population (Figure 1(b)). The CD8-enriched T cell γ-IFN response to the Sp17 peptides was abrogated by the removal of CD8-positive T cells or by the addition of the anti-HLA-A*0201 monoclonal antibody BB7.2 (Figure 1(c)). These results confirm the CD8-positive, MHC class I restricted nature of the response.

3.5. CTL and CD4 Th Responses to Both the Sp17 and PASD1 CTAs. Results of the Sp17 T cell responses reported here were compared to those obtained for the PASD1 antigen in two previous studies using cells from the same cohort of DLBCL patients [29, 30]. Cells from ten patients were able to mount CTL responses to both Sp17 and PASD1 CTAs (Supplementary Table 2). CD4 Th responses to both the PASD1 and Sp17 antigens were also detected in five of these patients.

4. Discussion

The Sp17 protein is a member of the CT-X group of CTAs, those whose members localize to the X chromosome [34]. Its restricted distribution in normal tissue but expression in myeloma [25] and in some solid tumours including ovarian cancer [21] and small cell lung carcinoma [22] highlighted Sp17 as a potential immunotherapeutic target in these diseases. We previously reported Sp17 to exhibit the broadest mRNA and protein expression profile in a wide range of haematological cell lines as well as protein expression in primary tumour biopsies from DLBCL [27]. This was of particular importance given previous reports of the paucity of CTA expression in B cell lymphomas [35, 36]. The potential of Sp17 as an immunotherapeutic target was further supported by studies of immunogenic Sp17 CTL epitopes in ovarian cancer [37–39] as well as in myeloma patients [24] and in healthy donors [23]. More recently, Mirandola et al. showed Sp17 to be aberrantly expressed in non-small cell lung cancer patients and it was also immunogenic in these patients [22]. The rationale for the current study was to further validate the Sp17 protein as a potential target in haematological malignancies by studying both its expression and presentation of T cell epitopes. Here, we explored the immunogenicity of Sp17 in a cohort of 31 DLBCL patients, T cell responses being used to demonstrate the presentation of distinct Sp17 epitopes. We have previously reported, in the same cohort of patients, the presence of both CTL and CD4 Th responses to another CTA, the PASD1 protein [29, 30], which is also a member of the CT-X group.

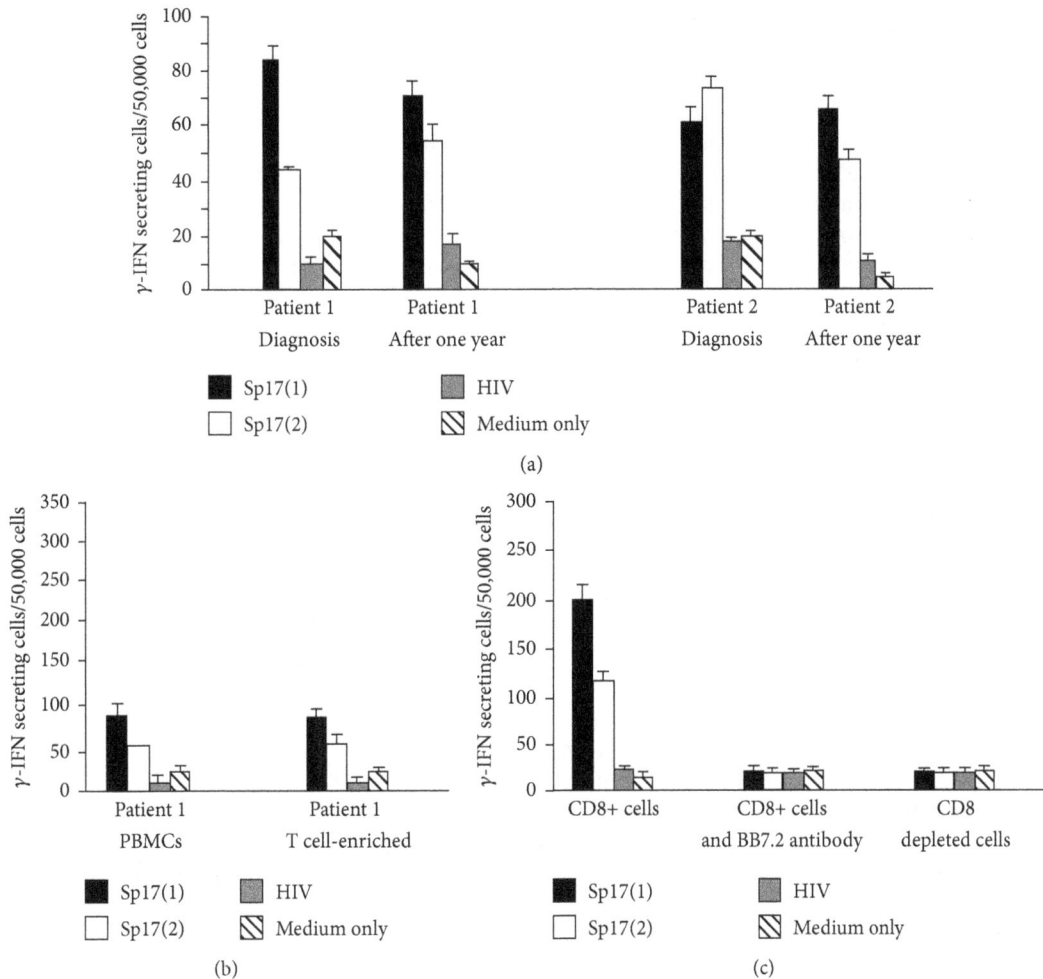

FIGURE 1: γ-IFN responses of patients 1 and 2 to Sp17 peptides. In (a) peripheral blood mononuclear cells (PBMCs) obtained from patients 1 and 2 at time of diagnosis after one year from start of treatment were maintained in short tern culture. A significant γ-IFN response to peptides Sp17(1) and Sp17(2) was observed in cells from both patients obtained at both time points ($P < 0.05$). No significant response was detected in cultures stimulated by the HIV peptide or containing medium only. (b) PBMCs from patient 1 after three rounds of peptide stimulation expanded in response to Sp17(1) and Sp17(2) peptides. (c) PBMCs from patient 1 were either enriched for CD8-positive cells using anti-CD8 antibody-coated magnetic beads or incubated with an anti-HLA-A*0201 monoclonal antibody (BB7.2). A significant γ-IFN response was observed only in the culture containing the CD*-positive cells in the absence of anti-MHC class I ($P < 0.05$). No significant responses were detected in the control cultures or the irrelevant peptides. The results are mean +/- SD and were obtained from triplicate ELISPOT cultures.

Cytotoxic T cells recognizing Sp17 peptides were detected in 13/31 (41%) of HLA-A*0201-positive DLBCL patients after only short-term culture. The magnitude of the CD8 T cell response to Sp17 varied between patients. These results compared favourably with those obtained for the MAGE-A(1–4), LAGE-1, PASD-1, and NY-ESO-1 CTAs in haematological malignancies [13, 29, 40] and for CEA, HER-2/neu, and MAGE-A3 in breast cancer [41]. Our data provide the first experimental validation that Sp17 epitopes are presented and recognized by a T cell response in patients with B cell lymphoma. Our demonstration of a γ-IFN response to Sp17 peptides by PBMCs from responder patients after only short-term culture also suggests that Sp17 peptide-specific CTL precursors were present in these individuals. Spontaneous immunity to CTAs, including MAGE-A3 and NY-ESO-1, has also been reported in multiple myeloma [13, 40]. Although

outside the scope of the current study investigating epitope presentation, Sp17 might also represent a potential vaccine candidate in DLBCL. To address this possibility, future studies to characterise the functional activity of these T cell populations (e.g., their cytolytic potential) would be needed.

Correlations have been reported between antibody responses to CTAs and prognosis in myeloma [40]. In the present study, a γ-IFN response to Sp17 peptides was detected in seven patients with good prognosis GCB-derived DLBCL in addition to the eight patients with poor-prognosis DLBCL (five patients with NGC-derived DLBCL and three patients with transformed DLBCL). These results suggest that Sp17 may be applicable as a therapeutic target regardless of DLBCL subtype. However, given the relatively small number of cases studied here, further study is required to draw any firm conclusions.

Our analysis of sequential blood samples from two DLBCL patients demonstrated a persistent CTL response to Sp17 peptides a year after diagnosis. Both patients remained in remission by the end of this study. Sustained CTL responses to TAAs have been previously reported in myeloma [13] and in anaplastic large cell lymphoma [33, 42]. The persistence of these T cell responses suggests the presence of memory T cells, which might be involved in protective immunity and which also represent potential populations of T cells that could be further stimulated following vaccination [43]. The presence of a significant γ-IFN response in these patients both at the time of diagnosis and after one year in remission also suggests the presence of a pool of memory CTL subsets. Such cells could play an important role not only in protective tumour immunity but also in the maintenance of memory CTL responses [44, 45].

A γ-IFN response to the Sp17(1) and Sp17(2) peptides was only detected in those patients who were HLA-A*0201-positive (except for patient 37). These results, combined with the abrogation of the γ-IFN response through depletion of CD8-positive cells or the addition of an anti-MHC class I reagent to CTL lines, provide further evidence for an MHC class I-dependent Sp17 CTL response.

Our study showed that while the Sp17(5) and Sp17(6) peptides were not immunogenic, Sp17(4) induced CD4 Th responses in 4/8 patients expressing Sp17. This is interesting since the responses were not restricted by the different HLA class II allele. The presence of such an epitope recognizable in the context of a variety of different MHC class II molecules could expand the population of patients for whom the peptide could be immunogenic beyond that determined by their MHC class I allele. Moreover, our study shows that CTL as well as CD4 Th responses to Sp17 were recorded in seven patients. A number of studies have demonstrated the potential of using peptide epitopes binding to both MHC class I and class II to achieve optimal immune responses on vaccination [46].

Sp17 represents a potential immunotherapeutic target and is therefore important to correlate the presence of CTL and CD4 γ-IFN responses with Sp17 protein expression in tumours. Immunohistochemical labelling with an anti-Sp17 monoclonal antibody confirmed Sp17 expression in 75% (9/12) of the patients tested who exhibited γ-IFN responses to Sp17 peptides. Previous studies [13, 40] were able to confirm NY-ESO-1 and MAGE protein expression in those myeloma patients who mounted CTL responses to these CTAs. The low levels and heterogeneity of Sp17 protein expression in the lymphoma cells may explain the absence of detectable Sp17 protein in two patients with a CTL response. Indeed, the biopsy from one patient (patient 5) was a very small bone marrow trephine containing very little lymphoma cells. Furthermore, we previously reported that Sp17 protein expression in DLBCL cell lines was commonly expressed only at low levels that were detectable by Western blotting and not by immunohistochemistry [27]. This may also be the case in primary DLBCL and provides a potential explanation as to why a small number of patients exhibited an anti-Sp17 immune response despite protein expression being undetectable by immunohistochemistry.

It is interesting to note that the majority of the patients with detectable CTL and CD4 Th responses to Sp17 were previously reported to show significant T cell responses to another CTA, the PASD1 protein [29, 30]. The results indicate that both proteins are expressed and immunogenic in this cohort of DLBCL patients. Previous studies have described the presence of more than one CTA antigen in both solid tumours and haematological malignancies such as myeloma and plasmacytoma [47, 48]. Intratumoural variation of CTA expression has been previously described in DLBCL [29], acute myeloid leukaemia [9], and myeloma [49]. The presence of more than one CTA within a tumour, combined with heterogeneity in their protein distribution, thus provides support for the inclusion of multiple CTAs in vaccine development. This approach should maximize the eradication of the tumour cells while minimizing tumour escape variants.

5. Conclusions

This study is the first to define immunogenic MHC-presented Sp17 peptides in DLBCL. We showed coordinated CTL and CD4 Th responses to Sp17 in DLBCL patients. The CTL response was MHC class I-restricted and was limited to patients expressing Sp17.

The current results support Sp17 as a potential immunotherapeutic target for patients with Sp17-positive DLBCL or other malignancies expressing this antigen. Since tumours may express more than one CTA, the inclusion of Sp17 in a polyepitope vaccine should increase the chances of successful treatment of patients expressing these antigens.

Conflicts of Interest

The authors declare no potential conflicts of interest.

Acknowledgments

This work was funded by the UK charity Bloodwise, Grants 04062 and 05037 (Kamel Ait-Tahar, Amanda P. Anderson, Alison H. Banham, and Karen Pulford). Graham P. Collins acknowledges support from the Blood Theme of the National Institute for Health Research Oxford Biomedical Research Centre.

References

[1] H. Stein, J. Chan, R. Warnke et al., "Diffuse large B-cell lymphoma, not otherwise specified, WHO Classification of tumours of haematopoietic and lymphoid tissues," in *International Agency for Research on Cancer*, pp. 233–237, Lyon, France, 2008.

[2] B. Coiffier, "Rituximab therapy in malignant lymphoma," *Oncogene*, vol. 26, no. 25, pp. 3603–3613, 2007.

[3] S. M. Ansell, A. M. Lesokhin, I. Borrello et al., "PD-1 blockade with nivolumab in relapsed or refractory Hodgkin's lymphoma," *The New England Journal of Medicine*, vol. 372, no. 4, pp. 311–319, 2015.

[4] A. L. Garfall, M. V. Maus, W.-T. Hwang et al., "Chimeric antigen receptor T cells against CD19 for multiple myeloma," *The New England Journal of Medicine*, vol. 373, no. 11, pp. 1040–1047, 2015.

[5] D. Atanackovic, J. Arfsten, Y. Cao et al., "Cancer-testis antigens are commonly expressed in multiple myeloma and induce systemic immunity following allogeneic stem cell transplantation," *Blood*, vol. 109, no. 3, pp. 1103–1112, 2007.

[6] D. L. Porter and J. H. Antin, "Donor leukocyte infusions in myeloid malignancies: new strategies," *Best Practice & Research Clinical Haematology*, vol. 19, no. 4, pp. 737–755, 2006.

[7] R. J. Inaoka, A. A. Jungbluth, S. Gnjatic et al., "Cancer/testis antigens expression and autologous serological response in a set of Brazilian non-Hodgkin's lymphoma patients," *Cancer Immunology, Immunotherapy*, vol. 61, no. 12, pp. 2207–2214, 2012.

[8] R. J. Inaoka, A. A. Jungbluth, O. C. G. Baiocchi et al., "An overview of cancer/testis antigens expression in classical Hodgkin's lymphoma (cHL) identifies MAGE-A family and MAGE-C1 as the most frequently expressed antigens in a set of Brazilian cHL patients," *BMC Cancer*, vol. 11, article no. 416, 2011.

[9] D. Atanackovic, T. Luetkens, B. Kloth et al., "Cancer-testis antigen expression and its epigenetic modulation in acute myeloid leukemia," *American Journal of Hematology*, vol. 86, no. 11, pp. 918–922, 2011.

[10] P. Srivastava, B. E. Paluch, J. Matsuzaki et al., "Immunomodulatory action of SGI-110, a hypomethylating agent, in acute myeloid leukemia cells and xenografts," *Leukemia Research*, vol. 38, no. 11, pp. 1332–1341, 2014.

[11] C. Pellat-Deceunynck, M.-P. Mellerin, N. Labarrière et al., "The cancer germ-line genes MAGE-1, MAGE-3 and PRAME are commonly expressed by human myeloma cells," *European Journal of Immunology*, vol. 30, no. 3, pp. 803–809, 2000.

[12] S. H. Lim, Z. Wang, M. Chiriva-Internati, and Y. Xue, "Sperm protein 17 is a novel cancer-testis antigen in multiple myeloma," *Blood*, vol. 97, no. 5, pp. 1508–1510, 2001.

[13] O. Goodyear, K. Piper, N. Khan et al., "CD8+T cells specific for cancer germline gene antigens are found in many patients with multiple myeloma, and their frequency correlates with disease burden," *Blood*, vol. 106, no. 13, pp. 4217–4224, 2005.

[14] F. De Carvalho, V. L. F. Alves, W. M. T. Braga, C. V. Xavier Jr., and G. W. B. Colleoni, "MAGE-C1/CT7 and MAGE-C2/CT10 are frequently expressed in multiple myeloma and can be explored in combined immunotherapy for this malignancy," *Cancer Immunology, Immunotherapy*, vol. 62, no. 1, pp. 191–195, 2013.

[15] B. J. Taylor, T. Reiman, J. A. Pittman et al., "SSX cancer testis antigens are expressed in most multiple myeloma patients: Co-expression of SSX1, 2, 4, and 5 correlates with adverse prognosis and high frequencies of SSX-positive PCs," *Journal of Immunotherapy*, vol. 28, no. 6, pp. 564–575, 2005.

[16] M. F. Gjerstorff, M. H. Andersen, and H. J. Ditzel, "Oncogenic cancer/testis antigens: prime candidates for immunotherapy," *Oncotarget*, vol. 6, no. 18, pp. 15772–15787, 2015.

[17] O. L. Caballero and Y.-T. Chen, "Cancer/testis (CT) antigens: Potential targets for immunotherapy," *Cancer Science*, vol. 100, no. 11, pp. 2014–2021, 2009.

[18] V. I. Seledtsov, A. G. Goncharov, and G. V. Seledtsova, "Clinically feasible approaches to potentiating cancer cell-based immunotherapies," *Human Vaccines & Immunotherapeutics*, vol. 11, no. 4, pp. 851–869, 2015.

[19] S. D. Xiang, Q. Gao, K. L. Wilson, A. Heyerick, and M. Plebanski, "Mapping T and B cell epitopes in sperm protein 17 to support the development of an ovarian cancer vaccine," *Vaccine*, vol. 33, no. 44, pp. 5950–5959, 2015.

[20] J.-X. Song, W.-L. Cao, F.-Q. Li, L.-N. Shi, and X. Jia, "Anti-Sp17 monoclonal antibody with antibody-dependent cell-mediated cytotoxicity and complement-dependent cytotoxicity activities against human ovarian cancer cells," *Medical Oncology*, vol. 29, no. 4, pp. 2923–2931, 2012.

[21] J. M. Straughn Jr., D. R. Shaw, A. Guerrero et al., "Expression of sperm protein 17 (Sp17) in ovarian cancer," *International Journal of Cancer*, vol. 108, no. 6, pp. 805–811, 2004.

[22] L. Mirandola, J. A. Figueroa, T. T. Phan et al., "Novel antigens in non-small cell lung cancer: SP17, AKAP4, and PTTG1 are potential immunotherapeutic targets," *Oncotarget*, vol. 6, no. 5, pp. 2812–2826, 2015.

[23] M. Chiriva-Internati, Z. Wang, E. Salati, D. Wroblewski, and S. H. Lim, "Successful generation of sperm protein 17 (Sp17)-specific cytotoxic T lymphocytes from normal donors: Implication for tumour-specific adoptive immunotherapy following allogeneic stem cell transplantation for Sp17-positive multiple myeloma," *Scandinavian Journal of Immunology*, vol. 56, no. 4, pp. 429–433, 2002.

[24] M. Chiriva-Internati, Z. Wang, S. Pochopien, E. Salati, and S. H. Lim, "Identification of a sperm protein 17 CTL epitope restricted by HLA-A1," *International Journal of Cancer*, vol. 107, no. 5, pp. 863–865, 2003.

[25] M. Chiriva-Internati, Z. Wang, Y. Xue, K. Bumm, A. B. Hahn, and S. H. Lim, "Sperm protein 17 (Sp17) in multiple myeloma: Opportunity for myeloma-specific donor T cell infusion to enhance graft-versus-myeloma effect without increasing graft-versus-host disease risk," *European Journal of Immunology*, vol. 31, no. 8, pp. 2277–2283, 2001.

[26] H. M. Lacy and R. D. Sanderson, "Sperm protein 17 is expressed on normal and malignant lymphocytes and promotes heparan sulfate-mediated cell-cell adhesion," *Blood*, vol. 98, no. 7, pp. 2160–2165, 2001.

[27] A. P. Liggins, S. H. Lim, E. J. Soilleux, K. Pulford, and A. H. Banham, "A panel of cancer-testis genes exhibiting broad-spectrum expression in haematological malignancies.," *Cancer immunity : a journal of the Academy of Cancer Immunology*, vol. 10, p. 8, 2010.

[28] F. Arnaboldi, A. Menon, E. Menegola et al., "Sperm Protein17 is an oncofetal antigen: A lesson from a murine model," *International Reviews of Immunology*, vol. 33, no. 5, pp. 367–374, 2014.

[29] K. Ait-Tahar, A. P. Liggins, G. P. Collins et al., "Cytolytic T-cell response to the PASD1 cancer testis antigen in patients with diffuse large B-cell lymphoma," *British Journal of Haematology*, vol. 146, no. 4, pp. 396–407, 2009.

[30] K. Ait-Tahar, A. P. Liggins, G. P. Collins et al., "CD4-positive T-helper cell responses to the PASD1 protein in patients with diffuse large B-cell lymphoma," *Haematologica*, vol. 96, no. 1, pp. 78–86, 2011.

[31] M. Bunce, C. M. O'Neill, M. C. N. M. Barnardo et al., "Phototyping: comprehensive DNA typing for HLA-A, B, C, DRB1, DRB3, DRB4, DRB5 & DQB1 by PCR with 144 primer mixes utilizing sequence-specific primers (PCR-SSP)," *Tissue Antigens*, vol. 46, no. 5, pp. 355–367, 1995.

[32] C. P. Hans, D. D. Weisenburger, T. C. Greiner et al., "Confirmation of the molecular classification of diffuse large B-cell lymphoma by immunohistochemistry using a tissue microarray," *Blood*, vol. 103, no. 1, pp. 275–282, 2004.

[33] K. Ait-Tahar, V. Cerundolo, A. H. Banham et al., "B and CTL responses to the ALK protein in patients with ALK-positive

ALCL," *International Journal of Cancer*, vol. 118, no. 3, pp. 688–695, 2006.

[34] F. Grizzi, L. Mirandola, D. Qehajaj, E. Cobos, J. A. Figueroa, and M. Chiriva-Internati, "Cancer-testis antigens and immunotherapy in the light of cancer complexity," *International Reviews of Immunology*, vol. 34, no. 2, pp. 143–153, 2015.

[35] S. Huang, K.-D. Preuss, X. Xie, E. Regitz, and M. Pfreundschuh, "Analysis of the antibody repertoire of lymphoma patients," *Cancer Immunology, Immunotherapy*, vol. 51, no. 11-12, pp. 655–662, 2002.

[36] X. Xie, H. H. Wacker, S. Huang et al., "Differential expression of cancer testis genes in histological subtypes of non-Hodgkin's lymphomas," *Clinical Cancer Research*, vol. 9, no. 1, pp. 167–173, 2003.

[37] M. Chiriva-Internati, J. A. Weidanz, Y. Yu et al., "Sperm protein 17 is a suitable target for adoptive T-cell-based immunotherapy in human ovarian cancer," *Journal of Immunotherapy*, vol. 31, no. 8, pp. 693–703, 2008.

[38] M. Chiriva-Internati, Y. Yu, L. Mirandola et al., "Cancer testis antigen vaccination affords long-term protection in a murine model of ovarian cancer," *PLoS ONE*, vol. 5, no. 5, Article ID e10471, 2010.

[39] S. D. Xiang, Q. Gao, K. L. Wilson, A. Heyerick, and M. Plebanski, "A nanoparticle based Sp17 peptide vaccine exposes new immuno-dominant and species cross-reactive B cell epitopes," *Vaccines*, vol. 3, no. 4, pp. 875–893, 2015.

[40] F. Van Rhee, S. M. Szmania, F. Zhan et al., "NY-ESO-1 is highly expressed in poor-prognosis multiple myeloma and induces spontaneous humoral and cellular immune responses," *Blood*, vol. 105, no. 10, pp. 3939–3944, 2005.

[41] M. Inokuma, C. Dela Rosa, C. Schmitt et al., "Functional T cell responses to tumor antigens in breast cancer patients have a distinct phenotype and cytokine signature," *The Journal of Immunology*, vol. 179, no. 4, pp. 2627–2633, 2007.

[42] L. Passoni, A. Scardino, C. Bertazzoli et al., "ALK as a novel lymphoma-associated tumor antigen: Identification of 2 HLA-A2.1-restricted CD8+ T-cell epitopes," *Blood*, vol. 99, no. 6, pp. 2100–2106, 2002.

[43] P. Baumgaertner, N. Rufer, E. Devevre et al., "Ex vivo detectable human CD8 T-cell responses to cancer-testis antigens," *Cancer Research*, vol. 66, no. 4, pp. 1912–1916, 2006.

[44] N. M. Provine, R. A. Larocca, M. Aid et al., "Immediate dysfunction of vaccine-elicited CD8+ T cells primed in the absence of CD4+ T cells," *The Journal of Immunology*, vol. 197, no. 5, pp. 1809–1822, 2016.

[45] S. Ostrand-Rosenberg, "CD4+ T lymphocytes: A critical component of antitumor immunity," *Cancer Investigation*, vol. 23, no. 5, pp. 413–419, 2005.

[46] G. Zeng, "MHC class II-restricted tumor antigens recognized by CD4+ T cells: New strategies for cancer vaccine design," *Journal of Immunotherapy*, vol. 24, no. 3, pp. 195–204, 2001.

[47] D. Atanackovic, I. Blum, Y. Cao et al., "Expression of cancer-testis antigens as possible targets for antigen-specific immunotherapy in head and neck squamous cell carcinoma," *Cancer Biology & Therapy*, vol. 5, no. 9, pp. 1218–1225, 2006.

[48] M. Condomines, D. Hose, P. Raynaud et al., "Cancer/testis genes in multiple myeloma: Expression patterns and prognosis value determined by microarray analysis," *The Journal of Immunology*, vol. 178, no. 5, pp. 3307–3315, 2007.

[49] M. V. Dhodapkar, K. Osman, J. Teruya-Feldstein et al., "Expression of cancer/testis (CT) antigens MAGE-A1, MAGE-A3, MAGE-A4, CT-7, and NY-ESO-1 in malignant gammopathies is heterogeneous and correlates with site, stage and risk status of disease." *Cancer immunity : a journal of the Academy of Cancer Immunology*, vol. 3, p. 9, 2003.

10

Prevalence and Factors Associated with Anemia among Pregnant Women Attending Antenatal Clinic at St. Paul's Hospital Millennium Medical College, Addis Ababa, Ethiopia

Angesom Gebreweld ⬥[1] **and Aster Tsegaye**[2]

[1]*Department of Medical Laboratory Sciences, College of Medicine and Health Science, Wollo University, Dessie, Ethiopia*
[2]*Department of Medical Laboratory Sciences, College of Health Science, Addis Ababa University, Ethiopia*

Correspondence should be addressed to Angesom Gebreweld; afsaha@gmail.com

Academic Editor: Elvira Grandone

Background. In pregnancy, anemia is an important factor associated with an increased risk of maternal, fetal, and neonatal mortality, poor pregnancy outcomes, and impaired cognitive development, particularly in developing countries like Ethiopia. This study aimed to assess prevalence and factors associated with anemia among pregnant women attending antenatal clinic at St. Paul's Hospital Millennium Medical College, Addis Ababa, Ethiopia. *Method.* A cross-sectional health facility based study was conducted on 284 pregnant women to assess prevalence and factors associated with anemia at St. Paul's Hospital Millennium Medical College from June to August 2014. Data on sociodemographic and clinical characteristics of the study participants were collected using a pretested structured questionnaire by interview and review of medical records. About 4 ml of venous blood was collected from each subject for peripheral blood film and complete blood counts (CBC). Binary Logistic regression analysis had been used to check for association between dependent and independent variables. In all cases, P value less than 0.05 was considered statistically significant. *Result.* The prevalence of anemia was found to be 11.6% (95 % CI; 7.8%-14.8%). Pregnant women in the second [AOR (95% CI), 6.72 (1.17-38.45), and P=0.03] and third trimester [AOR (95% CI), 8.31 (1.24-55.45), and P=0.029] were more likely to be anemic when compared to pregnant women in their first trimester. Pregnant women who did not receive iron/folic acid supplementation [AOR (95%CI), 4.03(1.49-10.92), and P=0.01] were more likely to be anemic when compared to pregnant women who did take supplementations. *Conclusion.* In this study the prevalence of anemia in pregnancy was low compared to the findings of others. Gestational age (trimester) and iron/folic acid supplementation were statistically associated with anemia. Therefore, iron supplementation and health education to create awareness about the importance of early booking for antenatal care are recommended to reduce anemia.

1. Background

Anemia is a decrease in the oxygen carrying capacity of the blood. It can arise if the hemoglobin (Hb) concentration of the red blood cells (RBCs) or the packed cell volume of RBCs (PCV) is below the lower limit of the reference interval for the individual's age, gender, geographical location, and physiological status [1, 2].

During pregnancy the total blood volume increases by about 1.5 liter [3]. The plasma volume increases more compared to red cell mass which leading to hemodilution and reduced hemoglobin concentration. This is termed physiological anemia of pregnancy [3, 4]. The World Health Organization (WHO) has suggested that anemia is present in pregnancy when Hb level is <11g/dl. It also classified anemia in pregnancy as mild (10.0-10.9 g/dl), moderate (7.0-9.9 g/dl), and severe (lower than 7.0 g/dl) based on the level of hemoglobin concentration [5].

Anemia is a public health problem in both developed and developing countries. It affects 1.62 billion people globally, which corresponds to 24.8% of the world population. Global prevalence of anemia in pregnant women is 41.8% and the highest proportions of pregnant women affected are in Africa (57.1%) [6, 7]. According to Ethiopia Demographic and Health Survey report of 2005, the prevalence of anemia in pregnant women is 30.6% [8].

Approximately 50% of cases of anemia are considered to be due to iron deficiency. Anemia resulting from iron deficiency in pregnancy is an important factor associated with an increased risk of maternal, fetal, and neonatal mortality; poor pregnancy outcomes such as low birth weight and preterm birth; impaired cognitive development, reduced learning capacity, and diminished school performance in children; and decreased productivity in adults, particularly in developing countries like Ethiopia. In neighboring Sudan, 20.3% of maternal deaths are associated with anemia [9–11].

In Ethiopia, different studies were conducted on prevalence of anemia among pregnant women, the prevalence range being from 9.7% in North Shoa Zone to 56.8% in Eastern Ethiopia [12, 13]. Studying the specific etiology and prevalence of anemia in a given setting and population group is very important to prevent or treat anemia [11]. However, there is very little data available in the study area. Therefore, this study is aimed to assess the prevalence and factors associated with anemia in pregnant women at St. Paul's Hospital Millennium Medical College, Addis Ababa, Ethiopia.

2. Methods

2.1. Study Setting and Design. A facility based cross-sectional study was conducted from June to August 2014 at St. Paul's Hospital Millennium Medical College (SPHMMC), Addis Ababa, Ethiopia. SPHMMC was built in 1969 by Emperor Haile Selassie as a source of medical care for underserved populations. It currently has 392 beds, with an annual average of 200,000 patients and a catchment population of more than 5 million.

2.2. Study Population. All pregnant women attending antenatal cares in SPHMMC that fulfills the inclusion criteria during the study period were considered as study participants. Written informed consent was obtained from all. Pregnant women with Hepatitis B Virus infection, with human immunodeficiency virus, and less than 18 years of age were excluded from the study.

2.3. Sampling Procedure. The required sample size for this study was calculated using a single population proportion formula with a 95% CI, 5% margin of error, and assumption that 21.3 % of pregnant women are anemic [14]. By adding 10% for nonresponse, a total of 284 pregnant women were enrolled from antenatal care clinic of obstetrics and gynecology department of SPHMMC. Systematic random sampling technique was used to recruit the study participants from their sequence of ANC visit during the study period.

2.4. Data Collection. Interviewer administered structured pretested questionnaire and review of medical records were used to collect data on the sociodemographic characteristics, obstetric and gynecological, diet, and clinical characteristics of the study participants. The interview and record review

were conducted by two trained ANC service provider nurses at ANC clinic of SPHMMC during ANC follow-up of the study participants. About 4 ml venous blood specimens were taken from each participant in K3-EDTA tubes for the hematological examinations. Automated hematology analyzer Cell-Dyn 1800 (Abbott Laboratories Diagnostics Division, USA) was used to determine complete blood count. Thin peripheral blood smears were prepared and stained by Wright's stain for red cells morphological study. Quality control materials were run alongside the study participant's sample to control performance of the hematological analyzer. All laboratory measurements were done by experienced laboratory technologists.

2.5. Data Analysis. Data from both questioner and laboratory were checked and cleaned for completeness and consistency. Data were then analyzed using Statistical Package for the Social Science (SPSS) Version 20 statistical software. Descriptive statistics such as frequency, percentage, and mean andstandard deviation were used to describe dependent and independent variables. Binary logistic regression analysis had been used to check for association between dependent and independent variables. In all cases P value less than 0.05 was considered statistically significant.

2.6. Ethical Considerations. Ethical clearance was obtained from both Research and Ethics Review Committee of the Department of Medical Laboratory Sciences, Addis Ababa University, and Institutional Review Board of SPHMMC. Written informed consent was obtained from each study participant after the purpose and importance of the study were explained. To ensure confidentiality, participants' data were linked to a code number. Any abnormal test results of participants were communicated to their attending physician.

3. Result

3.1. Characteristics of the Study Participants. A total of 284 pregnant women were included in the study. The mean age of the participants was 27.3 ± 4.5 years (range from 18-40). The majority of the study groups, 118 (41.5%), were in the age range of 26-30 years and 102 (35.9%) were in the weight group of 60-69 Kg. Most of the respondents, 261(91.9%), 164 (57.7%), and 115 (40.5%), were urban dwellers, house wives by occupation, and elementary school education level, respectively (Table 1).

Concerning obstetrical history and dietary habit, 170 (59.9%) were in their third trimester, 194 (68.3%) of the women had previous pregnancy, 166 (58.5%) were multigravida (2-4 pregnancy), 124 (43.7%) had no child, 28 (9.9%) had blood loss during the current pregnancy, 77 (27.1%) experienced abortion, and 166 (58.8%) had taken iron/folic acid supplementation. Out of the 284 participants, 160 (56.3%) had the habit of eating meat and animal products and 120 (42.3%) had the habit of eating fruit and vegetables once in week (Table 1).

3.2. Prevalence and Associated Risk Factors of Anemia. The mean $\pm$ SD hemoglobin concentration of the study

TABLE 1: Sociodemographic, obstetric, and other characteristics of pregnant women (N=284).

Variables	Frequency	Percentage (%)
Age group (years)		
≤20	16	5.6
21-25	93	32.7
26-30	118	41.5
31-35	43	15.1
≥36	14	4.9
weight group (kg)		
40-49	28	9.9
50-59	89	31.3
60-69	102	35.9
70-79	40	14.1
≥80	25	8.8
Occupation		
Farmer	16	5.6
Housewife	164	57.7
Government	24	8.5
Student	8	2.8
Private	72	25.4
Educational status		
Illiterate	42	14.8
Elementary	115	40.5
Secondary	54	19.0
Preparatory	23	8.1
University/college	50	17.6
Residence		
Rural	23	8.1
Urban	261	91.9
Trimester		
1st trimester	48	16.9
2nd trimester	66	23.2
3rd trimester	170	59.9
Previous Pregnancy		
No	90	31.7
Yes	194	68.3
Gravidity		
1	90	31.7
2-4	166	58.5
≥5	28	9.9
Number of child		
None	124	43.7
1	85	29.9
2	51	18.0
≥3	24	8.5
Space b/n the current pregnancy and the last child		
<1 year	122	43.0
1 year	12	4.2
2 year	21	7.4
3 year	33	11.6
4 year and above	96	33.8
Blood loss		
No	256	90.1
Yes	28	9.9

Table 1: Continued.

Variables	Frequency	Percentage (%)
Abortion		
No	207	72.9
Yes	77	27.1
Number of abortion		
None	207	72.9
Once	56	19.7
Two and above	21	7.4
Iron/folic acid Supplementation		
No	117	41.2
Yes	167	58.8
Meat and animal product		
No	12	4.2
Yes	272	95.8
Frequency of eating meat and animal product		
None	12	4.2
every day	37	13.0
every 2 days	22	7.7
once in week	160	56.3
once in month	53	18.7
Fruit and Vegetable		
No	3	1.1
Yes	281	98.9
Frequency of eating fruit and vegetable		
None	3	1.1
every day	100	35.2
every 2 days	58	20.4
once in week	120	42.3
once in month	3	1.1

participants was 13.0 ± 1.64 g/dl (ranges from 7.1-22.9 g/dl). In this study, the overall prevalence of anemia was 11.6% (95 % CI; 7.8%-14.8%) [15].

The rate of anemia was high in pregnant women who were in 26-30-year age range (15.3%), 60-69 weight group (17.6%), house wives (14.0%), elementary school (14.8%), and urban residents (12.6%) (Table 2).

Based on obstetric history and dietary habit, the prevalence of anemia was higher in pregnant women who were at the second trimester (16.7%), had previous history of pregnancy (12.4%), multigravida (12.7%), had one child (17.6%), had ≥ 4-year gap between the current and last child (16.7%), had history of abortion (14.3%), and did not take iron/folic acid supplementation (14.5%). The prevalence of anemia was also higher in those pregnant women who did not have a habit of eating meat and animal products (16.7%) and fruits and vegetables (33.3%) (Table 2).

All variables were analyzed using bivariate analysis to assess the association between the variables and anemia. Then, variables that show P value less than or equal to 0.3 in bivariate analysis were taken to multivariate analysis. Out of those variables treated under multivariate analysis,

trimester and iron/folic acid supplementations were statistically significantly associated with anemia. Pregnant women in the second [AOR (95% CI), 6.72 (1.17-38.45), and P=0.03] and third trimester [AOR (95% CI), 8.31 (1.24-55.45), and P=0.029] were more likely to be anemic when compared to pregnant women in their first trimester. Pregnant women who did not receive iron/folic acid supplementation [AOR (95%CI), 4.03(1.49-10.92), and P=0.01] were more likely to be anemic when compared to pregnant women who did take supplementations.

4. Discussion

The prevalence of anemia in the present study was 11.6% (95 % CI; 7.8%-14.8%) [15]. This prevalence was almost consistent with studies conducted in Awassa (15.1%), Gondar (16.6%), Debre Berhan (9.7%), Sudan (10%), Iran (13.6%), and Nakhon Sawan, Thailand (14.1%) [12, 16–20]. However, our finding is much lower than studies conducted in Pakistan (90.5%), India (87.2%), Malaysia (57.4%), Benin (68.3%), Nigeria (54.5%), Somali Region (56.8%), Walayita Sodo (40%), West Arsi zone (36.6%), and north western zone of Tigray (36.1%)

TABLE 2: Prevalence of anemia among pregnant women by sociodemographic, obstetric, and other characteristics of pregnant women (N=284).

Variables	Anemia status		AOR (95% CI)	P value
	Non-Anemic (%)	Anemic (%)		
Age group				
≤20	15 (93.8%)	1 (6.2%)	1	
21-25	86 (92.5%)	7 (7.5%)	1.53 (.16-14.70)	0.71
26-30	100 (84.7%)	18 (15.3%)	4.47 (.47-42.83)	0.19
31-35	37 (86.0%)	6 (14.0%)	5.58 (.457-68.10)	0.18
≥36	13 (92.9%)	1 (7.1%)	3.55 (.13-100.17)	0.46
weight group				
40-49	27 (96.4%)	1 (3.6%)	1	
50-59	81 (91.0%)	8 (9.0%)	2.34 (.25-21.85)	0.45
60-69	84 (82.4%)	18 (17.6%)	5.14 (.57-46.17)	0.14
70-79	36 (90.0%)	4 (10.0%)	1.38 (.12-16.30)	0.80
≥80	23 (92.0%)	2 (8.0%)	1.47 (.101-21.47)	0.78
Occupation				
Farmer	16 (100.0%)	0 (.0%)		
Housewife	141 (86.0%)	23 (14.0%)		
Government	22 (91.7%)	2 (8.3%)		
Student	7 (87.5%)	1 (12.5%)		
Private	65 (90.3%)	7 (9.7%)		
Educational status				
Not educated	40 (95.2%)	2(4.8%)		
Elementary	98(85.2%)	17 (14.8%)		
Secondary	48(88.9%)	6(11.1%)		
Preparatory	21 (91.3%)	2(8.7%)		
University/college	44 (88.0%)	6 (12.0%)		
Residence				
Rural	23 (100.0%)	0 (.0%)		
Urban	228 (87.4%)	33 (12.6%)		
Trimester				
1st trimester	46 (95.8%)	2(4.2%)	1	
2nd trimester	55(83.3%)	11(16.7%)	6.72 (1.17-38.45)	0.03**
3rd trimester	150 (88.2%)	20(11.8%)	8.31 (1.24-55.45)	0.03**
Previous Pregnancy				
No	81 (90.0%)	9 (10.0%)		
Yes	170(87.6%)	24(12.4%)		
Gravidity				
1	81 (90.0%)	9 (10.0%)		
2-4	145 (87.3%)	21 (12.7%)		
≥5	25 (89.3%)	3 (10.7%)		
Number of child				
None	112 (90.3%)	12 (9.7%)	1	
1	70 (82.4%)	15 (17.6%)	2.49 (.000)	0.99
2	47 (92.2%)	4 (7.8%)	6.81 (.000)	0.99
≥3	22 (91.7%)	2 (8.3%)	6.99 (.000)	0.99
Space b/n the current pregnancy and the last child				
0 year	110(90.2%)	12(9.8%)	1	
1 year	11(91.7%)	1(8.3%)	.00(.00)	0.99
2 year	20(95.2%)	1 (4.8%)	.00(.00)	0.99
3 year	30(90.9%)	3(9.1%)	.00(.00)	0.99
4 year and above	80 (83.3%)	16 (16.7%)	.00(.00)	0.99

TABLE 2: Continued.

Variables	Anemia status		AOR (95% CI)	P value
	Non-Anemic (%)	Anemic (%)		
Blood loss				
No	224(87.5%)	32(12.5%)	1	
Yes	27 (96.4%)	1(3.6%)	.29 (.03-2.52)	0.26
Abortion				
No	185(89.4%)	22 (10.6%)	1	
Yes	66 (85.7%)	11(14.3%)	2.06 (.82-5.15)	0.12
Number of abortion				
None	185 (89.4%)	22 (10.6%)		
Once	48 (85.7%)	8 (14.3%)		
Two and above	18 (85.7%)	3 (14.3%)		
Iron/folic acid Supplementation				
No	100 (85.5%)	17(14.5%)	4.03(1.49-10.92)	0.01**
Yes	151 (90.4%)	16 (9.6%)	1	
Meat and Animal Product				
No	11(84.6%)	2(15.4%)		
Yes	240 (88.6%)	31(11.4%)		
Frequency of eating meat and animal product				
every day	33 (89.2%)	4(10.8%)		
every 2 day	19(86.4%)	3(13.6%)		
once in week	139 (86.9%)	21 (13.1%)		
once in month	50 (94.3%)	3 (5.7%)		
none	10 (83.3%)	2 (16.7%)		
Fruit and Vegetable				
No	2 (66.7%)	1 (33.3%)		
Yes	249 (88.6%)	32 (11.4%)		
Frequency of eating fruit and vegetable				
every day	89 (89.0%)	11 (11.0%)		
every 2 day	51 (87.9%)	7 (12.1%)		
once in week	106 (88.3%)	14 (11.7%)		
once in month	3(100.0%)	0 (.0%)		
none	2 (66.7%)	1 (33.3%)		

**P < 0.05 (statistically significant association) for the Adjusted Odds Ratio (AOR).

[13, 21–28]. Our result is also lower than results reported from Uganda (22.1%), Southern Ethiopia (29%), Southeast Ethiopia (27.9%) Mekelle (19.7%), and Addis Ababa (21.3%) [14, 29–32].

The difference may be due to geographical variation, differences in socioeconomic status, and dietary habits of the study participants. The lower finding of our study also may be due to the governments' effort to achieve Millennium Development Goals (MDGs) since improving maternal health is one of the eight MDGs and targeted to reduce the maternal mortality ratio by three-quarters in 2015. The United Nations Population Fund (UNFPA) report showed a significant decline in the prevalence of anemia among all women from 20% to 13% between 2005 and 2011 in Ethiopia [33].

Only the association of gestational age (trimester) and iron/folic acid supplementations did reach to a statistically significance level. Pregnant women in second and third trimester were more likely to be anemic when compared to pregnant women in first trimester. This might be due to the higher maternal plasma volume increments (40–50%) relative to red cell mass (20–30%) and accounts for the fall in hemoglobin concentration [34]. Our study is similar with studies conducted in Malaysia [22], west Algeria [35], and Tikur Anbessa hospital [14].

The risk of developing anemia increased in pregnant women who did not receive iron supplementation during pregnancy when compared to those who received iron supplementation. This may be due to iron deficiencies developing during pregnancy because of the increased iron requirements to supply the expanding blood volume of the mother and the rapidly growing fetus and placenta. The study is in agreement with study conducted in Karnataka India, Uganda, and Eastern Ethiopia [13, 36, 37].

One of the limitation of this study is the cross-sectional nature of the study design; it did not reveal causal links between anemia and risk factors. Even though this study tried to address some important factors, other factors such as stool examination, malaria, inherited, or acquired disorders that affect hemoglobin or red blood cell synthesis were not addressed due to constraint of time and resource. The other limitation is that this study is done only at single hospital; hence, further studies should be conducted in different hospitals of Addis Ababa to have findings representing the whole population.

5. Conclusion

This study has revealed that the prevalence of anemia in pregnancy was low (11.62%) compared to the findings of other areas of Ethiopia. Gestational age (trimester) and iron/folic acid supplementation were statistically associated with anemia in this study. Therefore, iron supplementation and health education to create awareness about the importance of early booking for antenatal care are recommended to reduce anemia.

List of Abbreviations

ANC: Antenatal care
EDTA: Ethylenediaminetetraacetic acid
Hb: Hemoglobin
MDGs: Millennium Development Goals
RBC: Red blood cell
SPHMMC: St.Paul'sHospital MillenniumMedicalCollege
WHO: World Health Organization.

Disclosure

The funder has no role in the design of the study and collection, analysis, and interpretation of data and in writing the manuscript.

Conflicts of Interest

The authors declare no conflicts of interest.

Authors' Contributions

All authors participated in the study design, interpretation of the data, and writing of the paper and all authors have seen and approved the final version of the paper.

Acknowledgments

We would like to thank Wollo University and Addis Ababa University for their financial and material support for this project. St. Paul's Hospital Millennium College is gratefully acknowledged for the support given to undertake this study in the hospital. Our special thanks and appreciation go to all pregnant women who voluntarily participated in this study. This study was funded by Addis Ababa University.

References

[1] M. L. Turgeon, *Clinical Hematology: Theory and Procedures*, Wilkins, a Wolters Kluwer business, Philadelphia, Lippincott Williams, 5th edition, 2012.

[2] B. F. Rodak, G. A. Fritsma, and E. M. Keohane, *Hematology: Clinical Principles and Applications*, Elsevier Saunders, 4th edition, 2012.

[3] S. Chandra, A. K. Tripathi, S. Mishra, M. Amzarul, and A. K. Vaish, "Physiological changes in hematological parameters during pregnancy," *Indian Journal of Hematology and Blood Transfusion*, vol. 28, no. 3, pp. 144–146, 2012.

[4] S. Pavord and B. Hunt, *The Obstetric Hematology Manual*, Cambridge University Press, New York, NY, USA, 2018.

[5] WHO. Haemoglobin concentrations for the diagnosis of anaemia and assessment of severity. Vitamin and Mineral Nutrition Information System: Geneva, World Health Organization;2011. http://www.who.int/vmnis/indicators/haemoglobin.pdf.

[6] B. d. Benoist, E. McLean, I. Egll, and M. Cogswell, *Worldwide Prevalence of Anaemia 1993-2005: WHO Global Database on Anaemia*, World Health Organization, 2008.

[7] E. McLean, M. Cogswell, I. Egli, D. Wojdyla, and B. De Benoist, "Worldwide prevalence of anaemia, WHO Vitamin and Mineral Nutrition Information System, 1993–2005," *Public Health Nutrition*, vol. 12, no. 4, pp. 444–454, 2009.

[8] Central Statistical Agency, ORC Macro. Ethiopia demographic and health survey 2005. Addis Ababa, Ethiopia and Calverton, Maryland, USA: Cent Stat Agency ORC Macro. 2006.

[9] L. H. Allen, "Anemia and iron deficiency: effects on pregnancy outcome," *American Journal of Clinical Nutrition*, vol. 71, no. 5, pp. 1280s–1284s, 2000.

[10] A. A. Mohammed, M. H. Elnour, E. E. Mohammed, S. A. Ahmed, and A. I. Abdelfattah, "Maternal mortality in Kassala State - Eastern Sudan: Community-based study using Reproductive age mortality survey (RAMOS)," *BMC Pregnancy and Childbirth*, vol. 11, no. 1, pp. 102–107, 2011.

[11] WHO., WHO. The global prevalence of anaemia in 2011. World Health Organization Geneva; 2015.

[12] F. A. Yohannes Abere, "Pregnancy Anaemia Prevalence and Associated Factors among Women Attending Ante Natal Care in North Shoa Zone, Ethiopia," *Reproductive System & Sexual Disorders*, vol. 03, no. 03, 2014.

[13] K. A. Alene and A. Mohamed Dohe, "Prevalence of Anemia and Associated Factors among Pregnant Women in an Urban Area of Eastern Ethiopia," *Anemia*, vol. 2014, pp. 1–7, 2014.

[14] A. H. Jufar and T. Zewde, "Prevalence of anemia among pregnant women attending antenatal care at Tikur Anbessa Specialized Hospital," *Journal of Hematology Thromboembolic Diseases*, vol. 2, no. 1, pp. 1–6, 2014.

[15] A. Gebreweld, D. Bekele, and A. Tsegaye, "Hematological profile of pregnant women at St. Paul's Hospital Millennium Medical College, Addis Ababa, Ethiopia," *BMC Hematology*, vol. 18, no. 1, pp. 15–21, 2018.

[16] S. Gies, B. J. Brabin, M. A. Yassin, and L. E. Cuevas, "Comparison of screening methods for anaemia in pregnant women

in Awassa, Ethiopia," *Tropical Medicine & International Health*, vol. 8, no. 4, pp. 301–309, 2003.

[17] M. Melku, Z. Addis, M. Alem, and B. Enawgaw, "Prevalence and predictors of maternal anemia during pregnancy in Gondar, Northwest Ethiopia: an institutional based cross-sectional study," *Anemia*, vol. 2014, Article ID 108593, 9 pages, 2014.

[18] E. A. Abdelgader, TA. Diab, A. A. Kordofani, and S. E. Abdalla, "Hemoglobin level, RBCs Indices, and iron status in pregnant females in Sudan," *Basic Res J Med Clin Sci*, vol. 3, no. 2, pp. 8–13, 2014.

[19] E. Barooti, M. Rezazadehkermani, B. Sadeghirad, S. Motaghipisheh, S. Tayeri, and M. Arabi, "Prevalence of iron deficiency anemia among Iranian pregnant women; a systematic review and meta-analysis," *Journal of Reproduction & Infertility*, vol. 11, no. 1, pp. 17–24, 2010.

[20] B. Sukrat, P. Suwathanapisate, S. Siritawee, T. Poungthong, and K. Phupongpankul, "The prevalence of iron deficiency Anemia in pregnant women in Nakhonsawan, Thailand," *Journal of the Medical Association of Thailand*, vol. 93, no. 7, pp. 765–770, 2010.

[21] P. Lokare, P. Gattani, V. Karanjekar, and A. Kulkarni, "A study of prevalence of anemia and sociodemographic factors associated with anemia among pregnant women in Aurangabad city, India," *Annals of Nigerian Medicine*, vol. 6, no. 1, p. 30, 2012.

[22] R. N. Nik, N. S . Mohd, and Ismail I. M., "The Rate and Risk Factors for Anemia among Pregnant Mothers in Jerteh Terengganu, Malaysia," *Journal of Community Medicine & Health Education*, vol. 2, no. 150, pp. 2161-0711, 2012.

[23] N. Baig-Ansari, S. H. Badruddin, R. Karmaliani et al., "Anemia prevalence and risk factors in pregnant women in an urban area of Pakistan," *Food and Nutrition Bulletin*, vol. 29, no. 2, pp. 132–139, 2008.

[24] S. Ouédraogo, G. K. Koura, M. M. K. Accrombessi, F. Bodeau-Livinec, A. Massougbodji, and M. Cot, "Maternal anemia at first antenatal visit: Prevalence and risk factors in a malaria-endemic area in Benin," *The American Journal of Tropical Medicine and Hygiene*, vol. 87, no. 3, pp. 418–424, 2012.

[25] O. A. Olatunbosun, A. M. Abasiattai, E. A. Bassey, R. S. James, G. Ibanga, and A. Morgan, "Prevalence of anaemia among pregnant women at booking in the University of Uyo teaching hospital, Uyo, Nigeria," *BioMed Research International*, vol. 2014, Article ID 849080, 8 pages, 2014.

[26] L. Gedefaw, A. Ayele, Y. Asres, and A. Mossie, "Anemia and Associated Factors Among Pregnant Women Attending Antenatal Care Clinic in Wolayita Sodo Town, Southern Ethiopia," *Ethiopian Journal of Health Sciences*, vol. 25, no. 2, pp. 155–162, 2015.

[27] N. Obse, A. Mossie, and T. Gobena, "Magnitude of anemia and associated risk factors among pregnant women attending antenatal care in Shalla Woreda, West Arsi Zone, Oromia Region, Ethiopia," *Ethiopian Journal of Health Sciences*, vol. 23, no. 2, pp. 165–173, 2013.

[28] A. Gebre and A. Mulugeta, "Prevalence of anemia and associated factors among pregnant women in north western zone of tigray, northern ethiopia: A cross-sectional study," *Journal of Nutrition and Metabolism*, vol. 2015, Article ID 165430, 2015.

[29] G. Obai, P. Odongo, and R. Wanyama, "Prevalence of anaemia and associated risk factors among pregnant women attending antenatal care in Gulu and Hoima Regional Hospitals in Uganda: A cross sectional study," *BMC Pregnancy and Childbirth*, vol. 16, no. 1, 2016.

[30] R. S. Gibson, Y. Abebe, S. Stabler et al., "Zinc, gravida, infection, and iron, but not vitamin B-12 or folate status, predict hemoglobin during pregnancy in Southern Ethiopia," *Journal of Nutrition*, vol. 138, no. 3, pp. 581–586, 2008.

[31] F. Kefiyalew, E. Zemene, Y. Asres, and L. Gedefaw, "Anemia among pregnant women in Southeast Ethiopia: prevalence, severity and associated risk factors," *BMC Research Notes*, vol. 7, no. 1, pp. 771–778, 2014.

[32] A. Abriha, M. E. Yesuf, and M. M. Wassie, "Prevalence and associated factors of anemia among pregnant women of Mekelle town: A cross sectional study," *BMC Research Notes*, vol. 7, no. 1, 2014.

[33] Y. Mekonnen, *Trends in Maternal Health in Ethiopia; Challenges in achieving the Millennium Development Goal for maternal mortality In-depth Analysis of the Ethiopian Demographic and Health Surveys*, UNFPA, 2000.

[34] D. M. Townsley, "Hematologic complications of pregnancy," *Seminars in Hematology*, vol. 50, no. 3, pp. 222–231, 2013.

[35] A. Demmouche, S. Khelil, and S. Moulessehoul, "Anemia among pregnant women in the Sidi Bel Abbes Region (West Alegria): an epidemiologic study," *Journal of Blood Disorders & Transfusion*, vol. 2, no. 3, pp. 1–6, 2011.

[36] R. Viveki, A. Halappanavar, P. Viveki, S. Halki, V. Maled, and P. Deshpande, "Prevalence of anaemia and its epidemiological determinants in pregnant women," *Al Ameen J Med Sci*, vol. 5, no. 3, pp. 216–223, 2012.

[37] M. A. Mbule, Y. B. Byaruhanga, M. Kabahenda, and A. Lubowa, "Determinants of anaemia among pregnant women in rural Uganda.," *Rural and Remote Health*, vol. 13, no. 2, p. 2259, 2013.

11

Prevalence of Bleeding Symptoms among Adolescents and Young Adults in the Capital City of Saudi Arabia

Tarek Owaidah ⓘ,[1,2] Mahasen Saleh,[3] Hazzah Alzahrani,[4] Mahmood Abu-Riash,[4]
Ali Al Zahrani,[5] Mohammed Almadani,[6] Ayman Alsulaiman,[5] Abdulmajeed Albanyan,[2]
Khawar Siddiqui,[5] Khalid Al Saleh ⓘ,[2] and Abdulkareem Al Momen ⓘ[2]

[1]Department of Pathology and Laboratory Medicine, King Faisal Specialist Hospital and Research Centre, Riyadh, Saudi Arabia
[2]Center of Excellence in Thrombosis and Hemostasis, King Saud University, Riyadh, Saudi Arabia
[3]Pediatric Hematology, King Faisal Specialist Hospital and Research Centre, Riyadh, Saudi Arabia
[4]Oncology Center, King Faisal Specialist Hospital and Research Centre, Riyadh, Saudi Arabia
[5]Research Center, King Faisal Specialist Hospital and Research Centre, Riyadh, Saudi Arabia
[6]Ministry of Education, Riyadh, Saudi Arabia

Correspondence should be addressed to Tarek Owaidah; towaidah@kfshrc.edu.sa

Academic Editor: Elvira Grandone

Background. Bleeding disorders vary in prevalence. While some are rare, some can be common in both sexes. Most bleeding disorders manifest as chronic bleeding tendencies or as an increase in bleeding during surgical procedures or trauma. The consequences of bleeding can be as simple as iron deficiency or catastrophic, resulting in severe morbidity and mortality. Bleeding disorders typically affect both sexes except hemophilia A and B, which mainly affects males. *Method.* We conducted a questionnaire-based survey among adolescents and young adults (1901 [49%] boys, 1980 [51%] girls) in Riyadh city regarding bleeding symptoms. Of these, 1849 (47.6%) responded "Yes/Positive" for at least one question about the bleeding symptoms. *Results.* The most common bleeding symptom was epistaxis (19.7% of the sample population) detected in Phase I of the study. A tandem survey was conducted among 525 adolescents who had responded "Yes/Positive" to any one of the questions inquiring about bleeding symptoms. *Conclusion.* In this study, we report for the first time the prevalence of bleeding symptoms in a representative sample of Saudi adolescents and young adults.

1. Introduction

Bleeding disorders are a group of inherited disorders with different prevalence rates depending on many ethnicities. The most known inherited bleeding disorders are hemophilia A and B, which are relatively rare. Hemophilia A affects 1 : 5000–10,000 males, while hemophilia B affects 1 : 50,000–100,000 males. Hemophilia A and B can be very serious and life-threatening for individuals as well as a costly disease for families and countries [1]. von Willebrand disease (VWD) is another bleeding disorder, which is an inherited disorder that is caused by deficiency or dysfunction of VWF. VWD is a relatively common cause of bleeding, but the prevalence varies considerably among studies and depends strongly on the case definition that is used. The prevalence of VWD has been estimated in several countries on the basis of the number of symptomatic patients seen at hemostasis centers and ranges from about 23 to 110 per million population (0.0023–0.01%) [2]. It is also been estimated by screening populations for bleeding symptoms (population-based approach), with estimates reported at 0.6%, 0.8%, and 1.3% [3–7]. These international estimates of the prevalence of VWD do not address ethnicity or geographic variables as potential independent factors, though ethnic variation in VWF levels can influence the diagnosis of VWD [8–10]. Moreover, most mild bleeding disorders are often unrecognized, as patients bleed only during stress periods or with surgery and medical procedures [11, 12]. The most common result of these chronic bleeds is iron deficiency anemia, which is more common in women due to excessive menstrual bleeding.

The few studies estimating the prevalence of VWD by screening populations using formal standardized criteria reported a prevalence approaching 1%, with no ethnic differences [4, 6]. Platelet disorders are another group of bleeding disorders, in which bleeding can result from a decrease in platelet count (thrombocytopenia), with a reported incidence of 1.9 and 6.4 per 10 children/year. In adults, the incidence of idiopathic thrombocytopenic purpura is 3.3 per 10 adults/year [13, 14]. There are additional inherited platelet disorders with a generally unknown prevalence. Inherited thrombocytopathies are a heterogeneous group of platelet disorders present mainly with mucocutaneous bleeding of variable severity caused by defects in platelet adhesion, aggregation, granules, and signal transduction [15]. The diagnosis of more prevalent mild forms of inherited thrombocytopathies is difficult, even with extensive laboratory testing [16]. This could be due to the presence of a very broad range of candidate platelet proteins potentially implicated in the pathogenesis of nonsevere inherited thrombocytopathies, many of which are incompletely characterized [17]. Gresele et al. [18] estimated that only 40–60% of mild platelet disorders can be diagnosed at the level of the defective platelet pathway.

In the Kingdom of Saudi Arabia, no population-based screening studies have examined the prevalence of bleeding disorders, although several case reports and case-series have been published [19–23]. This is potentially important, as Arab populations may have a higher prevalence of bleeding disorders than in the West, primarily owing to the increased rate of consanguinity in Arab communities. The purpose of the current study was to conduct the first screening survey in the capital city of Riyadh focused on the prevalence of bleeding symptoms among adolescents and young adults.

2. Material and Methods

We conducted an epidemiological survey on a randomly selected Saudi national adolescent sample of intermediate and high school participants of both sexes in Riyadh using a semistructured validated condensed (MCMDM-1) VWD Bleeding Questionnaire. This questionnaire was selected owing to its capacity to generate quantifiable data from the entire study group [24]. Process of translation into Arabic and adaptation of MCMDM-1 through an expert committee for implementation has been published elsewhere [25]. A shorter questionnaire, derived from the same primary questions but with less detail, was extracted to be used as a primary screening tool for the initial phase of the study, whereas the original questionnaire was used in the second phase of the study only when participants gave a positive response to any primary question. The survey was conducted onsite by trained Arabic speaking interviewers. All questionnaires were coded for data entry. The process involved the following phases.

Phase I. Fifty schools (30 intermediate and 20 secondary) were randomly selected from a complete list of intermediate and secondary schools in Riyadh city (Table 1). We distributed invitations to the schools with the intention to have at least 100 participants from each school. An initial visit was paid to participating schools to explain the aim of the study and to distribute educational materials on bleeding disorders. Interviews were conducted after obtaining signed assents or consent, depending upon the age of the participant. The Phase I data were analyzed to identify participants who gave a positive response to any of the primary questions; these participants were considered to potentially have a bleeding tendency.

Phase II. Respondents with at least one positive response were contacted again for getting further details regarding symptoms and to assess potential recall bias. Their responses were recorded using a detailed questionnaire further probing on the bleeding type specific to the site of bleeding, based upon MCMDM-1.

2.1. Data Management and Quality Assurance. Arabic speaking trained individuals interviewed participants and collected data using specially designed Arabic-language Case Report Forms (CRF). Confidentiality was maintained by assigning each participant a unique identification number, which was entered into a computerized database. Data were validated for data entry errors by cross checking the improbable answers. Discrepancies were handled by reviewing the original forms. All data were transferred to IBM SPSS Statistics Version 20 (IBM Corp., Armonk, NY, USA) for final analysis.

Processed data are reported in percentages along with the denominator which defines the available data. To compare categorical data, Chi-Square or Fisher's exact test was used while Shapiro-Wilk test was utilized to test for the normality of continuous data. P value of less than 0.05 was considered as achieving statistical significance.

3. Results

3.1. Phase I. During Phase I, 3923 randomly selected students were approached and told about the study after providing written literature and assent forms with an invitation to be interviewed regarding bleeding tendency. Of these 98.9% (3881, male: 1901 [49%]; female: 1980 [51%]) gave assent to participate. Forty-two (42) refused to participate. Median age of the participants at the time of interview for available data was 18.2 years (n = 3322; range, 12.0–21.0 years; mean ± standard deviation: 17.8 ± 1.4 years; P value for normality < 0.001). There were 40 (1.2%) participants < 14 years, 1340 (40.3%) 14–17 years, and 1942 (58.5%) ≥ 18 years. Of 3881 participants who completed the survey, 1849 (47.6%) answered "yes/positive" to at least one of the eight questions (Table 2).

Of 72 (1.9%) participants who responded "Yes" to "Have you ever been diagnosed with any bleeding disorder?" question, eight reported having hemophilia, three platelets disorders, and none reported VWD; remaining participants did not disclose additional information. In response to a family history of any bleeding disorders, 237 out of 3730 (6.4%) participants who opted to answer, responded positively, 44 hemophilia, 22 platelet disorders, and 3 VWD; the remaining 167 did not provide any details or did not know the exact disorder.

TABLE 1: Sampling frame for determining the prevalence of bleeding symptoms.

	Intermediate schools			High schools		
	Number of participants	Number of schools	Number of clusters	Number of participants	Number of schools	Number of clusters
Boys	81,869	336	15	72,621	194	10
Girls	84,607	419	15	80,136	293	10
Total	166,476	755	30	152,757	487	20

TABLE 2: Responses to Phase I of the Survey ($n = 3881$).

Questions	Male n (total), %	Female n (total), %	Total n (total), %	P value
(1) Previous diagnosis of any bleeding disorder?				
Yes	42 (1901), 2.2	30 (1980), 1.5	72 (3881), 1.9	0.069
Did not reply	-	-	-	
(2) Previous episodes of epistasis?				
Yes	453 (1901), 23.8	311 (1980), 15.7	764 (3881), 19.7	<0.001
Did not reply	-	-	-	
(3) Bleeding under the skin?				
Yes	218 (1840), 11.8	406 (1931), 21.0	624 (3771), 16.5	<0.001
Did not reply	61	49	110	
(4) Postsurgery bleeding?				
Yes	97 (1834), 5.3	313 (1930), 16.2	410 (3764), 10.9	<0.001
Did not reply	67	50	117	
(5) Bleeding from the mouth?				
Yes	161 (1801), 8.9	188 (1928), 9.8	349 (3729), 9.4	0.399
Did not reply	100	52	152	
(6) Bleeding from the digestive system?				
Yes	107 (1834), 5.8	211 (1930), 10.9	318 (3764), 8.4	<0.001
Did not reply	67	50	117	
(7) Postdental extraction bleeding?				
Yes	314 (1823), 17.2	126 (1926), 6.5%	440 (3749), 11.7	<0.001
Did Not Reply	78	54	132	
(8) Muscular bleeding?				
Yes	94 (1725), 5.4	201 (1894), 10.6	295 (3619), 8.2	<0.001
Did Not Reply	176	86	262	
(9) Family history of bleeding disorders?				
Yes	146 (1821), 8.0	91 (1909), 4.8	237 (3730), 6.4	<0.001
Did Not Reply	80	71	151	
(10) Any other bleeding disorders? (for boys only)				
Yes	173 (1882), 9.2	-	173 (1882), 9.2	-
Did Not Reply	19	-	19	
(11) Heavy menstrual bleeding (girls only)				
Yes	-	330 (1980), 16.7	330 (1980), 16.7	-
Did Not Reply	-	-	-	
(12) Any Question 2 through 8 or 10				
Yes	832 (1901), 43.8	1017 (1980), 51.4	1849 (3881), 47.6	<0.001
Did Not Reply	-	-	-	

Responses left blank or *Did Not Reply* are not included in the final calculations.

TABLE 3: Responses to Phase II of the Survey ($n = 525$).

Symptom	Male n (total), %	Female n (total), %	Total n (total), %	P value
Oral cavity bleeding	144 (296), 48.6	134 (229), 58.5	278 (525), 52.9	0.028
Epistaxis	147 (296), 49.7	82 (229), 35.8	229 (525), 43.6	0.002
Cutaneous symptoms	52 (296), 17.6	102 (229), 44.5	154 (525), 29.3	<0.001
Menstrual bleeding	Not applicable	56 (229), 24.5	56 (229), 24.5	-
Minor wound bleeding	39 (296), 13.2	56 (229), 24.5	95 (525), 18.1	0.001
Bleeding during tooth extraction	25 (296), 8.4	42 (229), 18.3	67 (525), 12.8	0.001
Gastrointestinal bleeding	15 (296), 5.1	31 (229), 13.5	46 (525), 8.8	0.001
Muscle hematoma and hemarthrosis			24 (525), 4.6	
Spontaneous bleeding	3 (14), 21.4	6 (10), 60	9 (24), 37.5	0.092

Values are reported as n (N), %.

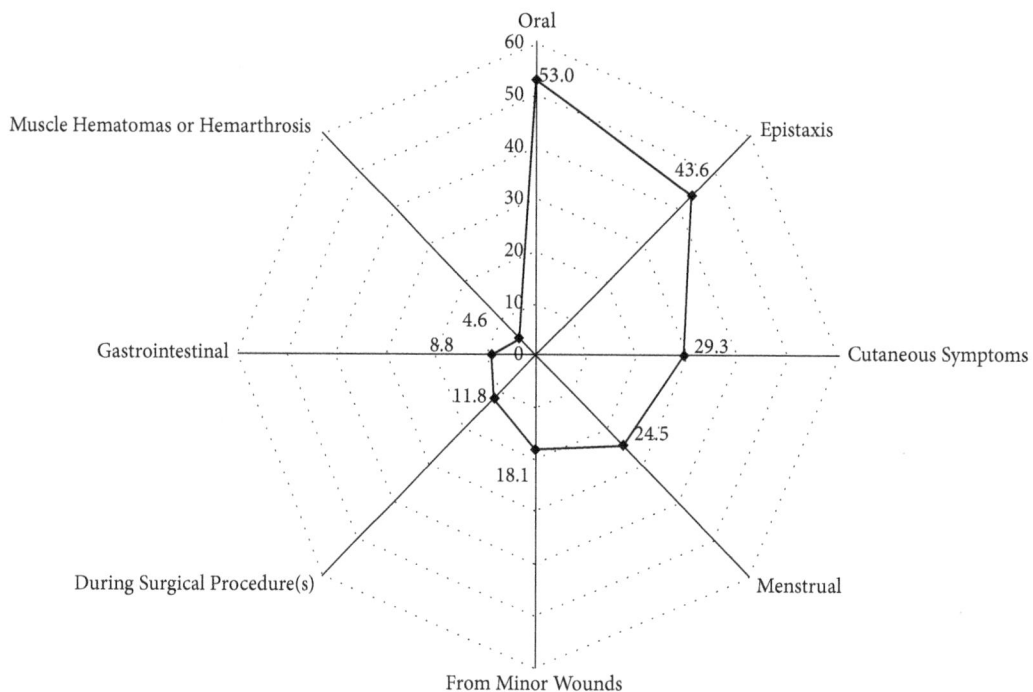

FIGURE 1: Prevalence of bleeding symptoms as reported by the participants.

3.2. Phase II. Of the 1849 (47.6%) participants who responded "yes" to at least one question in Phase I, only 525 (28.4%; male: 296 [56.4%]; female: 229 [43.6%]) replied to our call to participate in Phase II of the study and attend the second interview. Reasons for those participants of Phase I who had possibly exhibited bleeding symptoms during the interview, not completing the Phase II of the study, included wrong or changed phone numbers, participant moving out of the area, or incorrect contact details. Median age at the time of interview for this group of participants was 18.4 years (range: 12.5–20.9 years; mean ± standard deviation: 18.1 ± 1.4; P value for normality < 0.001). There were eight (1.8%) participants < 14 years, 140 (31.8%) 14–17 years, and 292 (66.4%) ≥ 18 years of age. Data on age at interview was available for 440 participants. A total of 442 participants of the Phase II of the study answered positive to any of the questions

inquiring about the symptoms pertaining to the bleeding disorders (Table 3); thus an overall prevalence of all bleeding symptoms was 84.2% (Figure 1).

3.3. Oral Cavity Bleeding. About fifty-three percent (278/525, 52.9%) of participants reported oral cavity bleeding. Of these, 85.3% (237/278) reported bleeding from the mouth while brushing their teeth, 20.5% (57/278) spontaneously from the gums, 11.2% (31/278) from lip or tongue bites, and 1.8% (5/278) from tooth eruption. In addition, 7.2% (20/278) reported having sought medical attention, 75% (15/20) sought consultation only, while one participant reported having undergone a blood transfusion. Oral cavity bleeding was significantly higher in girls (134/229, 58.5%) than in boys (144/296, 48.6%, $P = 0.028$). Similarly, oral bleeding from lip or tongue bites was significantly higher in girls (25/134, 18.7%) than in boys (6/144, 4.2%, $P < 0.001$).

3.4. Epistaxis. The next most common symptom was epistaxis, which was reported by 229 (43.6%) participants and was more predominant among boys (147/296, 49.7%) than girls (82/229, 35.8%, $P = 0.002$). Epistaxis mostly occurred 1–5 times yearly (118/228, 51.8%), lasted 1–10 minutes (111/223, 49.8%), and was spontaneous in 87.2% (197/226) of participants. It primarily occurred at a single nostril (149/225, 66.2%) and was not related to ingestion of any drugs (227/228, 99.6%), though 56.2% (127/226) reported a seasonal relationship. A majority (162/221, 73.3%) reported successful cessation of epistaxis with short compression, while some (57/221, 25.8%) reported spontaneous cessation, and a few (2/221, 0.9%) reported cessation following medical intervention. No significant dependence was found between the age of maximum severity (<14 years, 111/219, 50.7%; ≥14 years, 108/219, 49.3%). A small proportion of participants (36/227, 15.9%) reported that they had sought medical attention in the past due to epistaxis, including consultation only (66.7% [24/36]), cauterization (25.0% [9/36]), and packing (2.8% [1/36]). No participants reported needing blood transfusion.

There was a significant difference in the spontaneity of epistaxis between sexes (girls: 77.81 [95.1%]; boys: 120/145 [82.8%], $P = 0.007$). Moreover, 40.6% (58/143) of boys reported having experienced bleeding from both nostrils compared to 22% (18/82) of girls ($P = 0.005$).

3.5. Cutaneous Symptoms. Cutaneous symptoms were reported by 29.3% (154/525), most commonly occurring six times yearly (17/92, 18.5%) and ranging from one time (8/92, 8.7%) to 24 times (3/92, 3.2%). The most common manifestation was bruises (109/142, 76.8%), followed by hematoma (16/142, 11.3%); these were most commonly manifested at exposed sites (97/139, 69.8%). Only 14.2% (18/127) sought medical attention regarding this, nine of whom sought consultation only. Cutaneous symptoms occurred more commonly in girls (102/229, 44.5%) than in boys (52/296, 17.6%, $P < 0.001$). In addition, more boys (12/45, 26.7%) required medical attention than girls (6/82, 4.7%, $P = 0.006$).

3.6. Menstrual Bleeding. Heavy menstrual bleeding was reported by 24.5% (56/229) of female participants. Median duration of menstruation was 7 days (range: 3–15 days; mean: 6.5 days; P for normality < 0.001), and the median number of heavy days was 3 (range: 0–8; mean = 2.7, P for normality < 0.001). The most commonly reported duration of menstruation was 7 days (40.9% [90/220]), and the most commonly reported number of heavy days was 3 (36.9% [73/198]). Medical attention was sought by 21.4% (12/56); three had consultation only, and nine received iron supplements.

3.7. Minor Wound Bleeding. Bleeding from minor wounds was reported by 18.1% of participants (95/525), with 52.6% (41/78) reporting this occurred 6–12 times a year, and 25.6% (20/78) reporting >12 times a year. Average duration of a single episode was 1–10 minutes in 78.3% (65/83), > 10 minutes in 19.3% (16/83), and <1 minute in only 2.4% (2/83). Location of minor wounds was primarily exposed sites (89.6%, 69/77), and there was minimal or no trauma in 67.4% (64/95). Only 8.4% (8/95) needed medical attention, with

two participants needing surgical hemostasis. Bleeding from minor wounds was more common in girls (56/229, 24.5%) than in boys (39/296, 13.2%, $P = 0.001$).

3.8. Bleeding during Surgery/Tooth Extraction. Those who underwent at least one surgery of any type comprised 30.5% (160/525). Among these, 112 (70%) had one surgical episode, 33 (20.6%) had two, seven (4.4%) had three, three (1.9%) had four, four (2.5%) had five, and one (0.6%) had seven, thus totaling 238 reported surgical episodes. Among those who underwent any surgery, 24 (15%) reported at least one surgery followed by a bleeding episode and four (2.5%) reported two surgeries followed by bleeding episodes; thus 28/238 reported surgeries with a postsurgery bleeding episode alluding to a prevalence of 11.8%. Bleeding episode after first surgery was reported by almost one-quarter of the participants (39/160, 24.4%) and was significantly higher in girls (19/52, 36.5%) than in boys (20/108, 18.5%, $P = 0.018$). Types of surgeries included major abdominal surgery (4/160, 2.5%), major thoracic surgery (2/160, 1.2%), and molar extraction or dental surgery (28/160, 17.5%). Posttooth extraction bleeding was reported by 12.8% (67/525) of participants and was significantly higher in girls (42/229, 18.3%) than in boys (25/296, 8.4%, $P = 0.001$). No action was required to control the bleeding in 47 participants, resuturing was performed in nine, and only one required blood transfusion.

3.9. Gastrointestinal Bleeding. GI bleeding was reported by 8.8% (46/525) of participants. Six (6/16, 37.5%) reported having had GI bleeding at least once, four (25%) at least three times, two (12.5%) at least five times, two (12.5%) at least 10 times, one (6.2%) at least two times, and one (6.2%) at least 12 times. Of these, 39.1% (18/46) had hematemesis, 37% (17/46) had hematochezia, and 13% (6/46) had melena. In addition, 23.8% (10/42) had associated GI disease; of these, 30% (3/10) reported ulcer and 10% (1/10) angiodysplasia, while none reported portal hypertension. Moreover, 28.3% (13/46) mentioned that they sought medical attention for this, 84.6% (11/13) of whom had consultation only, while one female participant (7.7%) underwent a blood transfusion. GI bleeding was more common in girls (31/229, 13.5%) than in boys (15/296, 5.1%, $P = 0.001$).

3.10. Muscle Hematoma and Hemarthrosis. Muscle hematomas or hemarthrosis was reported by 4.6% (24/525), with spontaneous bleeding in 37.5% (9/24), which was higher in girls (6/10, 60%) than in boys (3/14, 21.4%, $P = 0.092$). Two of these participants (2/24, 8.3%) reported that they sought medical attention, one was given replacement therapy, and complete data was not available for the other. None received desmopressin or blood transfusion.

3.11. Other Types of Bleeding. A total of twelve (12/525, 2.3%) participants reported experiencing episodes of bleeding other than the above-mentioned types. Only two of these (2/12, 16.7%) went to see a medical practitioner; one was given replacement therapy and the other received consultation only. No data was available regarding the type of bleeding.

More than half (53.1%, $n = 279$) of the students (525) reported bleeding episodes from more than one group of sites. Majority of these (53%, $n = 148$) were females (P value: 0.001). Oral cavity bleeding with cutaneous symptoms was the most common (12.2%, 18 out of 148), followed by oral cavity bleeding with epistaxis (6.8%, 10 out of 148) and oral cavity bleeding with epistaxis and cutaneous symptoms (4.7%, 7 out of 148). Among boys reporting bleeding episodes observed from multiple sites ($n = 131$), oral cavity bleeding with epistaxis (31.3%, 41 out of 131) was the most frequently observed kind, followed by oral cavity bleeding with cutaneous symptoms (7.6%, 10 out of 131) and epistaxis with cutaneous symptoms (5.3%, 7 out of 131).

4. Discussion

To our knowledge, this is the first largest screening study attempting to address the estimation of prevalence of symptoms of bleeding disorders in the capital city of Saudi Arabia. Prior studies from Saudi Arabia reporting the same have been smaller, hospital-based studies. For instance, El-Bostany et al. [19] assessed the local prevalence of some inherited bleeding disorders in pediatric patients which involved 43 children with various bleeding manifestations recruited from a children's hospital in Cairo, Egypt, and Jeddah, Kingdom of Saudi Arabia. Of these, 12 (27.9%) had VWD, 11 (25.5%) had hemophilia A, three (7%) had hemophilia B, seven (16.3%) had platelet disorders, and 10 (23.3%) had bleeding of undiagnosed cause. In addition, Ahmed et al. [20] reported 34 cases of inherited bleeding disorders from Eastern Province of Saudi Arabia; of these, 15 had hemophilia, one had factor VII deficiency, one had factor X deficiency, 12 had Glanzmann thrombasthenia, and five had unidentified platelet function disorders. Moreover, Al-Sharif et al. [21] reported clinical phenotype of around 20 patients with factor XIII deficiency in the Riyadh region. Furthermore, Al-Fawaz et al. [22] conducted an 8-year retrospective analysis of patients referred for suspected inherited bleeding disorders in the Riyadh region and found 168 patients had bleeding symptoms that fulfilled the criteria for inherited bleeding disorders. Of these, 41 (24.4%) had hemophilia A, 16 (9.5%) had hemophilia B, 25 (14.9%) had VWD, 18 (10.7%) had Glanzmann thrombasthenia, 18 with Bernard-Soulier disease, five (3.0%) had factor XI deficiency, two (1.2%) had factor XII deficiency, four (2.4%) had factor V deficiency, four (2.4%) had factor VIII deficiency, one (0.6%) had factor VII deficiency, two (1.2%) had dysfibrinogenemia, and one (0.6%) had afibrinogenemia. Additionally, Islam and Quadri [23] conducted a 7-year retrospective review of all hospitals in Eastern Province of Saudi Arabia. They reported 54 patients diagnosed with hereditary coagulation factor deficiencies, including 42 hemophiliacs, 5 with probable factor XIII deficiency, and 7 with VWD. There are also rare reports from other Arab countries reporting small hospital-based studies [26–28].

In the current study, boys experienced epistaxis more frequently, which was more likely to be spontaneous, to occur at both nostrils, and to have seasonal differences; this may be explained by the more outdoor lifestyle in boys in a dry, hot environment, which leads to more nasal dryness and is one of the common causes of epistaxis in general [29–31]. In contrast, girls wear veils and are usually covered in the outdoor setting, which may reduce nasal dryness.

A study from Sweden among healthy university females showed a high prevalence of bleeding symptoms including menorrhagia. 73% of the participants had one bleeding symptom while 43% had more than one symptom [32]. Another study from Turkey done on female university residents showed 82/376 (22%) healthy females reporting menorrhagia, after excluding pelvic pathology out of 11/76 (14.5%) were found to have an underlying bleeding disorder [33].

This study provides insight into the existence of various bleeding disorders and highlights the need for a national surveillance system for identifying the individuals in the early age with such disorders. There is a need for genetic mapping of families suffering from bleeding diathesis in order to prevent further generations of Saudi nationals being affected. Specialized hematological investigations from a nationally representative sample would provide more insight into the nature and classification of the more prevalent disorders and guide treatment and prevention. Although every citizen has an easy access to the healthcare services in the Kingdom of Saudi Arabia, it is imperative to improve the quality of life of the affected individuals and families by raising awareness and reducing exposure to precipitating insults. Genetic counseling of the severely affected families is mandatory for genetically transmitted disorders.

It might be said that the participants in this sample were more aware of their health problems since they were residing in an urban area; the importance to search for the prevalence in other suburban and rural areas of the country is also highlighted, since consanguinity maybe more prevalent in those closed populations. Generally it was observed that girls reported higher prevalence of bleeding symptoms than boys. We believe this could be a reporting bias since girls are generally more self-caring than boys especially in the teenage years. Boys tend to ignore minor cuts and bruises and may attribute them to their typical physical activities.

5. Limitations

This report is limited by the lack of laboratory related data further identifying specific bleeding disorders. It was beyond the feasibility of the research with respect to logistics and financial support. It would be very interesting to observe the prevalent forms of bleeding disorders in a future report hence guiding the policy makers for efficient resource allocation.

6. Conclusion

This survey which is the first epidemiological study for bleeding symptoms in Saudi Arabia using standardized tool (MCMDM-1) that had highlighted the need to conduct a national survey in the Kingdom on broader representative sample with extensive laboratory test to explore the prevalence of different bleeding disorders. We also recommend that physicians be cautious of the existence of bleeding disorders in the community as minor symptoms can get easily ignored and lead to a catastrophe when challenged by trauma or surgery. Also, a sustainable public awareness program focusing the early diagnosis, treatment, and genetic counseling among the residents of the regions with high prevalence of bleeding disorders should be initiated.

Consent

Informed consent was obtained from the participants as per regulatory requirements of the relevant authorities in the Kingdom of Saudi Arabia.

Conflicts of Interest

The authors declare that they have no conflicts of interest with the funding institute.

Acknowledgments

The authors would like to thank King Abdulaziz City for Science and Technology (KASCT), Saudi Arabia, for providing the funding for this project, research Grant approval letter no. 408-34.

References

[1] W. F. O. Hemophilia, "World federation of hemophilia report on the annual global survey 2006," in *World Federation of Hemophilia 1425 René Lévesque Boulevard West, Suite 1010*, Montreal, Canada.

[2] W. L. Nichols, M. E. Rick, T. L. Ortel et al., "Clinical and laboratory diagnosis of von Willebrand disease: a synopsis of the 2008 NHLBI/NIH guidelines," *American Journal of Hematology*, vol. 84, no. 6, pp. 366–370, 2009.

[3] L. Hallberg, A. M. Högdahl, L. Nilsson, and G. Rybo, "Menstrual blood loss—a population study. Variation at different ages and attempts to define normality," *Acta Obstetricia et Gynecologica Scandinavica*, vol. 45, no. 3, pp. 320–351, 1966.

[4] F. Rodeghiero, G. Castaman, and E. Dini, "Epidemiological investigations of the prevalence of von Willebrand's disease," *Blood*, vol. 69, no. 2, pp. 454–459, 1987.

[5] J. E. Sadler, P. M. Mannucci, E. Berntorp et al., "Impact, diagnosis and treatment of von willebrand disease," *Thrombosis and Haemostasis*, vol. 84, no. 08, pp. 160–174, 2017.

[6] E. J. Werner, E. H. Broxson, E. L. Tucker, D. S. Giroux, J. Shults, and T. C. Abshire, "Prevalence of von Willebrand disease in children: a multiethnic study," *Journal of Pediatrics*, vol. 123, no. 6, pp. 893–898, 1993.

[7] A. S. Lukes, R. A. Kadir, F. Peyvandi, and P. A. Kouides, "Disorders of hemostasis and excessive menstrual bleeding: prevalence and clinical impact," *Fertility and Sterility*, vol. 84, no. 5, pp. 1338–1344, 2005.

[8] A. F. Fleming, "Ethnic variation in von Willebrand factor levels can influence the diagnosis of von Willebrand disease," *Clinical & Laboratory Haematology*, vol. 25, no. 6, p. 413, 2003.

[9] B. Friberg, A. K. Örnö, A. Lindgren, and S. Lethagen, "Bleeding disorders among young women: a population-based prevalence study," *Acta Obstetricia et Gynecologica Scandinavica*, vol. 85, no. 2, pp. 200–206, 2006.

[10] T. Quiroga, M. Goycoolea, O. Panes et al., "High prevalence of bleeders of unknown cause among patients with inherited mucocutaneous bleeding. A prospective study of 280 patients and 299 controls," *Haematologica*, vol. 92, no. 3, pp. 357–365, 2007.

[11] C. Biron-Andréani, B. Mahieu, A. Rochette et al., "Preoperative screening for von Willebrand disease type 1: low yield and limited ability to predict bleeding," *Journal of Laboratory and Clinical Medicine*, vol. 134, no. 6, pp. 605–609, 1999.

[12] M. Bowman, W. M. Hopman, D. Rapson, D. Lillicrap, M. Silva, and P. James, "A prospective evaluation of the prevalence of symptomatic von Willebrand Disease (VWD) in a pediatric primary care population," *Pediatric Blood & Cancer*, vol. 55, no. 1, pp. 171–173, 2010.

[13] D. R. Terrell, L. A. Beebe, S. K. Vesely, B. R. Neas, J. B. Segal, and J. N. George, "The incidence of immune thrombocytopenic purpura in children and adults: a critical review of published reports," *American Journal of Hematology*, vol. 85, no. 3, pp. 174–180, 2010.

[14] G. D'Andrea, M. Chetta, and M. Margaglione, "Inherited platelet disorders: thrombocytopenias and thrombocytopathies," *Blood Transfusion*, vol. 7, no. 4, pp. 278–292, 2009.

[15] M. V. Ragni, N. Machin, L. M. Malec et al., "Von Willebrand factor for menorrhagia: a survey and literature review," *Haemophilia*, vol. 22, no. 3, pp. 397–402, 2016.

[16] P. Noris, G. Biino, A. Pecci et al., "Platelet diameters in inherited thrombocytopenias: analysis of 376 patients with all known disorders," *Blood*, vol. 124, no. 6, pp. e4–e10, 2014.

[17] C. M. Kirchmaier and D. Pillitteri, "Diagnosis and management of inherited platelet disorders," *Transfusion Medicine and Hemotherapy*, vol. 37, no. 5, pp. 237–246, 2010.

[18] P. Gresele, P. Harrison, L. Bury et al., "Diagnosis of suspected inherited platelet function disorders: results of a worldwide survey," *Journal of Thrombosis and Haemostasis*, vol. 12, no. 9, pp. 1562–1569, 2014.

[19] E. A. El-Bostany, N. Omer, E. E. Salama, E. A. El-Ghoroury, and S. K. Al-Jaouni, "The spectrum of inherited bleeding disorders in pediatrics," *Blood Coagulation & Fibrinolysis*, vol. 19, no. 8, pp. 771–775, 2008.

[20] M. A. M. Ahmed, M. O. Al-Sohaibani, S. A. Al-Mohaya, T. Sumer, E. H. Al-Sheikh, and H. Knox-Macaulay, "Inherited bleeding disorders in the eastern province of saudi arabia," *Acta Haematologica*, vol. 79, no. 4, pp. 202–206, 1988.

[21] F. Z. Al-Sharif, M. D. Aljurf, A. M. Al-Momen et al., "Clinical and laboratory features of congenital factor XIII deficiency," *Saudi Medical Journal*, vol. 23, no. 5, pp. 552–554, 2002.

[22] I. M. Al-Fawaz, A. M. A. Gader, H. M. Bahakim, F. Al-Mohareb, A. K. Al-Momen, and M. S. Harakati, "Hereditary bleeding disorders in Riyadh, Saudi Arabia," *Annals of Saudi Medicine*, vol. 16, no. 3, pp. 257–261, 1996.

[23] S. I. A. Islam and M. I. Quadri, "Spectrum of hereditary coagulation factor deficiencies in Eastern Province, Saudi Arabia," *Eastern Mediterranean Health Journal*, vol. 5, no. 6, pp. 1188–1195, 1999.

[24] M. Bowman, G. Mundell, J. Grabell et al., "Generation and validation of the condensed MCMDM-1VWD bleeding questionnaire for von Willebrand disease," *Journal of Thrombosis and Haemostasis*, vol. 6, no. 12, pp. 2062–2066, 2008.

[25] S. S. Khawar, M. Abu-Riash, and A. Al-Suliman, "Translation and adaptation of english language questionnaire into arabic for implementation of a large survey on assessing the symptoms of bleeding disorders in Saudi Arabia," *Journal of Applied Hematology*, vol. 8, no. 4, 2017.

[26] S. S. Eid, N. R. Kamal, T. S. Shubeilat, and A. G. Wael, "Inherited bleeding disorders: a 14-year retrospective study," *Clinical Laboratory Science*, vol. 21, no. 4, pp. 210–214, 2008.

[27] G. M. Mokhtar, A. A. G. Tantawy, A. A. M. Adly, M. A. S. Telbany, S. E. E. Arab, and M. Ismail, "A longitudinal prospective study of bleeding diathesis in Egyptian pediatric patients: single-center experience," *Blood Coagulation & Fibrinolysis*, vol. 23, no. 5, pp. 411–418, 2012.

[28] A. S. Awidi, "A study of von Willebrand's disease in Jordan," *Annals of Hematology*, vol. 64, no. 6, pp. 299–302, 1992.

[29] M. Anie, G. Arjun, C. Andrews, and A. Vinayakumar, "Descriptive epidemiology of epistaxis in a tertiary care hospital," *International Journal of Advances in Medicine*, vol. 2, no. 3, pp. 255–259, 2015.

[30] A. Asghar, M. A. ul Haq, M. I. Anwar, and M. Awais, "Effects of extreme dry climate of sudan on Pakistani peacekeepers," *Pakistan Armed Forces Medical Journal*, vol. 67, no. 1, pp. 166–170, 2017.

[31] M. R. Chaaban, D. Zhang, V. Resto, and J. S. Goodwin, "Demographic, seasonal, and geographic differences in emergency department visits for epistaxis," *Otolaryngology—Head and Neck Surgery (United States)*, vol. 156, no. 1, pp. 81–86, 2017.

[32] B. Friberg, A. Kristin Örnö, A. Lindgren, and S. Lethagen, "Bleeding disorders among young women: a population-based prevalence study," *Acta Obstetricia et Gynecologica Scandinavica*, vol. 85, no. 2, pp. 200–206, 2006.

[33] T. Gursel, A. Biri, Z. Kaya, S. Sivaslioglu, and M. Albayrak, "The frequency of menorrhagia and bleeding disorders in university students," *Pediatric Hematology and Oncology*, vol. 31, no. 5, pp. 467–474, 2014.

12

The Effects of Sample Transport by Pneumatic Tube System on Routine Hematology and Coagulation Tests

Devi Subbarayan ⓘ, Chidambharam Choccalingam, and Chittode Kodumudi Anantha Lakshmi

Department of Pathology, Chettinad Health City and Research Institute, Kelambakkam, Chennai, Tamil Nadu, India

Correspondence should be addressed to Devi Subbarayan; sdevi2001@gmail.com

Academic Editor: Donna Hogge

Background. Automation helps improve laboratory operational efficiency and reduce the turnaround time. Pneumatic tube systems (PTS) automate specimen transport between the lab and other areas of the hospital. Its effect on complete blood count (CBC) and coagulation is still controversial. *Aim.* To study the effects of pneumatic tube system sample transport on complete blood count and coagulation parameters to compare them with hand delivered samples. *Methods.* 75 paired samples for complete blood count and 25 paired samples for coagulation analysis were compared between samples sent via pneumatic tube system and hand delivered system. *Results.* PTS showed significant decrease in red cell indices such as MCV and RDW and increase in MCHC. Other red cell parameters and WBC parameters showed no statistical significant difference. Statistically significant increase in platelet count was observed with PTS samples. However, these differences were clinically insignificant. No significant effect of PTS was found in PT and APTT samples compared to the hand delivered samples. *Conclusion.* Despite statistically significant changes in RBC parameters such as MCV, RDW, and MCHC and platelet count, these changes were clinically insignificant. Hence, blood samples for CBC and coagulation assay can safely be transported via our hospital's PTS. However, further studies on platelet count are warranted to ensure safe transport and accuracy of the results.

1. Introduction

To ensure the fastest possible turnaround time in laboratory analysis, the specimens should be delivered to the clinical laboratory quickly and safely. One such system used for sample transport is pneumatic tube system (PTS).

PTS automate specimen transport by vacuum and pressure between the lab and other areas of the hospital. During transport, the sample integrity can be affected by acceleration, deceleration forces, and radial gravity forces. Steige and Jones have stated that each pneumatic tube system must be individually evaluated because of the differences between each of pneumatic tube systems [1].

Previous studies have shown the changes in platelet aggregation and biochemical parameters such as elevated lactate dehydrogenase, alterations in serum potassium, serum haemoglobin, and arterial blood gas analysis due to PTS transport [2–6]. Few studies have shown shortening of activated partial thromboplastin time (APTT) and changes in mean platelet component (MPC) [3, 7]. Although the effect of PTS on biochemical changes and hemolysis has been studied widely, its effect on complete blood count (CBC) and coagulation samples is still controversial. Hence, we undertook this study to evaluate the effects of PTS on complete blood count and coagulation.

2. Aims And Objectives

This paper aims to study the effects of pneumatic tube system sample transport on complete blood count and coagulation parameters.

3. Materials And Methods

The study was carried out after obtaining ethical clearance from institutional ethical committee and written informed consent from the study subjects.

TABLE 1: Summary of the differences in CBC between pneumatic tube samples and hand delivered samples.

S. no.	Paired samples	Mean difference	Standard deviation of mean difference	95% confidence interval of mean difference		P value
				Lower	Upper	
1	RBC P-RBC M ($\times 10^{12}$/l)	-.03	.21	-.08	.01	.11
2	HB P-HB M (g/dl)	-.01	.24	-.06	.05	.84
3	MCV P-MCV M (fl)	-.82	1.9	-1.28	-.37	.001
4	MCH P-MCH M (pg)	.03	.41	-.06	.12	.500
5	MCHCP-MCHC M (g/dl)	.36	.84	.17	.56	<0.001
6	RDW P-RDW M (%)	-.33	.67	-.49	-.18	<0.001
7	WBC P-WBC M ($\times 10^9$/l)	.04	1.2	-.24	.32	.759
8	NE P-NE M (%)	-.45	2.94	-1.13	.21	.182
9	LY P-LY M (%)	.20	3.30	-.55	.96	.590
10	MO P-MO M (%)	.30	1.37	-.01	.62	.057
11	EO P-EO M (%)	.28	3.46	-.50	1.08	.472
12	BA P-BA M (%)	.01	.33	-.06	.08	.754
13	PLT P-PLT M ($\times 10^9$/l)	.13	.26	.07	.19	<0.001
14	MPV P-MPV M (fl)	-.18	.64	-.32	-.03	.017

P: pneumatic tube samples; M: hand delivered samples; RBC: red blood cells count; HB: hemoglobin; MCV: mean corpuscular volume; MCH: mean corpuscular hemoglobin; RDW: red cell distribution width; WBC: white blood cell count; NE: neutrophils; LY: lymphocytes; MO: monocytes; EO: eosinophils; BA: basophils; PLT: platelets; MPV: mean platelet volume.

75 randomly selected paired samples for CBC and 25 random paired samples for coagulation assay were collected during 2-month period from June 2017 to July 2017.

3.1. Sample Collection. Specimens were collected from outpatient collection center, ICUs, and wards. Specimens were collected by standard venipuncture under septic precautions.

75 duplicate venous samples of 3 ml blood were obtained in tripotassium ethylenediaminetetraacetic acid (K3-EDTA) vacutainer (Greiner Bio-One vacutainer). 25 duplicate samples of 2.7 ml blood were collected in 3.2% sodium citrate vacutainer (Becton Dickinson vacutainer) for coagulation. Collected samples were separated into two groups.

3.2. Sample Transport. Group 1 samples were immediately transported to the laboratory through PTS. The PTS used in this study was Swisslog's PTS (Swisslog Rohrpostsysteme GmbH, Hansacker 5-7, Westerstede, Germany). The system works electronically with TranspoNet software process to maximize its efficiency. Two types of carriers were used in this system: one for transportation of the sample which is leak proof provided with a special foam tube carriers and the other for sending request forms. The samples from various stations (ground floor, first floor, second floor, third floor, fourth floor, and fifth floor) to central collection laboratory are programmed at a speed of 5 m/s to reach the laboratory within 50 seconds, 53 seconds, 54 seconds, 56 seconds, 57 seconds, and 59 seconds, respectively.

Group 2 samples were hand delivered to the laboratory by personnel immediately.

CBC values were obtained from LH 780 automated analyzer (Beckman Coulter, India) using electrical impedance for total leukocyte count (TC), red blood cells count (RBC), and platelet count (PLT) and VCS (volume, conductance, and light scatter) technology for differential leukocyte count.

For coagulation studies, samples were immediately centrifuged at 2000 g at 15 mins at room temperature. Platelet-poor plasma was obtained. The PT and APTT assays were done on semiautomated photo optical coagulation analyzer (Sysmex CA-50) using reagents Thromborel S and Actin FSL, respectively.

CBC values and coagulation assays for PTS and hand delivered samples were entered in the data sheet.

3.3. Statistical Analysis. SPSS version 17.00 was used for statistical analysis. Mean, mean difference, standard deviation, and standard error of mean were calculated. All parameters between two groups were compared using paired t-test for statistical significance. P value < 0.05 was considered as statistically significant.

4. Results

75 paired samples for CBC were compared for PTS and hand delivered systems. The RBC parameters such as red blood corpuscle (RBC) count, hemoglobin (Hb), and mean cell hemoglobin (MCH) were comparable between two transport systems. However, there was a statistically significant decrease in MCV (mean corpuscular volume) and RDW (red cell distribution width) and increase in MCHC (mean corpuscular hemoglobin concentration) in PTS samples as compared to hand delivered samples (Table 1).

The estimated WBC parameters such as total count and differential count were similar between the two transport systems with no statistically significant difference.

TABLE 2: Summary of the differences in PT and APTT between pneumatic tube samples and hand delivered samples.

S. no.	Paired samples	Mean difference	Standard deviation	95% confidence interval of mean difference		P value
				Lower	Upper	
1	PT P-PT M (secs)	-.38	1.3	-.95	.18	.17
2	APTT P-APTT M (secs)	-.33	3.5	-1.7	1.1	.63

P: pneumatic tube samples; M: hand delivered samples; PT: prothrombin time; APTT: activated partial thromboplastin time.

Statistically significant elevation of platelet count was noted in PTS samples with mean difference of $0.135 \times 10^9/l$ with 95% confidence interval of 0.073–0.197. MPV showed statistically significant difference between the PTS and hand delivered system, wherein the mean difference was 0.18 with 95% confidence interval (0.32908–0.03359) (Table 1).

25 paired PTS and hand delivered samples were analyzed for PT and APTT. No statistically significant results were found for PT and APTT values between the two transport systems used (Table 2).

5. Discussion

PTS are widely used in hospitals to transport blood specimens to the clinical laboratory for most biochemical and hematological analyses. The present study aims to know the effects of transport of blood samples sent through Swisslog's PTS compared with hand delivered samples on complete blood count and coagulation using Beckman Coulter LH780 automated analyzer and Sysmex CA 50 semiautomated coagulation analyzer, respectively.

In the present study, the estimated RBC parameters such as RBC count, Hb, and MCH and WBC parameters such as total count and differential count were comparable between two transport systems (PTS and hand delivered samples). However, red cell indices such as MCV and RDW showed statistically significant decrease in PTS samples, while MCHC showed significant increase in PTS samples. Though there is significant statistical difference in these parameters, the present study observed mean difference percentage of 0.9%, 1%, and 2.1% for MCV, MCHC, and RDW, respectively, which is well below the clinically significant difference of 4-5% [8].

In this study, samples sent via PTS gave a statistically significant increase in platelet count which can be attributed to the fact that abrupt changes in force during transport can cause fragmentation of platelets. The present study observed increase in platelet count with significant decrease in MPV which had inverse relationship. However, though the present study observed statistically significant increase in platelet count, the mean difference (0.135 = 4.9%) is clinically insignificant. To be considered clinically significant, the difference should be 10–15% [8], which was not so in the present study.

Previous studies on CBC did not find any significant difference between the two transport systems [3, 7, 9–11]. Lee et al.'s study [12] demonstrated statistically significantly low MPV values with PTS samples compared to hand delivered samples. However, their study did not observe any significant difference in platelet count. Kratz et al. [7] showed statistically significant but clinically insignificant difference in MPC. So, this might turn out to be the first study that shows statistically significant effect of PTS on platelet count over hand delivered samples which may indicate the need for further studies.

The PT and APTT values were comparable between the two transport systems. Weaver et al. [3] observed statistically significant shortening of mean partial thromboplastin time (PTT) in samples sent through PTS. However, it was found to be clinically insignificant, since the difference was within the standard deviation of the method used. They did not find any significant difference for PT between these two systems. Kratz et al. [7] studied the effects of PTS on PT, PTT, and fibrinogen, and fibrin monomers showed no statistically significant difference.

There are few limitations in our study. The present study did not compare the effects of PTS at different levels of distance and also lack of significant number of samples with abnormal values to evaluate the effects of PTS in these cases, especially with abnormal platelet counts.

6. Conclusion

Based on the results, PTS showed significant decrease in red cell indices such as MCV and RDW and increase in MCHC. Samples sent via PTS gave statistically significant increase in platelet count. However, these differences were clinically insignificant. No significant effect of PTS was found in PT and APTT samples compared to the hand delivered samples. Hence, absence of clinically significant changes with samples sent via PTS in the present study concludes that blood samples for CBC and coagulation assay can safely be transported via our hospital's PTS.

Further studies on platelet counts and using different levels of distance should be done to ensure safe transport and accuracy of the results.

Conflicts of Interest

The authors declare that there are no conflicts of interest regarding the publication of this paper.

References

[1] H. Steige and J. D. Jones, "Evaluation of pneumatic tube system for delivery of blood specimens," *Clinical Chemistry*, vol. 17, pp. 1160–1164, 1971.

[2] A. A. Keshgegian and G. E. Bull, " Evaluation of a Soft-Handling Computerized Pneumatic Tube Specimen Delivery System: ," *American Journal of Clinical Pathology*, vol. 97, no. 4, pp. 535–540, 1992.

[3] D. K. Weaver, D. Miller, E. A. Leventhal, and V. Tropeano, "Evaluation of a computer directed pneumatic tube system for pneumatic transport of blood specimens," *American Journal of Clinical Pathology*, vol. 70, no. 3, pp. 400–405, 1978.

[4] P. O. Collinson, C. M. John, D. C. Gaze, L. F. Ferrigan, and D. G. Cramp, "Changes in blood gas samples produced by a pneumatic tube system," *Journal of Clinical Pathology*, vol. 55, no. 2, pp. 105–107, 2002.

[5] D. Astles Jr., B. Loun, F. A. Sedor, and J. G. Toffaletti, "Pneumatic transport exacerbates interference of room air contamination in blood gas samples," *Archives of Pathology & Laboratory Medicine*, vol. 120, pp. 642–647, 1996.

[6] T. Streichert, B. Otto, C. Schnabel et al., "Determination of hemolysis thresholds by the use of data loggers in pneumatic tube systems," *Clinical Chemistry*, vol. 57, no. 10, pp. 1390–1397, 2011.

[7] A. Kratz, R. O. Salem, and E. M. Van Cott, "Effects of a Pneumatic Tube System on Routine and Novel Hematology and Coagulation Parameters in Healthy Volunteers," in *Archives of Pathology & Laboratory Medicine*, vol. 131, pp. 293–296, 2007.

[8] B. De La Salle and D. J. Perry, "Quality Assuarance," in *Bain Barbara*, p. 542, Elsevier, London, UK, 12th edition, 2012.

[9] A. Z. Al-Riyami, M. Al-Khabori, R. M. Al-Hadhrami et al., "The pneumatic tube system does not affect complete blood count results; a validation study at a tertiary care hospital," *International Journal of Laboratory Hematology*, vol. 36, no. 5, pp. 514–520, 2014.

[10] F. Emel Koçak, M. Yöntem, Ö. Yücel, M. Çilo, Ö. Genç, and A. Meral, "The effects of transport by pneumatic tube system on blood cell count, erythrocyte sedimentation and coagulation tests," *Biochemia Medica*, vol. 23, no. 2, pp. 206–210, 2012.

[11] G. Kecskemétiné, Z. Csiki, M. Mile, K. S. Zsóri, and A. H. Shemirani, "The clinical significance of pneumatic tube transport system on platelet indices: EDTA or citrate anticoagulant?" *International Journal of Laboratory Hematology*, vol. 39, no. 4, pp. e102–e105, 2017.

[12] A. Lee, H. Suk Suh, C. Jeon, and S. Kim, "Effects of one directional pneumatic tube system on routine hematology and chemistry parameters; A validation study at a tertiary care hospital," *Practical Laboratory Medicine*, vol. 9, pp. 12–17, 2017.

13

Donor Specific Anti-HLA Antibody and Risk of Graft Failure in Haploidentical Stem Cell Transplantation

Piyanuch Kongtim,[1,2] Kai Cao,[3] and Stefan O. Ciurea[1]

[1]Department of Stem Cell Transplant and Cellular Therapy, The University of Texas MD Anderson Cancer Center, Houston, TX 77030, USA
[2]Division of Hematology, Department of Internal Medicine, Faculty of Medicine, Thammasat University, Pathumthani 12120, Thailand
[3]Department of Laboratory Medicine, The University of Texas MD Anderson Cancer Center, Houston, TX 77030, USA

Correspondence should be addressed to Stefan O. Ciurea; sciurea@mdanderson.org

Academic Editor: Suparno Chakrabarti

Outcomes of allogeneic hematopoietic stem cell transplantation (AHSCT) using HLA-half matched related donors (haploidentical) have recently improved due to better control of alloreactive reactions in both graft-versus-host and host-versus-graft directions. The recognition of the role of humoral rejection in the development of primary graft failure in this setting has broadened our understanding about causes of engraftment failure in these patients, helped us better select donors for patients in need of AHSCT, and developed rational therapeutic measures for HLA sensitized patients to prevent this unfortunate event, which is usually associated with a very high mortality rate. With these recent advances the rate of graft failure in haploidentical transplantation has decreased to less than 5%.

1. Introduction

Allogeneic hematopoietic stem cell transplantation (AHSCT) using one human leukocyte antigen (HLA) haplotype matched first-degree relative donor (haploidentical donor) represents an alternative treatment for patients with hematologic malignancies who lack HLA-matched related or unrelated donor. Historically, the main limitations of this treatment modality were high rate of graft failure (GF) and graft-versus-host disease (GVHD), which occur due to intense alloreactive reactions related to the major HLA mismatch between the recipient and the donor. Although several approaches have been developed which aimed to partially deplete T cells in the graft and decrease graft-versus-host alloreactivity, GF remains a major obstacle [1–3]. While increased rate of engraftment has occurred with the use of "megadoses" of hematopoietic stem cells (over 10 million $CD34^+$ cells/kg with a very low T cell content) (1×10^4 $CD3^+$ cells/kg) [4, 5], approximately 10–20% of patients still developed GF [6–8]. The increased risk of GF following haploidentical stem cell transplant (haploSCT) is due, in part, to an enhanced susceptibility of the graft to regimen-resistant host natural killer (NK) cell- and T lymphocyte-mediated rejection against mismatched donor cells [9, 10]. In addition to T cell- and NK-cell-mediated graft rejection (cellular rejection), antibody-mediated rejection (humoral rejection) occurring either by antibody-dependent cell-mediated cytotoxicity or complement mediated cytotoxicity has been described [11, 12]. Preformed donor-specific anti-HLA antibodies (DSAs) present at the time of transplant have been shown to be correlated with graft rejection and decrease survival in solid organ transplantation [13–16]. Therefore, lymphocyte crossmatch tests have been developed for prediction of graft rejection [17, 18] and became mandatory in solid organ transplant according to the American Society for Histocompatibility and Immunogenetics (ASHI). In AHSCT setting, there has been reported that a positive crossmatch for anti-donor lymphocytotoxic antibody associated strongly with GF, mainly in mismatched or haploSCT patients [19, 20]. Although a lymphocyte crossmatch is an effective tool to evaluate alloimmunization and potential donor-recipient incompatibility, the procedure is labor intensive and may detect non-HLA antibodies, which may not be associated with transplant outcome since there is no data to confirm the importance of these antibodies to date. Over the recent years, several methods have been developed to more precisely detect and characterize DSAs in AHSCT recipients [21, 22], and also the clear association between the presence of these antibodies and GF has been confirmed especially in mismatched and haploSCT patients [14, 23, 24]. Still, the mechanisms by which DSA may cause GF in AHSCT remain an area of active research.

Here we review the potential mechanisms and clinical importance of DSAs on GF in haploSCT, as well as treatment modalities used for DSA desensitization before transplant to abrogate the risk of GF and improve transplant outcomes.

2. Mechanisms of Graft Rejection in Haploidentical Stem Cell Transplantation

Engraftment failure rate has been approximately 4% in AHSCT using matched unrelated donors and about 20% in umbilical cord blood (UCB) or T cell-depleted haploSCT [25, 26]. The common cause of GF is host immunologic reaction against donor cells, so called graft rejection. Graft rejection following haploSCT is generally attributed to cytolytic host-versus-graft reaction mediated by host T and/or NK-cells that survived the conditioning regimen. However, antibody-mediated graft rejection (otherwise known as humoral rejection) has been increasingly recognized in the past decade.

2.1. Cellular-Mediated Graft Rejection. The resistance to engraftment of AHSCT was thought to be mediated primarily by recipient T lymphocytes which depends on the genetic disparity between the donor and recipient and the status of host antidonor reactivity [27]. This makes mismatched and haploSCT recipients likely more susceptible to develop graft rejection compared with matched AHSCT due to stronger alloreactive reactions in this setting. It has been found in animal model of stem cell transplantation that antidonor cytotoxic T cells sensitized to major and minor histocompatibility (MHC) antigens confer resistance against allogeneic bone marrow stem cells [28]. This finding also has been confirmed in clinical studies of AHSCT in patients with severe aplastic anemia, in which the presence of radioresistant antidonor cytotoxic T cell populations sensitized to donor MHC antigens through repeated blood transfusions is associated with a higher incidence of graft rejection and death [29]. Nevertheless, the molecular bases underlying T cell-mediated graft rejection remain incompletely defined.

NK-mediated graft rejection also has been demonstrated in animal models [9, 30, 31]. In preclinical models of bone marrow transplantation, radioresistant host NK-cells are also capable of lysing donor hematopoietic cell targets and rejecting bone marrow grafts, especially those that lack expression of MHC class I antigens [32]. Evidence that NK-cells mediate resistance to engraftment in clinical AHSCT is lacking, due in part to the difficulty of discriminating T cell- from NK-cell-mediated resistance in humans.

In haploSCT, the use of myeloablative conditioning chemotherapy and high-dose posttransplant cyclophosphamide can diminish these cellular-mediated immune reactions due to the fact that both human T cells and NK-cells are highly sensitive to cyclophosphamide, which is now commonly used after haploSCT to prevent GVHD [33].

2.2. Antibody-Mediated Graft Rejection. Antibody-mediated graft rejection has been a major obstacle and well recognized cause of rejection and organ dysfunction in solid organ transplants, especially in kidney transplantation, because transplanted kidneys are highly susceptible to antibody-mediated injury [34–36]. In animal models of AHSCT, preformed antibodies present at the time of marrow infusion in multitransfused mice, rather than primed T cells, have been shown to be a major barrier against marrow engraftment resulting in rapid graft rejection within a few hours in allosensitized recipients of MHC mismatched bone marrow transplantation while T cell-mediated graft rejection takes much longer [12, 37]. The risk of antibody-associated graft rejection in human depends on antigen density on the target and capacities of the antibody Fc-domain. While many types of preformed antibodies can be detected in alloimmunized stem cell transplant recipients, only antibodies against donor HLA antigens have been shown to have clinical significance [38–40].

3. Role of Complement System in DSA-Mediated Graft Rejection

Antibody-mediated BM failure after AHSCT can occur either by antibody-dependent cell-mediated cytotoxicity or by complement mediated cytotoxicity [41]. Evidence from studies in cardiac and renal transplant patients has shown that complement system is activated in the transplanted organ during rejection and can be detected by measuring the products of complement activation in the patients' blood and urine as well as in the transplanted organ itself [42–45]. In haploSCT setting, we recently found that DSAs that bind complement, detected by the C1q assay, the first component of the classical complement pathway, plays an important role in the development of graft rejection in haploSCT recipients. In this study, the presence of C1q-fixing DSA was found in 9 of 22 patients who had DSAs and was associated with a significantly higher rate of GF compared with patients who had DSAs but negative C1q. Moreover, 4 patients who became negative C1q after treatment with plasmapheresis and immunosuppressive therapies before transplant could engraft with donor cells successfully while 5 patients who remained positive C1q experienced GF [46]. Previous studies by Chen showed that there is no predictability by IgG mean fluorescence intensity (MFI) as to which of the antibodies will bind C1q because fixation is independent of MFI values [47]. However, most patients who had positive C1q in our study had higher median MFI of DSAs (all more than 5,000 MFI) compared with those who had negative C1q [46]. These results suggest that the possibility of complement fixation might depend on both ability and level of DSAs.

4. Prevalence and Risk Factors for the Development of DSAs in Haploidentical Stem Cell Transplantation

Anti-HLA antibodies can be found in healthy individuals as a consequence of allosensitization during pregnancy or related to either previous transplant with mismatched donor or multiple transfusions of blood products and the clinical significance of anti-HLA antibodies is well known in the field of transfusion medicine. The presence of anti-HLA antibodies in patients is one of the major causes of platelet refractoriness [57]. On the other hand, anti-HLA antibodies present in blood products have been shown to be a major cause of transfusion-related acute lung injury (TRALI) [58]. According to previous reports in healthy blood donors, anti-HLA antibodies could be identified up to 50% depending on sensitivity of the test used for screening [59–61]. The reported prevalence of anti-HLA antibodies is of approximately 20–25% in patients undergoing haploSCT [40, 48, 49].

Despite a high prevalence of anti-HLA antibodies reported in AHSCT patients, these anti-HLA antibodies might not be specific to donor HLA antigens. A delay in recognizing this as a major cause of GF in AHSCT could be because hematopoietic transplantation has been performed mostly with a high degree of HLA matching between the donor and recipient. The increasing use of mismatched donors (haploidentical, cord blood, and mismatched unrelated donors), in addition to improvements in detection techniques, has facilitated recognizing DSAs as a major cause of graft rejection in stem cell transplantation. With the use of highly sensitive solid-phase immunoassays, DSAs were identified in up to 24% of stem cell transplant recipients [3, 23, 24, 39, 48, 51, 62]. While, overall, in haploSCT the prevalence of DSAs may range between approximately 10 and 21% [22, 46, 48, 49], this proportion is highly dependent on the recipient's gender with very low prevalence in male recipients (5%) as compared with female recipients (86%) [43]. Anti-HLA antibodies detected in female patients are much more often DSAs in the settings of "child-to-mother" haploSCT compared to the settings of CBT [22, 50]. It is because those anti-HLA antibodies are the results of sensitization during pregnancies by offspring's HLA itself and it makes it often difficult to locate a donor who is not a target of anti-HLA antibodies. Thus it is particularly important to establish an effective desensitization protocol in the setting of haploSCT.

A few studies evaluated transplant outcomes in relation to non-donor-specific anti-HLA antibodies (non-DSAs) in various donor types of AHSCT [38–40]. Takanashi and colleagues reported a similar rate of engraftment in cord blood stem cell transplant recipients who had anti-HLA antibodies without the corresponding HLA in the transplanted cord blood compared with recipients without anti-HLA antibodies, while rate of engraftment in recipients who had anti-HLA antibodies corresponding with donor cord blood HLA (DSAs) was significantly lower [38]. Similar results were found in the study by the Eurocord group, which reported no difference in neutrophil engraftment after single or double UCB transplants in 32 recipients with non-DSAs,

compared to 158 patients without HLA antibodies [39]. Also, in a retrospective study of recipients of matched unrelated stem cell transplants, we found that alloimmunization as such did not cause a significant increase risk of GF unless antibodies were directed against the donor HLA antigens, suggesting that DSA is the key to the development of GF in AHSCT [40].

It is well recognized in solid organ transplantation that repeated transfusion is a major risk factor of developing DSAs [63, 64]. DSA developed after transfusion is also an important barrier of successful engraftment in patients with severe aplastic anemia [11] and other thalassemia or hemoglobinopathies [65].

Additionally, there is a strong evidence to suggest that female sex and pregnancy confer a significant risk for allosensitization, and this risk is further increased with a higher number of pregnancies. Our group has formerly observed a striking association between the sex of patients who experience GF and the development of allosensitization. In our study of haploSCT, we found that all patients who developed DSAs were multiparous young women with a median of 3 pregnancies; 30% of women versus 12% of men had DSAs ($P < 0.0001$) and 7 of 8 patients with DSAs were women, all of whom except 1 had at least 2 prior pregnancies. When the presence of DSAs was evaluated in women with no pregnancies compared with the male recipients, no significant association was identified. Although the majority of allosensitized individuals in this study were women, 12% of patients with anti-HLA antibodies were men, suggesting that other factors are associated with the development of anti-HLA antibodies in these patients, most likely related to transfusion of blood products [22].

5. Testing for Anti-HLA Antibodies

5.1. DSA Testing. Pretransplant sera of patient are tested for anti-HLA class I and class II antibodies using multianalyte bead assays performed on the Luminex platform including LABScreen® PRA, LABScreen Mixed methods for screening; the binding level of DSA is determined by the LABScreen Single Antigen bead assay (One Lambda, Part of Thermo Fisher Scientific, Canoga Park, California, USA) per manufacturer's instructions and results are expressed as mean fluorescence intensity (MFI). Briefly, $5\,\mu$L of mixed beads, HLA class I and class II single antigen beads, is added to $20\,\mu$L of sample serum and incubated for 30 min at room temperature (RT) in the dark with gentle shaking. After washing with wash buffer three times, $100\,\mu$L of goat anti-human IgG secondary antibody conjugated with R-phycoerythrin (PE) is added and the samples are incubated in the dark for 30 min at RT. After washing three times, the samples are read on Luminex-based LABScan™ 100 flow analyzer. Antibody specificity and binding level are analyzed and determined through HLA Visual or HLA Fusion software from the manufacturer.

5.2. C1q Testing. Complement binding antibodies are detected for patients with DSA using the C1q assay. The complement component (C1q) bound by the antigen-antibody complex is detected with R-PE labeled anti-C1q antibody.

Fluorescence intensity is measured using Luminex-based LABScan 100 flow analyzer. DSA specificity and binding level are determined by the C1qScreen™ assay per manufacturer's instructions [One Lambda, Part of Thermo Fisher Scientific (Canoga Park, California, USA)]. Briefly, 5 μL of human C1q and 5 μL of HLA class I and class II single antigen beads are added to 5 μL of heat-inactivated sample serum and incubated for 20 min in dark at RT, followed by adding 5 μL of R-PE labeled anti-C1q antibody and incubation for 20 min in dark at RT. The samples are read and C1q specific antibody specificity and binding levels are analyzed and determined.

6. DSA and Haploidentical Stem Cell Transplant Outcomes

Multiple investigators have demonstrated that DSAs are associated with primary GF in either mismatched related (haploidentical), matched, and mismatched unrelated donor or UCB transplants (Table 1). This association appears more discernable in haploSCT presumably due to the close relationship and higher likelihood of sharing the mismatched HLA antigens with DSAs against the immediate family.

Back in 2009, our group initially showed that DSAs are associated with primary GF in AHSCT with mismatched donors [22]. We tested 24 consecutive patients including a total of 28 haploSCTs with "megadoses" of $CD34^+$ stem cells for the presence of DSAs determined by a highly sensitive and specific solid-phase/single antigen assay. DSAs were detected in 5 patients (21%). Three out of 4 (75%) patients with DSAs prior to transplant failed to engraft, compared with only 1 out of 20 (5%) without DSAs ($P = 0.008$). All 4 patients who experienced primary GF had second haploSCT and 1 patient who had persistent high titer of DSAs developed a second GF, while 2 out of 3 engrafted patients had the absence of DSAs [22]. Patients in this study had DSAs directed against high-expression HLA loci, including class I HLA antigens (HLA-A and HLA-B) and class II (HLA-DRB1) antigens. In a later study, we found that anti-HLA antibodies directed against low-expression loci (HLA-DPB1 and HLA-DQB1) are also associated with graft rejection, however, to a lower extent. In our large prospectively tested patients for HLA antibodies of 592 matched unrelated AHSCT recipients, anti-HLA antibodies that were not reactive with donor loci were identified in 116 patients (19.6%), whereas DSAs were found only in 8 patients (1.4%) in this population, all directed against the HLA-DPB1 molecule. Overall, GF occurred in 19 of 592 patients (3.4%), including 16 of 584 (2.7%) patients without DSAs compared with 3 of 8 (37.5%) patients with DSAs ($P = 0.0014$). As noted above, we have found that the presence of anti-HLA antibodies in the absence of DSAs did not predict graft failure. In multivariate analysis, DSA was the only factor that predicted GF in these patients [40]. Recently we reported outcomes of 122 patients receiving haploSCT including 22 patients with DSAs. Results from this study were consistent with the previous reports, a significantly higher proportion of DSA-positive patients experienced GF (32%) compared with DSA negative patients (4%; $P < 0.001$) [46].

In another study in haploSCT by Yoshihara and colleagues, the authors tested anti-HLA antibodies in 79 patients receiving haploSCT. Among 79 screened patients, 16 (20.2%) were anti-HLA antibodies-positive, including 5 non-DSA-positive and 11 DSA-positive patients. The cumulative incidence of donor neutrophil engraftment was significantly lower in DSA-positive patients than in DSA-negative patients (61.9 versus 94.4%, $P = 0.026$) [48]. Furthermore the most recent study by Chang and colleagues also confirmed a significantly higher rate of primary graft rejection (20% versus 0.3%) and poor graft function (27.3% versus 1.9%) in haploSCT who developed DSAs before transplant compared with recipients without DSAs.

The clinical importance of DSAs has also been confirmed in other donor types of AHSCT. In a retrospective case controlled study by Spellman and colleagues, they have demonstrated that the prevalence of DSAs was higher in a group of mismatched unrelated donor-recipients who suffered graft rejection than in a control group that engrafted. Among the 37 recipients who failed to engraft, 9 (24%) had DSAs against HLA-A, HLA-B, or HLA-DP, whereas DSA was identified in only 1 of 78 patients in the control group who successfully engrafted [23].

Same results have also been demonstrated in some studies in patients receiving umbilical cord stem cell transplant as summarized in Table 1.

Besides GF, some investigators have shown that patients with DSAs had significantly lower event-free survival as well as overall survival compared with those without DSAs [24, 39, 50]. Though the results from these studies have clearly confirmed that the presence of DSAs influences graft outcomes and survival in haploSCT, we need to bear in mind that different cut-off levels of DSAs as well as different methods of DSAs detection were used in these studies. The definition of a threshold for DSAs, according to MFI, is a premise for analyzing the association of DSAs with GF. In a case-control study conducted by us, MFI of 500 or more was considered positive [40], while, in haploSCT, MFI values of more than 1500 or 5000 were defined as significant by our group [22] and by Yoshihara et al. [48], respectively. An important difference between these two studies is that our study was done in patients treated with a T cell-depleted graft, while the second one was done in patients treated with a T cell replete graft with ATG or intensified GVHD prophylaxis. It is possible that stem cells without T cells are more exposed to the HLA antigens as the only targets available for the DSAs and by the lack of contribution of donor T cells to engraftment and eradication of recipient's alloreactive T cells. Recently, Chang and colleagues also showed that positive DSA at MFI of 10,000 or more was correlated to primary graft rejection while MFI of 2,000 or more was strongly associated with primary poor graft function [49]. So far the conclusion from these published studies is that a very strong titer of DSA, which may be revealed by serum dilution or titration for those false-low or false negative antibodies defined by the MFI in the solid-phase immunoassays, poses an absolute contraindication to transplantation (in the absence of treatment), whereas very weak antibodies may be considered as a relative contraindication for transplantation. Although the standard cut-off level of DSAs that is considered safe for transplant

TABLE 1: DSAs and transplant outcomes.

Reference	Donor	Test	N	%Anti-HLA+	%DSA+	Graft outcome (DSA+/DSA−)	Comment
Ciurea et al. 2009 [22]	TCD HaploSCT	Luminex SA	24	NA	21	GF was 75% versus 5% ($P = 0.008$)	
Spellman et al. 2010 [23]	MMUD	FlowPRA, Luminex SA	115	37	8.7	24% of GF group had DSAs versus 1% of control group that had DSAs	
Ciurea et al. 2011 [3]	MUD, 1 Ag MMUD	Luminex SA	592	21	1.4	GF was 37.5% versus 2.7% ($P = 0.0014$)	
Yoshihara et al. 2012 [48]	HaploSCT	Luminex SA	79	20	14	GF was 27% versus 4% CI of neutrophil engraftment was 61.9% versus 94.4%, ($P = 0.026$)	(i) 5 patients were desensitized and 3/5 engrafted (ii) 67, 5, and 7 patients were antibody-negative, non-DSA-positive, and DSA-positive after desensitization
Ciurea et al. 2015 [46]	HaploSCT	Luminex SA	122	NA	18	GF was 32% versus 4% ($P < 0.001$)	
Chang et al. 2015 [49]	HaploSCT	NA	345	25.2	11.3	Primary graft rejection was 20% versus 0.3% ($P = 0.002$) Primary poor graft function was 27.3% versus 1.9% ($P = 0.003$)	
Takanashi et al. 2010 [50]	Single UCB	FlowPRA, Luminex SA	386	23.1	5	CI of neutrophil engraftment was 32% versus 83% ($P < 0.0001$)	Patients with DSA had significantly lower EFS and OS compared with no DSA
Brunstein et al. 2011 [51]	Double UCB	Luminex SA	126	41	24% had DSAs target to 1 UCB, 12% had DSA target to both UCB	GF was 17% versus 22%	
Cutler et al. 2011 [24]	Double UCB	Luminex SA	73	NA	24.6	GF was 18.2% and 57% in patients who had DSAs against 1 and 2 UCB, respectively, versus 5.5% in patients without DSAs ($P = 0.01$)	The rates of death or relapse within 100 days for the group of patients without DSAs, with DSAs against a single UCB unit, or DSAs against both UCB units were 23.6%, 36.4%, and 71.4%, respectively ($P = 0.01$)
Ruggeri et al. 2013 [39]	Single UCB, double UCB	Luminex SA	294	21	4.7	GF was 56% versus 23%	The presence of DSA was associated with lower survival (42% versus 29%; $P = 0.07$).

MMUD: mismatched unrelated donor; MUD: matched unrelated donor; GF: graft failure; DSA: donor specific antibody; TCD HaploSCT: T cell-depleted haploidentical stem cell transplant; UCB: umbilical cord blood; EFS: event-free survival; OS: overall survival; NA: not available.

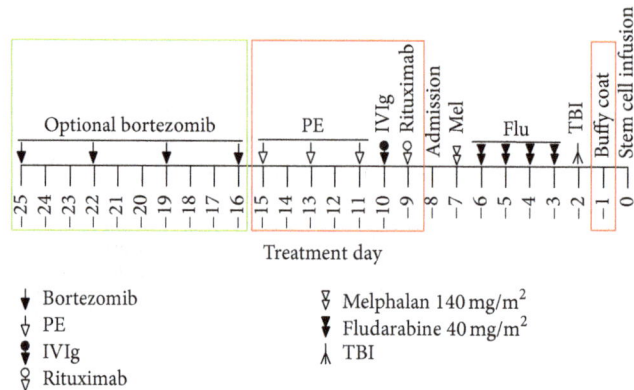

FIGURE 1: Desensitization approach for patients with DSAs undergoing haploidentical stem cell transplantation at MD Anderson Cancer Center.

still needs to be determined, it is likely that other transplant factors need to be taken into consideration.

7. Desensitization Therapy for Allosensitized Recipients

Preformed antibodies present at the time of stem cell infusion are unaffected by standard transplantation conditioning regimens or T cell or B-cell immunosuppressive or modulatory strategies given in the peritransplantation period. To reduce the risk of GF, a number of studies have reported beneficial effects of a variety of interventions used to reduce total anti-HLA antibody load, predominantly by using a combined approach [66]. Reversal of DSAs mediated graft rejection and reduction in antibody load by using plasmapheresis, intravenous immunoglobulin (IVIg), cyclophosphamide, polyclonal anti-lymphocyte antibodies, monoclonal antibodies to CD20$^+$ B lymphocytes (rituximab), and proteasome inhibitor against alloantibody producing plasma cells (bortezomib) have been described in solid organ transplant. However, their effectiveness is modest [67–71]. These treatment modalities also have been used to desensitize DSAs in haploSCT and mismatched AHSCT recipients with a variety of graft outcomes as summarized in Table 2. The first case was reported by Barge and colleagues in 1989; a patient with positive crossmatch test with donor lymphocytes was treated with plasmapheresis before haploSCT but did not result in a negative crossmatch before transplant and subsequently developed GF [41]. Maruta et al. confirmed that repeated high-volume plasmapheresis does not effectively eliminate preformed anti-HLA antibodies and applied adsorption of HLA-antibodies to irradiated donor lymphocytes before marrow transplantation for a successful engraftment [52]. We were the first to use a combined approach using plasmapheresis, IVIg, and rituximab with mixed results: out of the first 4 patients treated with this approach 2 achieved a significant reduction in antibody levels and engrafted the donor cells whereas the other 2 patients maintained high levels of DSAs and experienced primary GF [22]. Yoshihara et al. have tried 3 desensitization approaches for 5 patients who were to receive both bone marrow and peripheral blood stem

cell grafts from haploidentical donors. Treatment regimen in this study was a combination of plasmapheresis, rituximab, antibody adsorption with platelets, and administration of the proteasome inhibitor, bortezomib. One of the 2 patients treated with plasmapheresis and rituximab received plasmapheresis on day −11 and the other received plasmapheresis on days −17, −15, and −13. Both were given a single dose of rituximab at 375 mg/mm^2. DSA reduction was achieved in only 1 of 2 patients. However, both engrafted. Some of the most impressive reductions of DSAs were achieved by using 40 units of platelet transfusion from healthy donors selected to have the HLA antigens corresponding to the DSAs [48]. In a more recent study, in addition to 3 doses of alternating plasmapheresis every other day followed by 1 dose of IVIg and rituximab, we added an irradiated buffy coat infusion on day −1 prepared from 1 unit of blood on day −2 instead of using platelet transfusion to try to block remaining circulating antibodies after treatment as platelet has only class I HLA antigens on their surface (Figure 1) [46]. Moreover, in this study we have also found that what is more important appears to be the absence of C1q after treatment (conversion from C1q positivity to negativity) not merely the reduction of antibody levels. All 5 patients who remained C1q positive after treatment with plasmapheresis, IVIg, and rituximab with or without buffy coat prepared from donors experienced engraftment failure, whereas all 4 patients who became C1q negative after treatment/before transplant engrafted the donor cells. Although antibody level did not significantly change early on, all patients eventually clear the antibodies completely in the first few weeks after transplant [46]. These results suggested to us that a reduction to noncomplement binding level of DSAs should be the goal of treatment rather than clearing of the noncomplement binding DSAs, which appear to clear more slowly in the immediate posttransplant period and became undetectable in all patients within the first few weeks after transplant, similar to prior experience [72]. Although our experience is limited, this approach has been very successful as none of the patients treated as such experienced primary GF. A different approach was developed by the John Hopkins group from solid organ transplants, using a combination of repeated

TABLE 2: DSA desensitization in haploidentical and mismatched related AHSCT.

Reference	Donor type (N)	Anti-HLA abs test	Desensitization method	MFI after treatment	Graft outcome
Barge et al. 1989 [41]	Haplo (N = 1)	CDC	Plasmapheresis	NA	Graft failure
Maruta et al. 1991 [52]	Mismatched related (N = 1)	AHG-CDC	CyA, methylpred, Plasmapheresis, DLI	Negative XM	Engrafted
Braun et al. 2000 [53]	Haplo (N = 1)	FCXM	Staphylococcal protein A immunoadsorption	Negative XM	Engrafted
Ottinger et al. 2002 [20]	Mismatched related (N = 2)	DTT-CDC	Plasmapheresis, mismatched platelet transfusion	1 patient with negative XM, 1 patient with positive XM	Patient with negative XM after treatment engrafted, while patients with positive XM had GF
Pollack and Ririe 2004 [54]	Mismatched HLA-A68 related (N = 1)	FCXM	Platelet transfusion, plasmapheresis, IVIg	Negative XM	Engrafted
Narimatsu et al. 2005 [55]	Mismatched related (N = 1)	AHG-LCT	Rituximab, platelet transfusion	Negative AHG-LCT	Engrafted
Ciurea et al. 2009 [22]	Haplo (N = 4)	Luminex MFI >500	Rituximab, plasmapheresis	1 negative, 1 low titer, 2 high titers	Patients with DSAs negative and low titer after treatment engrafted; 2 patients with high titer had GF
Yoshihara et al. 2012 [48]	Haplo (N = 5)	Luminex MFI >500	Plasmapheresis + rituximab (N = 2), platelet transfusion (N = 2), bortezomib + dexa (N = 1)	1 patient had temporary DSA reduction and 1 patient had significant reduction after plasmapheresis; 2 patients had a significant reduction post platelet transfusion; 1 patient had moderate DSA reduction after bortezomib and dexa	All patients engrafted
Ciurea et al. 2015 [46]	Haplo (N = 12)	Luminex MFI >500	Plasmapheresis + rituximab + IVIg (N = 5), PE + rituximab + IVIg + donor buffy coat infusion (N = 7)	No significant change of MFI before transplant All patients cleared DSA after transplant	5 patients with C1q positive after treatment had GF while patients who became C1q negative engrafted
Leffell et al. 2015 [56]	Haplo (N = 13) MMUD (N = 2)	Luminex MFI >1000	Plasmapheresis + IVIg	Mean reduction of DSAs after treatment was 64.4%. 1 patient failed to reduce DSAs to the level that was thought to be safe for transplant	All 14/14 transplanted patients engrafted

MFI: mean fluorescence intensity; CDC: complement mediated cytotoxic; XM: crossmatch, FCXM: flow cytometric crossmatch, GF: graft failure; AHG-LCT: anti-human immunoglobulin lymphocytotoxicity test; NA: not available; MMUD: mismatched unrelated donor.

plasmapheresis, IVIg, and immunosuppressive medications. This group treated 15 mismatched AHSCT patients including 13 haploSCTs with alternate day of single volume plasmapheresis followed by 100 mg/kg of IVIg, tacrolimus (1 mg/day, i.v.), and mycophenolate mofetil (1 g twice daily) starting 1-2 weeks before the beginning of transplant conditioning, depending on patient's starting DSA levels. Reduction of DSA to the level that was thought safe for transplant was seen in 14 of 15 patients, all of these 14 patients engrafted with donor cells [56]. Even though, the majority of these studies have been anecdotal and included only a few patients but taken together have indicated that reduction of DSA to low levels can permit successful engraftment.

8. Conclusions

In the past 5 years much has been learned about the risks posed by DSAs in the development of primary GF in AHSCT with mismatched donors. These findings have impacted donor selection and helped the development of preventive treatments for allosensitized patients, who now can more safely undergo a transplant with a major HLA mismatched donor. Future studies will explore the pathogenesis of antibody-mediated rejection and develop effective therapies for allosensitized recipients.

Conflict of Interests

The authors declare that there is no conflict of interests regarding the publication of this paper.

References

[1] R. J. O'Reilly, C. Keever, N. A. Kernan et al., "HLA nonidentical T cell depleted marrow transplants: a comparison of results in patients treated for leukemia and severe combined immunodeficiency disease," *Transplantation Proceedings*, vol. 19, no. 6, supplement 7, pp. 55–60, 1987.

[2] R. C. Ash, M. M. Horowitz, R. P. Gale et al., "Bone marrow transplantation from related donors other than HLA-identical siblings: effect of T cell depletion," *Bone Marrow Transplantation*, vol. 7, no. 6, pp. 443–452, 1991.

[3] S. O. Ciurea, V. Mulanovich, Y. Jiang et al., "Lymphocyte recovery predicts outcomes in cord blood and T cell-depleted haploidentical stem cell transplantation," *Biology of Blood and Marrow Transplantation*, vol. 17, no. 8, pp. 1169–1175, 2011.

[4] F. Aversa, A. Tabilio, A. Velardi et al., "Treatment of high-risk acute leukemia with T-cell-depleted stem cells from related donors with one fully mismatched hla haplotype," *The New England Journal of Medicine*, vol. 339, no. 17, pp. 1186–1193, 1998.

[5] E. Bachar-Lustig, N. Rachamim, H.-W. Li, F. Lan, and Y. Reisner, "Megadose of T cell-depleted bone marrow overcomes MHC barriers in sublethally irradiated mice," *Nature Medicine*, vol. 1, no. 12, pp. 1268–1273, 1995.

[6] P. Lang, J. Greil, P. Bader et al., "Long-term outcome after haploidentical stem cell transplantation in children," *Blood Cells, Molecules, and Diseases*, vol. 33, no. 3, pp. 281–287, 2004.

[7] F. Ciceri, M. Labopin, F. Aversa et al., "A survey of fully haploidentical hematopoietic stem cell transplantation in adults with high-risk acute leukemia: a risk factor analysis of outcomes

for patients in remission at transplantation," *Blood*, vol. 112, no. 9, pp. 3574–3581, 2008.

[8] L.-P. Koh, D. A. Rizzieri, and N. J. Chao, "Allogeneic hematopoietic stem cell transplant using mismatched/haploidentical donors," *Biology of Blood and Marrow Transplantation*, vol. 13, no. 11, pp. 1249–1267, 2007.

[9] W. J. Murphy, V. Kumar, and M. Bennett, "Acute rejection of murine bone marrow allografts by natural killer cells and T cells. Differences in kinetics and target antigens recognized," *Journal of Experimental Medicine*, vol. 166, no. 5, pp. 1499–1509, 1987.

[10] C. Bordignon, N. A. Kernan, C. A. Keever et al., "The role of residual host immunity in graft failures following T-cell-depleted marrow transplants for leukemia," *Annals of the New York Academy of Sciences*, vol. 511, pp. 442–446, 1987.

[11] R. P. Warren, R. Storb, P. L. Weiden, P. J. Su, and E. D. Thomas, "Lymphocyte-mediated cytotoxicity and antibody-dependent cell-mediated cytotoxicity in patients with aplastic anemia: distinguishing transfusion-induced sensitization from possible immune-mediated aplastic anemia," *Transplantation Proceedings*, vol. 13, no. 1, part 1, pp. 245–247, 1981.

[12] H. Xu, P. M. Chilton, M. K. Tanner et al., "Humoral immunity is the dominant barrier for allogeneic bone marrow engraftment in sensitized recipients," *Blood*, vol. 108, no. 10, pp. 3611–3619, 2006.

[13] N. Suciu-Foca, E. Reed, C. Marboe et al., "The role of anti-HLA antibodies in heart transplantation," *Transplantation*, vol. 51, no. 3, pp. 716–724, 1991.

[14] P. I. Terasaki and M. Ozawa, "Predicting kidney graft failure by HLA antibodies: a prospective trial," *American Journal of Transplantation*, vol. 4, no. 3, pp. 438–443, 2004.

[15] Q. Mao, P. I. Terasaki, J. Cai et al., "Extremely high association between appearance of HLA antibodies and failure of kidney grafts in a five-year longitudinal study," *American Journal of Transplantation*, vol. 7, no. 4, pp. 864–871, 2007.

[16] R. M. McKenna, S. K. Takemoto, and P. I. Terasaki, "Anti-HLA antibodies after solid organ transplantation," *Transplantation*, vol. 69, no. 3, pp. 319–326, 2000.

[17] A. Ting, T. Hasegawa, S. Ferrone, and R. A. Reisfeld, "Presensitization detected by sensitive crossmatch tests," *Transplantation Proceedings*, vol. 5, no. 1, pp. 813–817, 1973.

[18] A. A. Zachary, L. Klingman, N. Thorne, A. R. Smerglia, and G. A. Teresi, "Variations of the lymphocytotoxicity test. An evaluation of sensitivity and specificity," *Transplantation*, vol. 60, no. 5, pp. 498–503, 1995.

[19] C. Anasetti, D. Amos, P. G. Beatty et al., "Effect of HLA compatibility on engraftment of bone marrow transplants in patients with leukemia or lymphoma," *The New England Journal of Medicine*, vol. 320, no. 4, pp. 197–204, 1989.

[20] H. D. Ottinger, V. Rebmann, K. A. Pfeiffer et al., "Positive serum crossmatch as predictor for graft failure in HLA-mismatched allogeneic blood stem cell transplantation," *Transplantation*, vol. 73, no. 8, pp. 1280–1285, 2002.

[21] R. Pei, J.-H. Lee, N.-J. Shih, M. Chen, and P. I. Terasaki, "Single human leukocyte antigen flow cytometry beads for accurate identification of human leukocyte antigen antibody specificities," *Transplantation*, vol. 75, no. 1, pp. 43–49, 2003.

[22] S. O. Ciurea, M. de Lima, P. Cano et al., "High risk of graft failure in patients with anti-HLA antibodies undergoing haploidentical stem-cell transplantation," *Transplantation*, vol. 88, no. 8, pp. 1019–1024, 2009.

[23] S. Spellman, R. Bray, S. Rosen-Bronson et al., "The detection of donor-directed, HLA-specific alloantibodies in recipients of unrelated hematopoietic cell transplantation is predictive of graft failure," *Blood*, vol. 115, no. 13, pp. 2704–2708, 2010.

[24] C. Cutler, H. T. Kim, L. Sun et al., "Donor-specific anti-HLA antibodies predict outcome in double umbilical cord blood transplantation," *Blood*, vol. 118, no. 25, pp. 6691–6697, 2011.

[25] S. M. Davies, C. Kollman, C. Anasetti et al., "Engraftment and survival after unrelated-donor bone marrow transplantation: a report from the national marrow donor program," *Blood*, vol. 96, no. 13, pp. 4096–4102, 2000.

[26] P. Rubinstein, C. Carrier, A. Scaradavou et al., "Outcomes among 562 recipients of placental-blood transplants from unrelated donors," *The New England Journal of Medicine*, vol. 339, no. 22, pp. 1565–1577, 1998.

[27] N. A. Kernan, N. H. Collins, L. Juliano, T. Cartagena, B. Dupont, and R. J. O'Reilly, "Clonable T lymphocytes in T cell-depleted bone marrow transplants correlate with development of graft-v-host disease," *Blood*, vol. 68, no. 3, pp. 770–773, 1986.

[28] H. Nakamura and R. E. Gress, "Graft rejection by cytolytic T cells. Specificity of the effector mechanism in the rejection of allogeneic marrow," *Transplantation*, vol. 49, no. 2, pp. 453–458, 1990.

[29] K. Doney, W. Leisenring, R. Storb, and F. R. Appelbaum, "Primary treatment of acquired aplastic anemia: outcomes with bone marrow transplantation and immunosuppressive therapy," *Annals of Internal Medicine*, vol. 126, no. 2, pp. 107–115, 1997.

[30] G. Cudkowicz and M. Bennett, "Peculiar immunobiology of bone marrow allografts. I. Graft rejection by irradiated responder mice," *Journal of Experimental Medicine*, vol. 134, no. 1, pp. 83–102, 1971.

[31] R. Kiessling, P. S. Hochman, O. Haller, G. M. Shearer, H. Wigzell, and G. Cudkowicz, "Evidence for a similar or common mechanism for natural killer cell activity and resistance to hemopoietic grafts," *European Journal of Immunology*, vol. 7, no. 9, pp. 655–663, 1977.

[32] Y. Huang, F. Rezzoug, P. M. Chilton, H. Leighton Grimes, D. E. Cramer, and S. T. Ildstad, "Matching at the MHC class I K locus is essential for long-term engraftment of purified hematopoietic stem cells: a role for host NK cells in regulating HSC engraftment," *Blood*, vol. 104, no. 3, pp. 873–880, 2004.

[33] D. Ross, M. Jones, K. Komanduri, and R. B. Levy, "Antigen and lymphopenia-driven donor T cells are differentially diminished by post-transplantation administration of cyclophosphamide after hematopoietic cell transplantation," *Biology of Blood and Marrow Transplantation*, vol. 19, no. 10, pp. 1430–1438, 2013.

[34] D. Glotz, J.-P. Haymann, N. Sansonetti et al., "Suppression of HLA-specific alloantibodies by high-dose intravenous immunoglobulins (IVIg). A potential tool for transplantation of immunized patients," *Transplantation*, vol. 56, no. 2, pp. 335–337, 1993.

[35] D. Morioka, H. Sekido, K. Kubota et al., "Antibody-mediated rejection after adult ABO-incompatible liver transplantation remedied by gamma-globulin bolus infusion combined with plasmapheresis," *Transplantation*, vol. 78, no. 8, pp. 1225–1228, 2004.

[36] S. K. Takemoto, A. Zeevi, S. Feng et al., "National conference to assess antibody-mediated rejection in solid organ transplantation," *American Journal of Transplantation*, vol. 4, no. 7, pp. 1033–1041, 2004.

[37] P. A. Taylor, M. J. Ehrhardt, M. M. Roforth et al., "Preformed antibody, not primed T cells, is the initial and major barrier to bone marrow engraftment in allosensitized recipients," *Blood*, vol. 109, no. 3, pp. 1307–1315, 2007.

[38] M. Takanashi, K. Fujiwara, H. Tanaka, M. Satake, and K. Nakajima, "The impact of HLA antibodies on engraftment of unrelated cord blood transplants," *Transfusion*, vol. 48, no. 4, pp. 791–793, 2008.

[39] A. Ruggeri, V. Rocha, E. Masson et al., "Impact of donor-specific anti-HLA antibodies on graft failure and survival after reduced intensity conditioning-unrelated cord blood transplantation: a Eurocord, Société Francophone d'Histocompatibilité et d'Immunogénétique (SFHI) and Société Française de Greffe de Moelle et de Thérapie Cellulaire (SFGM-TC) analysis," *Haematologica*, vol. 98, no. 7, pp. 1154–1160, 2013.

[40] S. O. Ciurea, P. F. Thall, X. Wang et al., "Donor-specific anti-HLA Abs and graft failure in matched unrelated donor hematopoietic stem cell transplantation," *Blood*, vol. 118, no. 22, pp. 5957–5964, 2011.

[41] A. J. Barge, G. Johnson, R. Witherspoon, and B. Torok-Storb, "Antibody-mediated marrow failure after allogeneic bone marrow transplantation," *Blood*, vol. 74, no. 5, pp. 1477–1480, 1989.

[42] J. Damman, M. A. Seelen, C. Moers et al., "Systemic complement activation in deceased donors is associated with acute rejection after renal transplantation in the recipient," *Transplantation*, vol. 92, no. 2, pp. 163–169, 2011.

[43] T. F. Müller, M. Kraus, C. Neumann, and H. Lange, "Detection of renal allograft rejection by complement components C5A and TCC in plasma and urine," *Journal of Laboratory and Clinical Medicine*, vol. 129, no. 1, pp. 62–71, 1997.

[44] T. R. Welch, L. S. Beischel, and D. P. Witte, "Differential expression of complement C3 and C4 in the human kidney," *The Journal of Clinical Investigation*, vol. 92, no. 3, pp. 1451–1458, 1993.

[45] K. Keslar, E. R. Rodriguez, C. D. Tan, R. C. Starling, and P. S. Heeger, "Complement gene expression in human cardiac allograft biopsies as a correlate of histologic grade of injury," *Transplantation*, vol. 86, no. 9, pp. 1319–1321, 2008.

[46] S. O. Ciurea, P. F. Thall, D. R. Milton et al., "Complement-binding donor-specific anti-HLA antibodies and risk of primary graft failure in hematopoietic stem cell transplantation," *Biology of Blood and Marrow Transplantation*, vol. 21, no. 8, pp. 1392–1398, 2015.

[47] G. Chen, F. Sequeira, and D. B. Tyan, "Novel C1q assay reveals a clinically relevant subset of human leukocyte antigen antibodies independent of immunoglobulin G strength on single antigen beads," *Human Immunology*, vol. 72, no. 10, pp. 849–858, 2011.

[48] S. Yoshihara, E. Maruya, K. Taniguchi et al., "Risk and prevention of graft failure in patients with preexisting donor-specific HLA antibodies undergoing unmanipulated haploidentical SCT," *Bone Marrow Transplantation*, vol. 47, no. 4, pp. 508–515, 2012.

[49] Y. J. Chang, X. Y. Zhao, L. P. Xu et al., "Donor-specific anti-human leukocyte antigen antibodies were associated with primary graft failure after unmanipulated haploidentical blood and marrow transplantation: a prospective study with randomly assigned training and validation sets," *Journal of Hematology & Oncology*, vol. 8, article 84, 2015.

[50] M. Takanashi, Y. Atsuta, K. Fujiwara et al., "The impact of anti-HLA antibodies on unrelated cord blood transplantations," *Blood*, vol. 116, no. 15, pp. 2839–2846, 2010.

[51] C. G. Brunstein, H. Noreen, T. E. DeFor, D. Maurer, J. S. Miller, and J. E. Wagner, "Anti-HLA antibodies in double umbilical

cord blood transplantation," *Biology of Blood and Marrow Transplantation*, vol. 17, no. 11, pp. 1704–1708, 2011.

[52] A. Maruta, H. Fukawa, H. Kanamori et al., "Donor-HLA-incompatible marrow transplantation with an anti-donor cytotoxic antibody in the serum of the patient," *Bone Marrow Transplantation*, vol. 7, no. 5, pp. 397–400, 1991.

[53] N. Braun, C. Faul, D. Wernet et al., "Successful transplantation of highly selected CD34+ peripheral blood stem cells in a HLA-sensitized patient treated with immunoadsorption onto protein A," *Transplantation*, vol. 69, no. 8, pp. 1742–1744, 2000.

[54] M. S. Pollack and D. Ririe, "Clinical significance of recipient antibodies to stem cell donor mismatched class I HLA antigens," *Human Immunology*, vol. 65, no. 3, pp. 245–247, 2004.

[55] H. Narimatsu, A. Wake, Y. Miura et al., "Successful engraftment in crossmatch-positive HLA-mismatched peripheral blood stem cell transplantation after depletion of antidonor cytotoxic HLA antibodies with rituximab and donor platelet infusion," *Bone Marrow Transplantation*, vol. 36, no. 6, pp. 555–556, 2005.

[56] M. S. Leffell, R. J. Jones, and D. E. Gladstone, "Donor HLA-specific Abs: to BMT or not to BMT?" *Bone Marrow Transplant*, vol. 50, no. 6, pp. 751–758, 2015.

[57] S. J. Stanworth, C. Navarrete, L. Estcourt, and J. Marsh, "Platelet refractoriness—practical approaches and ongoing dilemmas in patient management," *British Journal of Haematology*, vol. 171, no. 3, pp. 297–305, 2015.

[58] P. Álvarez, R. Carrasco, C. Romero-Dapueto, and R. L. Castillo, "Transfusion-Related Acute Lung Injured (TRALI): current concepts," *The Open Respiratory Medicine Journal*, vol. 9, pp. 92–96, 2015.

[59] R. R. Vassallo, S. Hsu, M. Einarson, J. Barone, J. Brodsky, and G. Moroff, "A comparison of two robotic platforms to screen plateletpheresis donors for HLA antibodies as part of a transfusion-related acute lung injury mitigation strategy," *Transfusion*, vol. 50, no. 8, pp. 1766–1777, 2010.

[60] T. L. Densmore, L. T. Goodnough, S. Ali, M. Dynis, and H. Chaplin, "Prevalence of HLA sensitization in female apheresis donors," *Transfusion*, vol. 39, no. 1, pp. 103–106, 1999.

[61] R. M. Kakaiya, D. J. Triulzi, D. J. Wright et al., "Prevalence of HLA antibodies in remotely transfused or alloexposed volunteer blood donors," *Transfusion*, vol. 50, no. 6, pp. 1328–1334, 2010.

[62] D. E. Gladstone, A. A. Zachary, E. J. Fuchs et al., "Partially mismatched transplantation and human leukocyte antigen donor-specific antibodies," *Biology of Blood and Marrow Transplantation*, vol. 19, no. 4, pp. 647–652, 2013.

[63] W. W. Hancock, W. Gao, N. Shemmeri et al., "Immunopathogenesis of accelerated allograft rejection in sensitized recipients: humoral and nonhumoral mechanisms," *Transplantation*, vol. 73, no. 9, pp. 1392–1397, 2002.

[64] A. Vongwiwatana, A. Tasanarong, L. G. Hidalgo, and P. F. Halloran, "The role of B cells and alloantibody in the host response to human organ allografts," *Immunological Reviews*, vol. 196, pp. 197–218, 2003.

[65] N. Ben Salah, W. El Borgi, F. Ben Lakhal et al., "Anti-erythrocyte and anti-HLA immunization in hemoglobinopathies," *Transfusion Clinique et Biologique*, vol. 21, no. 6, pp. 314–319, 2014.

[66] K. Marfo, A. Lu, M. Ling, and E. Akalin, "Desensitization protocols and their outcome," *Clinical Journal of the American Society of Nephrology*, vol. 6, no. 4, pp. 922–936, 2011.

[67] R. M. Ratkovec, E. H. Hammond, J. B. O'Connell et al., "Outcome of cardiac transplant recipients with a positive donor-specific crossmatch—preliminary results with plasmapheresis," *Transplantation*, vol. 54, no. 4, pp. 651–655, 1992.

[68] B. A. Pisani, G. M. Mullen, K. Malinowska et al., "Plasmapheresis with intravenous immunoglobulin G is effective in patients with elevated panel reactive antibody prior to cardiac transplantation," *The Journal of Heart and Lung Transplantation*, vol. 18, no. 7, pp. 701–706, 1999.

[69] O. Grauhan, C. Knosalla, R. Ewert et al., "Plasmapheresis and cyclophosphamide in the treatment of humoral rejection after heart transplantation," *Journal of Heart and Lung Transplantation*, vol. 20, no. 3, pp. 316–321, 2001.

[70] D. A. Baran, S. Lubitz, S. Alvi et al., "Refractory humoral cardiac allograft rejection successfully treated with a single dose of rituximab," *Transplantation Proceedings*, vol. 36, no. 10, pp. 3164–3166, 2004.

[71] J. J. Everly, R. C. Walsh, R. R. Alloway, and E. S. Woodle, "Proteasome inhibition for antibody-mediated rejection," *Current Opinion in Organ Transplantation*, vol. 14, no. 6, pp. 662–666, 2009.

[72] R. M. Fasano, E. Mamcarz, S. Adams et al., "Persistence of recipient human leucocyte antigen (HLA) antibodies and production of donor HLA antibodies following reduced intensity allogeneic haematopoietic stem cell transplantation," *British Journal of Haematology*, vol. 166, no. 3, pp. 425–434, 2014.

Efficacy and Safety of Manual Partial Red Cell Exchange in the Management of Severe Complications of Sickle Cell Disease in a Developing Country

B. F. Faye,[1] D. Sow,[1] M. Seck,[1] N. Dieng,[1] S. A. Toure,[1] M. Gadji,[1] A. B. Senghor,[2] Y. B. Gueye,[2] D. Sy,[2] A. Sall,[1] T. N. Dieye,[1] A. O. Toure,[1] and S. Diop[1]

[1]Hematology, Cheikh Anta Diop University, BP 5005, Dakar, Senegal
[2]Centre National de Transfusion Sanguine, BP 5002, Dakar, Senegal

Correspondence should be addressed to B. F. Faye; blaisefelixfaye@yahoo.fr

Academic Editor: Angela Panoskaltsis-Mortari

Introduction. The realization of red cell exchange (RCE) in Africa faces the lack of blood, transfusion safety, and equipment. We evaluated its efficacy and safety in severe complications of sickle cell disease. *Patients and Method.* Manual partial RCE was performed among sickle cell patients who had severe complications. Efficacy was evaluated by clinical evolution, blood count, and electrophoresis of hemoglobin. Safety was evaluated on adverse effects, infections, and alloimmunization. *Results.* We performed 166 partial RCE among 44 patients including 41 homozygous (SS) and 2 heterozygous composites SC and 1 S/β0-thalassemia. The mean age was 27.9 years. The sex ratio was 1.58. The regression of symptoms was complete in 100% of persistent vasoocclusive crisis and acute chest syndrome, 56.7% of intermittent priapism, and 30% of stroke. It was partial in 100% of leg ulcers and null in acute priapism. The mean variations of hemoglobin and hematocrit rate after one procedure were, respectively, +1.4 g/dL and +4.4%. That of hemoglobin S after 2 consecutive RCE was −60%. Neither alloimmunization nor viral seroconversion was observed. *Conclusion.* This work shows the feasibility of manual partial RCE in a low-resource setting and its efficacy and safety during complications of SCD outside of acute priapism.

1. Introduction

Transfusion therapy is the cornerstone of the management of sickle cell disease (SCD) [1]. It reduces significantly the morbidity and mortality [1–3]. In the study *"stroke with transfusions changing to hydroxyurea (SWiTCH)"* chronic transfusion proved to be the best preventive option of stroke among sickle cell patients who had a cerebral vasculopathy [4, 5]. The National Heart Lung and Blood Institute (NHLBI) guidelines, 2014, strongly recommend transfusion, in particular red cell exchange (RCE), in several other indications such as acute chest syndrome (ACS), stroke, hepatic sequestration, and multisystem organ failure [6]. However transfusion increases blood viscosity particularly in patients whose rate of hemoglobin is higher than 10 g/dL. Thus it can participate in the occurrence of vasoocclusive complications [1, 2, 7]. Also, chronic transfusion therapy exposes to the risk of iron

overload [1, 7] while no iron chelator treatment is available now in our country. Partial RCE consists on replacing a part of the blood of sickle cell patients by another from donors who are free of SCD [8]. It reduces the hemoglobin S (HbS) rate, brings normal hemoglobin without increasing the hemoglobin rate where hyperviscosity is a risk, and decreases iron overload [2, 8]. The method can be automated using cytapheresis or manual based on the realization of a bleeding followed by a transfusion of red blood cells [2]. The automated RCE has already proved its efficacy and safety in the developed countries [2, 3, 9]. One of the major limits for its use is the high cost of its equipment which makes it unavailable in centers with limited resources [9, 10]. In the comparative study of Koehl et al. the cost of automated RCE was 74 times higher than the manual method relating to equipment cost [11]. Manual method however has the advantage of being more accessible and not expensive and requires few tools [10]. In our clinical unit, the cost of one session of partial RCE is only 11.4 euros (7500 frs CFA). Its procedure differs from one center to another and depends largely on local resources [9]. The aim of this study was to evaluate the feasibility, efficacy, and safety of an easy protocol of manual partial RCE in adult sickle cell patients with severe complications.

2. Patients and Method

We conducted a prospective study from 11/01/2012 to 02/28/2015 (28 months).

2.1. Patients. All types of SCD in patients older than 16 years with severe complications were included. RCE was performed in the first time of the management in patients with stroke, severe ACS, and acute priapism. In those with persistent vasoocclusive crisis (PVOC), recurrent priapism, or leg ulcer, it was done after failure of the medical treatment.

Patients with a hemoglobin rate lower than 6 g/dL and those with cardiac failure or severe renal deficiency were not included.

2.2. Method

2.2.1. Setting. The Clinical Hematology Department is a public center located in the National Blood Transfusion Center, next to the blood donation department and his medical laboratory. It includes a medical consultation unit where about 20 patients are checked daily and an inpatient unit of 20 beds. It is the national reference center for adult SCD, malignant hemopathies, and hemophilia. It also welcomes students of the Faculty of Medicine and Pharmacy during their training. Pre- and posttransfusion tests are performed in the medical laboratory of the National Blood Transfusion Center.

2.2.2. Pretherapeutic Assessment. It included a clinical examination, blood count, blood group determination, electrophoresis of hemoglobin, serology of HIV, hepatitis B, hepatitis C, and syphilis.

2.2.3. Characteristics of the Red Cell Units. The red cell units used had approximately a volume of 250 mL, an hematocrit rate about 60%, and an hemoglobin content greater than 45 g. They were preserved in citrate, phosphate, dextrose, and adenine (CPDA). All the units underwent the following tests: ABO and Rhesus group, serology of HIV, hepatitis B, hepatitis C, and syphilis which were negatives, and the sickling-test which was negative too indicating the absence of HbS.

2.2.4. Partial RCE Procedure. All procedures were performed on peripheral venous of the upper limbs by nurses who had been trained in partial manual RCE by the medical team. Each procedure was performed by one nurse. The procedure began with a bleeding in free flow in a blood bag. Its total volume was according to the baseline hemoglobin rate. It was 250 mL when the hemoglobin rate was between

6 and 8 g/dL; 500 mL, 750 mL, and 1000 mL, respectively, for 8.1–10 g/dL, 10.1–12 g/dL, and higher than 12 g/L. It was followed by an intravenous hydration using isotonic saline. Its volume was equal to the bleeding one in order to prevent hypovolemia. In patients whose total volume of the bleeding was 750 mL or 1000 mL, we removed at first 500 mL of blood, gave 500 mL saline, and then removed 250 mL or 500 mL, respectively, to prevent hypovolemia. Then a transfusion of 2 units of red blood cell was done. Finally a last saline hydration with the same volume than the transfusion was carried out in order to prevent hyperviscosity. When after RCE, the hematocrit was higher than 40% or the hemoglobin rate higher than 12 g/dL, an additional bleeding of 500 mL was carried out in order to return below these limits. One procedure of RCE was performed for each episode of recurrent priapism and PVOC. Two consecutive RCE were done at the day of the admission for stoke, severe ACS, and acute priapism. For leg ulcers, one procedure was performed every 4 weeks.

2.2.5. The Monitoring for Adverse Transfusion Reactions. We monitored the blood pressure, pulse, respiratory rate, temperature, oxygen saturation, and consciousness before RCE, every 30 min during the procedure and at the end. At least twice daily after RCE, clinical examination was done for evaluate the evolution of symptoms and screen adverse events. Additional tests depended on the type of reactions suspected.

2.2.6. Evaluation of Efficacy and Safety. The main symptoms evaluated were bone pain in PVOC; chest pain, dyspnea, and oxygen saturation in severe ACS; paralysis, alteration of consciousness, and convulsions in stroke; painful erection in priapism; size reduction in leg ulcers. The regression of symptoms was considered as complete when they disappeared within 4 hours after RCE for acute priapism, 1 day for recurrent priapism, 3 days for PVOC, severe ACS, and stroke, and 1 month for leg ulcer. A blood count was done after every RCE and an electrophoresis of hemoglobin was done after two consecutive RCE. Red cell antibodies screening was performed by the gel card method of the Biorad kit. Serology of HIV, hepatitis B, hepatitis C, and syphilis were tested at the end of the study.

2.2.7. Statistical Study. Data analysis was done using SPSS software version 18. Descriptive study was conducted by calculating frequencies and proportions for qualitative variables. For quantitative data, we calculated the averages with their 95% confidence intervals.

3. Results

A total of 166 partial RCE was performed in 44 sickle cell patients including 41 homozygous (SS) and two heterozygous composites SC and one S/β0-thalassemia. They were from a cohort of 1120 patients (3.9%). The sex ratio was 1.58; the mean age was 27.9 years [95% IC: 25.8–30].

TABLE 1: Indications and clinical evolution of patients after RCE.

Indications	Number of patients (N = 44)	Number of RCE per patient	Total number of RCE (N = 166)	Regression of symptoms Complete (%)	Partial (%)	Mean delay before regression (day)
Recurrent priapism[*]	12	5	60	56,7	43,3	1
Acute priapism[***]	6	2	12	0	0	NA
PVOC[*]	8	5	40	100	0	2,4
Leg ulcer[**]	6	5	30	0	100	21
Stroke[***]	10	2	20	30	70	3,2
Severe ACS[***]	2	2	4	100	0	1,7

[*] Clinical evaluation after one RCE; the other episodes had occurred several months later.
[**] Clinical evaluation conducted monthly during 5 months.
[***] Clinical evaluation conducted after 2 consecutive RCE performed the day of admission.

TABLE 2: Evaluation of the blood count parameters after one RCE and hemoglobin fractions after 2 consecutive RCE performed the day of admission.

Parameters	Values Baseline Mean	95% CI	Final Mean	95% CI	Mean variation
Blood count before and after one RCE (N = 166)					
Red cells count (10^{12}/L)	3,1	2,9–3,3	3,3	3,1–3,4	+0,2
Hemoglobin rate (g/dL)	8,9	8,6–9,1	10,3	8,5–12,2	+1,4
Hematocrit (%)	26,2	24,7–27,8	30,6	23,3–37,6	+4,4
White cells count (10^9/L)	11,5	10,7–12,2	11,6	10,4–12,7	+0,1
Platelets count (10^9/L)	443	414–473	433	401–475	−10
Fractions of hemoglobin before and after 2 RCE performed the day of admission (N = 12)					
Hemoglobin S (%)	84,8	80,5–89	24,8	20,6–32	−60
Hemoglobin A (%)	0	—	64	58–70	+64
Hemoglobin F (%)	10,2	8,0–12,5	6	3,0–7,5	−4,2
Hemoglobin A2 (%)	3,3	2,9–3,7	2,3	1,9–3,0	−1

3.1. Indications. The main indications were recurrent priapism (36.1%), PVOC (24%), and chronic leg ulcer (18%) (Table 1).

3.2. RCE Parameters. The average duration of RCE was 170 minutes [95% IC: 167–175] per procedure. The average volume of bleeding was 475 mL [95% IC: 439.5–510.5]. That of the transfused blood was 556.6 mL [95% IC: 540.4–572.8] corresponding to 2 red cell units. The total of red blood cell units was 332 with an average of 7.5 units per patient [95% IC: 5.8–10].

3.3. Efficacy of RCE. Regression of symptoms was complete in 100% of cases of PVOC and severe ACS, 56.7% of recurrent priapism, and 30% of stroke. It was partial in 100% of leg ulcers, 70% of stroke, and 43.3% of recurrent priapism. Zero percent (0%) of acute priapism cases had obtained regression; thus they were transferred to the urological emergencies (Table 1). The mean variations of the hemoglobin rate and hematocrit after each procedure were, respectively, +1.4 g/dL

and +4.4%. That of HbS after 2 consecutive RCE was −60% (Table 2).

3.4. Safety of RCE. There were no difficulties of venous access which limited the performing or continuation of RCE. Minor adverse events had occurred in 6 cases (3.6%) such as dizziness, headaches, fever, urticaria (1 case for each of them), and itching (2 cases). Neither alloimmunization nor seroconversion to the HIV, HBV, HCV, and syphilis was observed.

4. Discussion

This work shows that given proper training, despite a low-resource setting, manual partial RCE can be safely and successfully performed in the management of several complications of SCD outside the acute priapism. It allows a significant reduction of the hemoglobin S (HbS) rate and brings normal hemoglobin without increasing the hemoglobin rate where hyperviscosity is a risk. This efficacy was variable according to indications. Several authors found variation of the efficacy of partial RCE according to the methods used and the indications [2, 8, 12, 13].

In the cases of PVOC and recurrent priapism, one procedure was performed for each episode because it allowed a favorable evolution. So the variation of HbS rate was not evaluated. In these indications, the clinical evolution is the decisive parameter for the assessment of efficacy. Correlation between the rate of HbS and clinical improvement is not perfect [9]. Two consecutive RCE was done in the vital emergency situations such as severe ACS and stroke to exchange large volumes of blood in order to obtain a significant reduction of HbS level [9]. They were done in two times to prevent adverse events related to a large volume of bleeding. In these cases erythrocytapheresis would be more suitable because it could be performed safely under isovolemia [2, 9]. The efficacy of RCE was less remarkable in stroke (only 30% of complete clinical regression) although HbS had reached the recommended rate of 30% [14]. This could be related to the severity of the cerebral injuries before treatment. Regarding the healing of leg ulcers, it was only partial in 100% of the cases. Minniti et al. found that there is no controlled data that shows the efficacy of chronic transfusion in the healing of chronic leg ulcers in SCD likely due to their multifactorial origin [15].

As for the acute priapism, RCE failed in 100% of the cases. With respect to this outcome, we acknowledge that transfusion is not effective for the treatment of acute priapism according to the 2014 NIH guidelines [6]. The interest of the RCE in the management of the priapism remains controversial [14]. In a literature review conducted by Kato [16], he found that RCE and other drug treatments were not efficient in this indication and delayed the urologic management. However Ballas and Lyon had obtained clinic regression by cytapheresis by maintaining an HbS rate lower than 30% [17].

Concerning the biological response, the average rate of hemoglobin after one RCE (10.3 g/dL) and that of HbS after two consecutive RCE (24.8%) were according to recommendations. The suggested goal is a hemoglobin rate close to but not greater than 10 g/dL and the HbS rate lower than 30% in stroke and lower than 50% in other complications [2, 9, 14].

About safety, a low rate of minor acute adverse events (3,6%) had occurred. Indeed during RCE, acute complications are usually rare and transitory [12, 18].

No infection by HIV, HBV, and HCV was observed. In Senegal the safety against infections related to transfusion has improved thanks to the efficient strategies in medical selection of blood donors [19, 20] and better techniques in the screening of infectious diseases [21]. Despite these advances, the risk of infections related transfusion remains high in Senegal and in Africa in general. So it limits the indications of chronic transfusion in these countries [7, 19, 21–24].

No case of alloimmunization was observed either. It could partly be due to a better homogeneity between the blood group antigens in donors and patients. In a systematic review and meta-analysis done by Ngoma et al. about red blood cell alloimmunization in transfused patients in sub-Saharan Africa, overall proportions of alloimmunization were 6.7 (95% CI: 5.7–7.8) per 100 transfused patients [25]. In Europe

where black sickle cell patients usually receive blood from white donors, the risk of alloimmunization is higher due to a greater antigenic difference [1, 7, 23]. Michot et al. found in their cohort that the prevalence of the alloimmunization was 33% [26]. However, Venkateswaran et al. had shown that when the RCE is done with Rhesus and Kell system matched, it does not increase the risk of allo- or autoimmunization more than simple chronic transfusion despite the exposure to a larger number of red cell units [27].

5. Conclusion

This work shows that, given proper training, despite a low-resource setting, manual partial RCE can be safely and successfully performed in the management of several complications of SCD. Its efficacy is variable according to indications. It allows a significant reduction of the hemoglobin S (HbS) rate and brings normal hemoglobin without increasing the hemoglobin rate where hyperviscosity is a risk. However it should not delay the urologic management in acute priapism. A larger study should better evaluate the quality of this treatment and the associated difficulties such as iron overload.

Conflicts of Interest

The authors declare that there are no conflicts of interest regarding the publication of this paper.

References

[1] S. T. Chou, "Transfusion therapy for sickle cell disease : a balancing act.," *Hematology. American Society of Hematology. Education Program*, pp. 439–446, 2013.

[2] P. S. Swerdlow, "Red cell exchange in sickle cell disease," *Hematology. American Society of Hematology. Education Program*, pp. 48–53, 2006.

[3] D. A. Tsitsikas, B. Sirigireddy, R. Nzouakou et al., "Safety, tolerability, and outcomes of regular automated red cell exchange transfusion in the management of sickle cell disease," *Journal of Clinical Apheresis*, vol. 31, no. 6, pp. 545–550, 2016.

[4] R. E. Ware and R. W. Helms, "Stroke with transfusions changing to hydroxyurea (SWITCH)," *Blood*, vol. 119, no. 17, pp. 3925–3932, 2012.

[5] R. E. Ware, B. R. Davis, W. H. Schultz et al., "Hydroxycarbamide versus chronic transfusion for maintenance of transcranial doppler flow velocities in children with sickle cell anaemia-TCD With Transfusions Changing to Hydroxyurea (TWiTCH) : a multicentre, open-label, phase 3, non-inferiority trial," *The Lancet*, vol. 387, pp. 661–670, 2016.

[6] B. P. Yawn, G. R. Buchanan, A. N. Afenyi-Annan et al., "Management of sickle cell disease: summary of the 2014 evidence-based report by expert panel members," *JAMA*, vol. 312, no. 10, pp. 1033–1048, 2014.

[7] W. S. Dzik, D. Kyeyune, G. Otekat et al., "Transfusion medicine in sub-saharan Africa: conference summary," *Transfusion Medicine Reviews*, vol. 29, no. 3, pp. 195–204, 2015.

[8] H. C. Kim, "Red cell exchange: Special focus on sickle cell disease," *Hematology. American Society of Hematology. Education Program*, vol. 2014, no. 1, pp. 450–456, 2014.

[9] M. De Montalembert, "Échanges érythrocytaires chez les patients drépanocytaires," *Hématologie*, vol. 13, pp. 243–249, 2007.

[10] K. H. M. Kuo, R. Ward, B. Kaya, J. Howard, and P. Telfer, "A comparison of chronic manual and automated red blood cell exchange transfusion in sickle cell disease patients," *British journal of haematology*, vol. 170, no. 3, pp. 425–428, 2015.

[11] B. Koehl, J. Sommet, L. Holvoet et al., "Comparison of automated erythrocytapheresis versus manual exchange transfusion to treat cerebral macrovasculopathy in sickle cell anemia," *Transfusion*, vol. 56, no. 5, pp. 1121–1128, 2016.

[12] A. E. Dokekias and G. B. Basseila, "Résultats des échanges transfusionnels partiels chez 42 patients drépanocytaires homozygotes au CHU de Brazzaville," *Transfusion Clinique et Biologique*, vol. 17, pp. 232–241, 2010.

[13] H. S. Mian, R. Ward, P. Telfer, B. Kaya, and K. H. M. Kuo, "Optimal manual exchange transfusion protocol for sickle cell disease: a retrospective comparison of two comprehensive care centers in the United Kingdom And Canada," *Hemoglobin*, vol. 39, no. 5, pp. 310–315, 2015.

[14] S. T. Chou and R. M. Fasano, "Management of patients with sickle cell disease using transfusion therapy: guidelines and complications," *Hematology/Oncology Clinics of North America*, vol. 30, no. 3, pp. 591–608, 2016.

[15] C. P. Minniti, J. Eckman, P. Sebastiani, M. H. Steinberg, and S. K. Ballas, "Leg ulcers in sickle cell disease," *American Journal of Hematology*, vol. 85, no. 10, pp. 831–833, 2010.

[16] G. J. Kato, "Priapism in sickle-cell disease: a hematologist's perspective," *The Journal of Sexual Medicine*, vol. 9, no. 1, pp. 70–78, 2012.

[17] S. K. Ballas and D. Lyon, "Safety and efficacy of blood exchange transfusion for priapism complicating sickle cell disease," *Journal of Clinical Apheresis*, vol. 31, no. 1, pp. 5–10, 2016.

[18] M. N. Aloni, M. N. Aloni, P.-Q. Lê et al., "A pilot study of manual chronic partial exchange transfusion in children with sickle disease," *Hematology*, vol. 20, no. 5, pp. 284–288, 2015.

[19] J.-J. Lefrère, H. Dahourouh, A. E. Dokekias et al., "Estimate of the residual risk of transfusion-transmitted human immunodeficiency virus infection in sub-Saharan Africa: a multinational collaborative study," *Transfusion*, vol. 51, no. 3, pp. 486–492, 2011.

[20] M. Seck, B. Dièye, Y. B. Guèye, B. F. Faye, A. B. Senghor, and S. A. Toure, "Évaluation de l'efficacité de la sélection médicale des donneurs de sang dans la prévention des agents infectieux," *Transfusion Clinique et Biologique*, vol. 23, pp. 98–102, 2016.

[21] A. O. Touré-Fall, T. N. Dièye, A. Sall, M. Diop, M. Seck, and S. Diop, "Risque résiduel de transmission du VIH et du VHB par transfusion sanguine entre 2003 et 2005 au Centre national de transfusion sanguine de Dakar (Sénégal)," *Transfusion Clinique et Biologique*, vol. 16, pp. 439–443, 2009.

[22] T. N. Williams, "Sickle cell disease in Sub-Saharan Africa," *Hematology/Oncology Clinics of North America*, vol. 30, no. 2, pp. 343–358, 2016.

[23] S. Diop, S. O. Mokono, M. Ndiaye, A. O. Touré Fall, D. Thiam, and L. Diakhaté, "La drépanocytose homozygote après l'âge de 20 ans: suivi d'une cohorte de 108 patients au CHU de Dakar," *La Revue de Médecine Interne*, vol. 24, pp. 711–715, 2003.

[24] A. Diarra, A. Guindo, B. Kouriba et al., "Sécurité transfusionnelle et drépanocytose à Bamako, Mali. Séroprévalence des infections à VIH, VHB, VHC et allo-immunisation anti-Rh et Kell chez les drépanocytaires," *Transfusion Clinique et Biologique*, vol. 20, pp. 476–481, 2013.

[25] A. M. Ngoma, P. B. Mutombo, K. Ikeda, K. E. Nollet, B. Natukunda, and H. Ohto, "Red blood cell alloimmunization in transfused patients in sub-Saharan Africa: a systematic review and meta-analysis," *Transfusion and Apheresis Science*, vol. 54, no. 2, pp. 296–302, 2016.

[26] J.-M. Michot, F. Driss, C. Guitton et al., "Immunohematologic tolerance of chronic transfusion exchanges with erythrocytapheresis in sickle cell disease," *Transfusion*, vol. 55, no. 2, pp. 357–363, 2015.

[27] L. Venkateswaran, J. Teruya, C. Bustillos, D. Mahoney, and B. U. Mueller, "Red cell exchange does not appear to increase the rate of allo- and auto-immunization in chronically transfused children with sickle cell disease," *Pediatric Blood and Cancer*, vol. 57, no. 2, pp. 294–296, 2011.

15

Review on Haploidentical Hematopoietic Cell Transplantation in Patients with Hematologic Malignancies

William A. Fabricius and Muthalagu Ramanathan

Division of Hematology-Oncology, Bone Marrow Transplant Service, Department of Medicine,
University of Massachusetts Medical School, 55 Lake Avenue N., Worcester, MA 01655, USA

Correspondence should be addressed to Muthalagu Ramanathan; muthalagu.ramanathan@umassmemorial.org

Academic Editor: Franco Aversa

Allogenic hematopoietic cell transplantation (HSCT) is typically the preferred curative therapy for adult patients with acute myeloid leukemia, but its use has been reduced as a consequence of limited donor availability in the form of either matched-related donors (MRD) or matched-unrelated donors (MUD). Alternative options such as unrelated umbilical cord blood (UCB) transplantation and haploidentical HSCT have been increasingly studied in the past few decades to overcome these obstacles. A human leukocyte antigen- (HLA-) haploidentical donor is a recipient's relative who shares an exact haplotype with the recipient but is mismatched for HLA genes on the unshared haplotype. These dissimilarities pose several challenges to the outcomes of the patient receiving such a type of HSCT, including higher rates of bidirectional alloreactivity and graft failure. In the past 5 years, however, several nonrandomized studies have shown promising results in terms of graft success and decreased rates of alloreactivity, in part due to newer grafting techniques and graft-versus-host disease (GVHD) prophylaxis. We present here a summary and review of the latest results of these studies as well as a brief discussion on the advantages and challenges of haploidentical HSCT.

1. Introduction

A human leukocyte antigen- (HLA-) haploidentical donor is one who shares, by inheritance, precisely one HLA haplotype with the recipient and is mismatched for HLA genes on the unshared haplotype. HLA-haploidentical donors can be biological parents, biological children, full or half siblings, and collateral related donors.

Allogeneic hematopoietic cell transplantation (HSCT) is the treatment of choice with the intention of cure for some malignant and nonmalignant hematologic disorders. The hematopoietic stem cells required for this procedure are usually obtained from the bone marrow or peripheral blood of a related or unrelated donor. Historically, the best results of allogeneic HSCT have been observed when the stem cell donor is a HLA-matched sibling, but, unfortunately, an HLA-matched sibling donor (MSD) can be found in only approximately 30 percent of patients or less. For patients who lack an HLA-matched sibling, alternative sources of donor grafts can be found in suitably HLA-matched adult unrelated donors

(MUD), unrelated umbilical cord blood (UCB) donors, and partially HLA-mismatched-unrelated donors (mMUD) or HLA-haploidentical related donors [1].

The major challenge of HLA-haploidentical HSCT is the intense bidirectional alloreactivity leading to high incidences of graft rejection and graft-versus-host disease (GVHD). Advances in graft techniques and in pharmacologic prophylaxis of GVHD have reduced the risks of graft failure and GVHD after HLA-haploidentical HSCT and have made this stem cell source a viable alternative for patients lacking an HLA-matched donor [2].

Historically, a MSD has been preferred over other donor sources due to improved clinical outcomes following transplant, such as improved graft failure and less GVHD, and the speed and cost-effectiveness of the search. But when a MSD is not available or suitable, the transplant center usually proceeds with an unrelated donor search and alternative donor sources (HLA-haploidentical HSCT, UCB transplant) are considered if there is an urgent need to proceed to transplantation or if a preliminary search indicates a low likelihood of finding an eight of eight allele-MUD. Unfortunately, despite an increasing number of volunteers in the unrelated donor registries, unrelated adult donor HSCT is performed in only around 35% of patients for whom an unrelated donor search has been activated [3].

2. Literature Review

In the past year, two large retrospective studies comparing outcomes of patients receiving haploidentical HSCT versus MSD HSCT and MUD HSCT, respectively, have been published showing promising results regarding grafting success, overall survival, and complications such as GVHD and fatal graft failure.

The first one, a large, retrospective, study published in 2015 by a Swedish group with international collaboration [9], compared data collected from 10,679 AML patients who underwent HSCT from a MSD ($n = 9,815$) and haploidentical donor ($n = 864$) between 2007 and 2012. This study showed no statistically significant difference in probability of relapse between both groups but the leukemia-free survival was superior in the MSD group when compared to haploidentical transplantation group who received either T cell-replete or T cell depleted grafts. The authors acknowledge, however, that this was a retrospective study and the different study groups were not strictly matched. Since the risk of relapse was similar in both haploidentical donor grafts and MSD grafts, we could infer a similar graft-versus-leukemia effect in both groups.

A second retrospective study that compared adults with AML who received haploidentical donor transplantation ($n = 192$), with 8/8 HLA-MUD ($n = 1982$) transplantation, showed that survival for patients with AML after haploidentical transplantation with posttransplant cyclophosphamide (PTCy) was comparable with MUD transplantation [8]. The haploidentical recipients considered in this study received calcineurin inhibitor, mycophenolate, and PTCy for graft-versus-host disease (GVHD) prophylaxis; 104 patients received myeloablative and 88 received reduced intensity conditioning (RIC) regimens. MUD transplant recipients received CNI with mycophenolate or methotrexate for GVHD prophylaxis; 1245 patients received myeloablative and 737 received RIC regimens. In the myeloablative setting, day 30 neutrophil recovery was lower after haploidentical compared to MUD transplants (90% versus 97%, $p = 0.02$). Corresponding engraftment rates after RIC transplants were however 93% and 96% ($p = 0.25$), respectively. In the myeloablative setting, 3-month acute grade 2–4 (16% versus 33%, $p < 0.0001$) and 3-year chronic GVHD (30% versus 53%, $p < 0.0001$) were lower after haploidentical, due to in vivo T cell depletion with PTCy, in comparison to MUD transplants. Similar differences were observed after RIC transplants, 19% versus 28% ($p = 0.05$) and 34% versus 52% ($p = 0.002$). Among patients receiving myeloablative and RIC regimens, there was no statistically significant difference in survival (3-year OS was 45% versus 50% ($p = 0.38$) for the myeloablative regimen group and 46% versus 44% for the RIC group ($p = 0.71$)).

In a retrospective comparative study published in 2014, Raiola et al. [6] reported data from 459 consecutive patients with hematologic malignancies, with a median age of 44 years (range of 15–71 years), who received allogeneic HSCT between January 2006 and July 2012, with grafts from MSD ($n = 176$), MUD ($n = 43$), mMUD ($n = 43$), and UCB ($n = 105$) of HLA-haploidentical family donors ($n = 92$). GVHD prophylaxis varied based on the source of donor graft: cyclosporine and methotrexate for the MSD recipients and ATG for the MUD, mMUD, and UCB recipients. PTCy, cyclosporine, and mycophenolate were used for the haploidentical transplant group.

This report showed a comparable time (16–18 days) to engraftment for all groups with the exception of UCB group that took 23 days on average to achieve absolute neutrophil count >500 ($p = 0.001$). Cumulative incidence of developing CMV antigenemia was highest in the haploidentical group: 58% in the MSD group, 60% in the MUD group, 68% in UCB group, and 74% in the haploidentical group ($p = 0.004$ for the latter). On the other hand, the cumulative incidence of transplant-related mortality (TRM) at 1000 days favored the haploidentical group: 24% for the MSD group, 33% for the MUD group, 35% for the UCB group, and 18% for the haploidentical group ($p = 0.02$). Rates of acute and chronic GVHD, relapse, and OS were comparable across all donor types.

A prospective, multicenter, nonrandomized study conducted by Wang et al. [7] between 2010 and 2013 was published in 2015 comparing results of patients with AML in complete first remission (CR1) that underwent haploidentical donor HSCT versus patients that received MSD HSCT. In this trial, 450 patients were assigned to undergo haploidentical HSCT (231 patients) or MSD HSCT (219 patients) according to donor availability. GVHD prophylaxis regimen consisted of cyclosporine A, mycophenolate mofetil, and short-term methotrexate.

The outcomes were comparable across the haploidentical and MSD HSCT groups, the 3-year disease-free survival (DFS) rate was 74% and 78% ($p = 0.34$), the overall survival (OS) rate was 79% and 82% ($p = 0.36$), cumulative incidences of relapse were 15% and 15% ($p = 0.98$), and the nonrelapse-mortality rates (NRM) were 13% and 8% ($p = 0.13$), respectively. All patients in both groups achieved donor-cell engraftment. The median time to achieve neutrophil engraftment was 2 days shorter after haploidentical HSCT ($p = 0.004$); meanwhile, platelet engraftment was achieved 3 days shorter after MSD HSCT. The cumulative incidences for grades 3 to 4 acute GVHD at 100 days were, however, 10% (95% CI, 6–14) for the haploidentical transplant group and 3% (95% CI, 1–5) for the MSD group ($p = 0.004$). The cumulative rates of severe chronic GVHD at 1 year were 12% (95% CI, 8–16) and 2% (95% CI, 0–4), respectively ($p < 0.001$), as well. In sum, the results of this study showed comparable DFS, OS, and relapse in haploidentical and MSD HSCT for AML patients in CR1. The fact that both study groups received the same GVHD regimen might explain, on the other hand, the higher incidences of acute and chronic GVHD for the haploidentical group as well as the noticeable lower incidence for the MSD group compared to prior, although retrospective, studies.

Currently, there are no published randomized studies comparing HLA-haploidentical HSCT versus UCB. However, the United States Blood and Marrow Transplant Clinical Trials Network (CTN) is conducting a phase III randomized trial of RIC and transplantation for patients with acute leukemia in complete remission or with lymphoma, comparing double UCB versus HLA-haploidentical bone marrow transplantation (BMT CTN 1101; NCT01597778). For patients who are not eligible or referred for this trial, the choice between the two graft sources remains a matter of clinician preference.

3. Donor Selection Criteria for Haploidentical HSCT

Most patients will have more than one HLA-haploidentical first-degree relative willing and able to donate, so the appropriate selection of the donor should follow several criteria in order to achieve the best results for a successful grafting, best graft versus leukemic effect , and to minimize graft rejection and GVHD.

A study by Kasamon et al. [10] published in 2010 showed that increasing HLA disparity between donor and recipient had no detrimental impact on the outcome of 185 hematologic malignancy patients treated with nonmyeloablative conditioning, T cell-replete bone marrow transplantation, and GVHD prophylaxis including high-dose cyclophosphamide. In this study, the presence of an HLA-DRB1 antigen mismatch in the graft-versus-host direction actually was associated with a lesser risk of relapse and increased survival.

No significant difference in overall or disease-free survival between recipients of grafts from MSD versus HLA-haploidentical donors was shown by three subsequent retrospective small studies, supporting the hypothesis that these transplantation platforms have nullified the detrimental impact of HLA mismatching on outcome. For GVHD prophylaxis, the patients received PTCy in two of these studies [6, 11] and the GIAC (granulocyte-colony stimulating factor filgrastim, intensified immunosuppression, antithymocyte globulin, and combination of peripheral blood stem cell and bone marrow allografts; see below) protocol in the other one [12].

Most selection criteria for a haploidentical stem cell donor are common to other graft types, such as ABO blood type, cytomegalovirus (CMV) serostatus of the donor and recipient, sex mismatch, and donor age and parity. There are, however, criteria that are unique to HLA-mismatched HSCT, which include donor-specific HLA antibodies, donor relationship, donor-recipient HLA mismatch, noninherited maternal antigens, and natural killer cell alloreactivity.

Absolute contraindication to the use of a specific HLA-haploidentical donor is determined by donor fitness and the presence of strong anti-donor HLA antibodies, if any, in the recipient against the donor.

4. Haploidentical Stem Cell Transplantation Strategies

Given the lack of large randomized comparative studies and scarcity of large prospective studies, the decision of how to plan this type of HSCT is mainly based on the expertise of practicing clinicians. Over the past few years, several strategies to HLA-haploidentical HSCT were developed. The approaches most commonly used are as follows.

4.1. T Cell Depletion (TCD) with "Megadose" CD34+ Cells. This modality has been associated with increased nonrelapse mortality (NRM) due to infectious complications secondary to slow immune reconstitution. It is recommended that centers, choosing this modality, have a predefined immunotherapy strategy readily available to hasten immune reconstitution and reduce the risk of infections. Initial studies of TCD required negative selection of CD3+ cells and later studies used grafts with CD34+ positive selection [13–15]. These studies using "megadose" CD34+ grafts with intensive conditioning and no additional postgrafting GVHD prophylaxis showed engraftment rates of 90 to 95% and rates of acute and chronic GVHD of <10% [16–19]. The conditioning regimen used with this approach evolved with time from TBI (8 Gy in single fraction) followed by thiotepa, cyclophosphamide, and rabbit ATG, up to newer regimens that replaced fludarabine and thymoglobulin, respectively, with cyclophosphamide and alemtuzumab [20].

Methods used to improve immune reconstitution after TCD haploidentical HSCT include CD3/CD19 negative selection [21, 22]; depletion of alpha/beta but not gamma/delta T cells [23, 24]; the infusion of cytotoxic T cell lines with viral-specificity for the prevention or treatment of viral infections [25]; and reintroduction of lower levels of both conventional and regulatory T cells [26]. Another approach infuses donor lymphocytes expressing suicide genes that could be activated in case GVHD occurs [27–29].

4.2. The "GIAC" Strategy. This modality is based on GCSF-stimulation of the donor with filgrastim ("G"), intensified immunosuppression posttransplantation ("I"), antithymocyte globulin (ATG—"A") added to conditioning to help prevent GVHD and aid engraftment, and combination ("C") of peripheral blood stem cell and bone marrow allografts. Although relatively inexpensive and not requiring significant expertise in graft manipulation, there is limited experience with this approach outside of China. When compared with high-dose, posttransplantation cyclophosphamide, GIAC appears to be associated with higher rates of acute and chronic GVHD. Conditioning is usually a modified busulfan plus cyclophosphamide regimen with antithymocyte globulin (ATG), cytarabine, and semustine (Me-CCNU).

In the original study presenting this alternative strategy [12], engraftment occurred in all 171 patients, with the cumulative incidences of acute GVHD grades 2–4 of 55% and grades 3-4 of 23%. The cumulative incidences of chronic GVHD and extensive chronic GVHD at two years were 74 and 47%, respectively. The two-year probabilities of nonrelapse mortality (NRM), relapse, and disease-free survival (DFS) were 20, 12, and 68% for standard-risk-disease patients and 31, 39, and 42% for high-risk-disease patients, respectively. Subsequent publications also indicated that this GIAC protocol could achieve complete engraftment, acceptable NRM, and favorable DFS after T cell-replete haploidentical HSCT [7, 30, 31]. Unfortunately, increased incidence of severe acute and chronic GVHD has been noted with this approach. In trying to improve these results, Italian investigators presented a report in 2013 modifying this approach through using only BM allografts and adding basiliximab [32] which allowed them to achieve a lower rate of chronic GVHD, which was 17% including both forms, limited and extensive. Furthermore, in this population, a cumulative incidence of only 5% was noted for the extensive form of GVHD. The rate of neutrophil engraftment in this approach was 93%, with only one patient having failed grafting, and the NRM was 36%.

4.3. High-Dose, Posttransplantation Cyclophosphamide (PTCy).

PTCy is comparatively inexpensive as it does not include graft manipulation. PTCy can also be safely used in the myeloablative conditioning setting with peripheral blood progenitor cells as a donor source. Following an initial phase I/II study and subsequent modifications to include a non-myeloablative conditioning regimen of low-dose cyclophosphamide, and low-dose total body irradiation (TBI), a GVHD prophylaxis regimen was established consisting of posttransplant cyclophosphamide at 50 mg/kg given on each of days +3 and +4 and mycophenolate mofetil and calcineurin inhibitor tacrolimus administered for 30 and 180 days, respectively [33, 34].

According to recent publications, this strategy has shown very little negative impact of the extent of human leukocyte antigen (HLA) disparity on acute GVHD or progression-free survival (PFS) [10].

In the large retrospective study mentioned above by Ciurea et al. [8] utilizing PTCy as a GVHD prophylaxis strategy, the day 30 neutrophil recovery was slightly lower in the haploidentical compared with MUD transplants (90% versus 97%, $p = 0.25$). However, this haploidentical engraftment success rate does not vary significantly compared with the other haploidentical approaches which were about 93% in the GIAC and 90–95% in the TCD groups. The study by Ciurea et al., as well, showed no evidence of posttransplantation lymphoproliferative disease within the first posttransplant year among patients treated with PTCy [8].

Recently, a longer follow-up of a cohort of more than 370 patients showed very similar outcomes to prior studies with cumulative incidences of NRM and severe acute GVHD at six months of 8 and 4%, respectively [35]. The cumulative incidence of chronic GVHD was 13% at two years. PFS and OS rates at three years were 40 and 50%, respectively. When a disease risk index was applied to stratify across all histologies, three-year OS rates ranged from 35 to 71%. Relapse and OS estimates were comparable to those seen with HLA-matched HCST. These outcomes were also seen in two parallel studies sponsored by the Bone Marrow Transplant Clinical Trials Network (BMT CTN): a multicenter phase II

trial of haploidentical HSCT (CTN 0603) and transplantation of double UCB units for high-risk hematologic malignancies after RIC.

However, higher rates of leukemia relapse have been suggested as a disadvantage in haploidentical HSCT with PTCy by data from certain studies. In the retrospective study published in 2010 by Kasamon et al. [10], higher doses of PTCy were associated with higher relapse risk, probably explained by the deleterious cytotoxic effect of cyclophosphamide on the allografts, thus impairing the antitumor effect of the latter. Five years later, in 2015, such higher risk of relapse in haploidentical PTCy regimens was also noted by Ciurea et al. [8] within the group that got RIC. Although there were no differences in survival in the RIC group, haploidentical transplantation showed a statistically significant increased risk of relapse, compared to MUD transplantation, of 58% (46–68) versus 42% (38–45), respectively. After myeloablative conditioning, a nonsignificant increase in risk of relapse was noted in the haploidentical transplantation group versus the MUD transplantation group of 44% (34–53) versus 39% (37–42), respectively.

4.4. Other Strategies.

Other approaches are also being studied to improve the outcomes of haploidentical HSCT. One of them is the use of CD45RA depletion. This strategy has been developed over the idea that T cell depletion results in a profound and often prolonged immunocompromised state and increased risk for graft failure. Because naïve T cells are believed to be amongst the most alloreactive T cell subsets and can be identified by CD45RA expression, allogeneic HSCT using CD45RA depletion is currently being studied as an option in haploidentical donors. A recent small study [36] involved 8 children with relapsed or refractory solid tumors who were transplanted following myeloablative conditioning. Each patient received two cell products. The haploidentical donor apheresis product from the first day of collection was depleted using the CD3 Microbead reagent and from the second day was depleted after labeling with the CD45RA Microbead reagent. The products showed a median CD34 recovery of 59.2% with CD45RA depletion, compared to 82.4% using CD3 depletion. Median CD3+ T cell dose after CD45RA reduction was 99.2×10^6 cells/kg, yet depletion of CD3+ CD45RA+ cells exceeded 4.5 log. CD45RA depletion also resulted in substantial depletion of B-cells (median 2.45 log). Patients received the CD3-depleted HSCT infusion on day 0 and the CD45RA-depleted infusion on day +1. All eight patients engrafted within 14 days and rapidly achieved 100% donor chimerism. No acute GVHD or secondary graft failure was observed.

Another study [37] published by the same group later in 2015 presented results from 17 patients with poor-prognosis hematologic malignancy, who received haploidentical donor transplantation with CD45RA-depleted progenitor cell grafts following a novel RIC regimen without TBI or serotherapy. The group achieved significant depletion of CD45RA+ T cells and B-cells, with preservation of abundant memory T cells, in all 17 products. Neutrophil engraftment was rapidly observed on median day +10 and full donor chimerism on median day +11 posttransplantation. There was no infection-related mortality in this heavily pretreated population, and no patient developed acute GVHD despite infusion of a median of >100 million per kilogram of haploidentical T cells.

5. Discussion: Advantages and Limitations of Haploidentical Donors

When compared with the other stem cell sources, the *major advantages* of the HLA-haploidentical donor option include the following:

(a) Increased availability of highly motivated donors: patients have an average of 2.7 potential HLA-haploidentical donors among first-degree relatives. In comparison, only approximately 30 percent of patients will have a HLA-matched sibling, and availability of an unrelated donor genotypically matched at eight of eight alleles (HLA-A, HLA-B, HLA-C, and HLA-DRB1) ranges from 16 to 75 percent depending upon the recipient's ethnic background. A recent study published in 2014 was able to determine that the likelihood of finding an available 8/8 HLA-matched donor for HSCT in the US Registry showed a wide range depending on racial and/or ethnic background. This varied from 75% for white patients of European descent versus 46% for white patients of Middle Eastern or North African descent and even lower rates were noted for black Americans of all ethnic backgrounds, whose probabilities were 16 to 19%, whereas among Hispanics, Asians, Pacific Islanders, and Native Americans, such likelihood ranged between 27% and 52% [3].

(b) Immediate availability: an HLA-haploidentical donor can be identified and mobilized in two weeks to one month while the time to identify and mobilize an adult unrelated donor can be longer than three months for up to 25 percent of patients.

(c) Adequate doses of hematopoietic stem cells (HSCs): HLA-haploidentical grafts have sufficient doses of HSCs for transplantation and of memory T cells for immune reconstitution. In contrast, the total dose of nucleated cells in a single umbilical cord blood unit may be suboptimal for engraftment in larger adults in addition to delayed immune reconstitution.

(d) Lower cost of graft acquisition: the costs of acquiring grafts for adult unrelated donors and umbilical cord blood are substantially higher than those of related donors.

(e) Immediate availability of the donor for repeated donations of HSCs or lymphocytes to treat relapse. In contrast, umbilical cord blood is a nonrecurring source of cells.

(f) Graft-versus-leukemia effect: for patients with high-risk acute leukemia, HLA-haploidentical HSCT may be associated with a stronger graft-versus-leukemia effect compared with HLA-matched sibling HSCT, resulting in a lower cumulative incidence of relapse [38] and an improved overall survival [39].

The *major disadvantages* of HLA-haploidentical HSCT are due to the higher frequency of host and donor T cells reactive to HLA alloantigens resulting in intense bidirectional alloreactivity [40]:

(a) Higher rate of fatal graft rejection.

(b) Severe or fatal GVHD in the absence of effective prophylactic measures.

(c) Attempts at T cell depletion of the donor graft and posttransplant cyclophosphamide successfully reducing the incidence of acute GVHD, but at the cost of increased incidence of graft rejection and relapse, hence without improvement of leukemia-free survival [41].

(d) Increased nonrelapse mortality (NRM) due to infectious complications secondary to slow immune reconstitution, mostly seen in T cell depleted strategies. Fortunately in the last decade, numerous advances in graft engineering and pharmacologic management of alloreactivity have decreased the incidences of GVHD and nonrelapse mortality and improved OS, PFS, and immune reconstitution, making this graft source an acceptable option for patients without an HLA-matched sibling or unrelated donor (Table 1) [6–8, 10, 35].

6. Conclusion

HLA-haploidentical hematopoietic cell transplantation is a viable treatment option for either patients who lack an HLA-identical matched sibling donor or those for whom a matched-unrelated donor cannot be found or mobilized in a timely fashion. There are no published randomized comparisons of haploidentical HSCT versus matched sibling, umbilical cord blood, or matched or mismatched-unrelated donor HSCT. Thus, the choice between these alternative graft sources depends ultimately on the urgency of the transplant and on each institutional preference.

The major advantage of haploidentical HSCT is the almost universal availability of highly motivated donors who can be mobilized in a short time at a relatively low cost. The major challenge in haploidentical transplant is from bidirectional alloreactivity that leads to graft rejection and fatal GVHD. This can be largely overcome by the use of in vivo or in vitro T cell depletion strategies, which however entails a higher risk for severe infections and relapse.

Selection of the optimal donor needs to take into consideration donor health, age, and gender, relationship to the patient, HLA mismatch in host-versus-graft and graft-versus-host directions, ABO blood type, and CMV serostatus. Other factors that can be considered include noninherited maternal antigen (NIMA) matching and natural killer cell alloreactivity as predicted by donor killer immunoglobulin receptor (KIR) haplotype matching with recipient KIR ligand.

Haploidentical HSCT regimens differ according to each center and clinician: these regimens include the use of either in vitro T cell-depleted (TCD) "megadose" stem cell graft with no pharmacologic prophylaxis of GVHD or in vivo T

TABLE 1: Comparative summary of haploidentical (HAPLO) versus matched sibling donor (MSD), matched-unrelated donor (MUD), and unrelated cord blood (UCB) hematopoietic stem cell transplantation outcomes in patients with acute myelogenous leukemia (AML).

	HAPLO	MSD	MUD	UCB
Donor availability [3]	(~50–70%)	(~15–20%)	(~20–30%)	(~50%)
Time to transplant	(~10–20 days)	(~10–20 days)	(~2–12 months)	(~2–4 weeks)
Stem cell dose (CD34+/kg) [4, 5]	$\sim 6\text{--}8 \times 10^6$	$\sim 6\text{--}8 \times 10^6$	$\sim 6\text{--}8 \times 10^6$	$\sim 3\text{--}5 \times 10^5$
Days to engraftment [6] ($p < 0.001$)	18 d	18 d	17 d	23 d
Acute GVHD, cumulative				
Grades 2–4 ($p < 0.01$) [6]	14%	31%	21%	19%
Grades 3-4 ($p = 0.10$) [6]	4%	7%	3%	1%
Grades 3-4 ($p = 0.004$) [7]	10%	3%	—	—
Grades 3-4, myeloablative conditioning ($p = 0.02$) [8]	7%	—	13%	—
Grades 3-4, reduced intensity conditioning ($p < 0.0001$) [8]	2%	—	11%	—
Chronic GVHD				
Cumulative, moderate-severe ($p = 0.053$) [6]	15%	29%	22%	23%
Cumulative, at 1 year, severe ($p = 0.001$) [7]	12%	2%	—	—
Myeloablative conditioning, at 36 months ($p = 0.0001$) [8]	30%	—	53%	—
Reduced intensity conditioning, at 36 months ($p \leq 0.002$) [8]	34%	—	52%	—
Relapse rate				
3 y, cumulative ($p = 0.98$) [7]	15%	15%	—	—
4 y, cumulative ($p = 0.89$) [6]	35%	40%	23%	30%
Early disease (CR1, CR2) ($p = 0.09$) [6]	18%	36%	20%	24%
Advanced disease (>CR2) ($p = 0.60$) [6]	47%	47%	28%	40%
Disease-free survival				
Cumulative 3 y DFS ($p = 0.34$) [7]	74%	78%	—	—
Cumulative 4 y DFS ($p = 0.20$) [6]	43%	32%	36%	33%
Overall survival				
3 y OS ($p = 0.36$) [7]	79%	82%	—	—
4 y OS ($p = 0.10$) [6]	52%	45%	43%	34%
Relapse-related mortality [6]	26% ($n = 24$)	26% ($n = 48$)	21% ($n = 9$)	29% ($n = 29$)
Transplantation-related mortality ($p = 0.10$) [6]	18%	24%	33%	35%
Immune reconstitution: CD4+ count at posttransplant day +100 ($p < 0.1$) [6]	190/μL	229/μL	106/μL	63/μL
Cumulative incidence of CMV antigenemia ($p = 0.004$) [6]	74%	58%	60%	68%
Infection incidence at posttransplant day +100 [6]				
Bacterial	25%	23%	36%	39%
Fungal	11%	4%	14%	14%
Rate of fatal infections [6]	11% ($n = 10$)	4% ($n = 7$)	14% ($n = 6$)	17% ($n = 18$)

Data obtained from retrospective comparative studies by Raiola et al. [6], Ciurea et al. [8], and Gragert et al. [3] and a prospective study by Wang et al. [7]. The prospective study by Wang et al. [7] was the only one which used the same GVHD regimen for both the HAPLO and the MSD groups. ~: approximate; 3 y: 3 years; 4 y: 4 years; CR1: first complete remission; CR2: second complete remission; DFS: disease-free survival; OS: overall survival.

cell depletion using the GIAC strategy or PTCy strategy or CD45RA depletion discussed above. The excellent outcomes recently seen in haploidentical transplants have largely been made possible by the use of in vivo T cell depletion GVHD regimens such as cyclophosphamide posttransplant as well as effective immune reconstitution platforms. In summary, haploidentical stem cell transplantation, with outcomes comparable to any other graft source, is here to stay and sure to change the future landscape of transplantation.

Conflict of Interests

The authors declare no conflict of interests.

References

[1] N. Bejanyan, H. Haddad, and C. Brunstein, "Alternative donor transplantation for acute myeloid leukemia," *Journal of Clinical Medicine*, vol. 4, no. 6, pp. 1240–1268, 2015.

[2] C. G. Kanakry, M. J. de Lima, and L. Luznik, "Alternative donor allogeneic hematopoietic cell transplantation for acute myeloid leukemia," *Seminars in Hematology*, vol. 52, no. 3, pp. 232–242, 2015.

[3] L. Gragert, M. Eapen, E. Williams et al., "HLA match likelihoods for hematopoietic stem-cell grafts in the U.S. registry," *The New England Journal of Medicine*, vol. 371, no. 4, pp. 339–348, 2014.

[4] J. Mehta, O. Frankfurt, J. Altman et al., "Optimizing the CD34 + cell dose for reduced-intensity allogeneic hematopoietic stem

cell transplantation," *Leukemia and Lymphoma*, vol. 50, no. 9, pp. 1434–1441, 2009.

[5] J. N. Barker, A. Scaradavou, and C. E. Stevens, "Combined effect of total nucleated cell dose and HLA match on transplantation outcome in 1061 cord blood recipients with hematologic malignancies," *Blood*, vol. 115, no. 9, pp. 1843–1849, 2010.

[6] A. M. Raiola, A. Dominietto, C. di Grazia et al., "Unmanipulated haploidentical transplants compared with other alternative donors and matched sibling grafts," *Biology of Blood and Marrow Transplantation*, vol. 20, no. 10, pp. 1573–1579, 2014.

[7] Y. Wang, Q.-F. Liu, L.-P. Xu et al., "Haploidentical vs identical-sibling transplant for AML in remission: a multicenter, prospective study," *Blood*, vol. 125, no. 25, pp. 3956–3962, 2015.

[8] S. O. Ciurea, M. J. Zhang, A. A. Bacigalupo et al., "Haploidentical transplant with posttransplant cyclophosphamide vs matched unrelated donor transplant for acute myeloid leukemia," *Blood*, vol. 126, no. 8, pp. 1033–1040, 2015.

[9] O. Ringden, M. Labopin, M. Ciceri et al., "Is there a stronger graft-versus-leukemia effect using HLA-haploidentical donors compared with HLA-identical siblings?" *Leukemia*, 2015.

[10] Y. L. Kasamon, L. Luznik, M. S. Leffell et al., "Nonmyeloablative HLA-haploidentical bone marrow transplantation with high-dose posttransplantation cyclophosphamide: effect of HLA disparity on outcome," *Biology of Blood and Marrow Transplantation*, vol. 16, no. 4, pp. 482–489, 2010.

[11] A. Bashey, X. Zhang, C. A. Sizemore et al., "T-cell-replete HLA-haploidentical hematopoietic transplantation for hematologic malignancies using post-transplantation cyclophosphamide results in outcomes equivalent to those of contemporaneous HLA-matched related and unrelated donor transplantation," *Journal of Clinical Oncology*, vol. 31, no. 10, pp. 1310–1316, 2013.

[12] D.-P. Lu, L. Dong, T. Wu et al., "Conditioning including antithymocyte globulin followed by unmanipulated HLA-mismatched/haploidentical blood and marrow transplantation can achieve comparable outcomes with HLA-identical sibling transplantation," *Blood*, vol. 107, no. 8, pp. 3065–3073, 2006.

[13] F. Aversa, A. Tabilio, A. Terenzi et al., "Successful engraftment of T-cell-depleted haploidentical "three-loci" incompatible transplants in leukemia patients by addition of recombinant human granulocyte colony-stimulating factor-mobilized peripheral blood progenitor cells to bone marrow inoculum," *Blood*, vol. 84, no. 11, pp. 3948–3955, 1994.

[14] F. Aversa, A. Tabilio, A. Velardi et al., "Treatment of high-risk acute leukemia with T-cell-depleted stem cells from related donors with one fully mismatched HLA haplotype," *The New England Journal of Medicine*, vol. 339, no. 17, pp. 1186–1193, 1998.

[15] F. Aversa, A. Terenzi, A. Tabilio et al., "Full haplotype-mismatched hematopoietic stem-cell transplantation: a phase II study in patients with acute leukemia at high risk of relapse," *Journal of Clinical Oncology*, vol. 23, no. 15, pp. 3447–3454, 2005.

[16] F. Ciceri, M. Labopin, F. Aversa et al., "A survey of fully haploidentical hematopoietic stem cell transplantation in adults with high-risk acute leukemia: a risk factor analysis of outcomes for patients in remission at transplantation," *Blood*, vol. 112, no. 9, pp. 3574–3581, 2008.

[17] P. Lang, J. Greil, P. Bader et al., "Long-term outcome after haploidentical stem cell transplantation in children," *Blood Cells, Molecules, and Diseases*, vol. 33, no. 3, pp. 281–287, 2004.

[18] T. Klingebiel, J. Cornish, M. Labopin et al., "Results and factors influencing outcome after fully haploidentical hematopoietic stem cell transplantation in children with very high-risk acute

lymphoblastic leukemia: impact of center size: an analysis on behalf of the Acute Leukemia and Pediatric Disease Working Parties of the European Blood and Marrow Transplant group," *Blood*, vol. 115, no. 17, pp. 3437–3446, 2010.

[19] I. Walker, N. Shehata, G. Cantin et al., "Canadian multicenter pilot trial of haploidentical donor transplantation," *Blood Cells, Molecules, and Diseases*, vol. 33, no. 3, pp. 222–226, 2004.

[20] M. F. Martelli, M. Di Ianni, L. Ruggeri et al., "HLA-haploidentical transplantation with regulatory and conventional T-cell adoptive immunotherapy prevents acute leukemia relapse," *Blood*, vol. 124, no. 4, pp. 638–644, 2014.

[21] E. K. Waller, C. R. Giver, H. Rosenthal et al., "Facilitating T-cell immune reconstitution after haploidentical transplantation in adults," *Blood Cells, Molecules, and Diseases*, vol. 33, no. 3, pp. 233–237, 2004.

[22] W. A. Bethge, C. Faul, M. Bornhäuser et al., "Haploidentical allogeneic hematopoietic cell transplantation in adults using CD3/CD19 depletion and reduced intensity conditioning: an update," *Blood Cells, Molecules, and Diseases*, vol. 40, no. 1, pp. 13–19, 2008.

[23] M. Schumm, P. Lang, W. Bethge et al., "Depletion of T-cell receptor alpha/beta and CD19 positive cells from apheresis products with the CliniMACS device," *Cytotherapy*, vol. 15, no. 10, pp. 1253–1258, 2013.

[24] I. Airoldi, A. Bertaina, I. Prigione et al., "$\gamma\delta$ T-cell reconstitution after HLA-haploidentical hematopoietic transplantation depleted of TCR-$\alpha\beta^+$/CD19$^+$ lymphocytes," *Blood*, vol. 125, no. 15, pp. 2349–2358, 2015.

[25] K. Perruccio, A. Tosti, E. Burchielli et al., "Transferring functional immune responses to pathogens after haploidentical hematopoietic transplantation," *Blood*, vol. 106, no. 13, pp. 4397–4406, 2005.

[26] M. F. Martelli, M. Di Ianni, L. Ruggeri et al., "'Designed' grafts for HLA-haploidentical stem cell transplantation," *Blood*, vol. 123, no. 7, pp. 967–973, 2014.

[27] C. Bonini, G. Ferrari, S. Verzeletti et al., "HSV-TK gene transfer into donor lymphocytes for control of allogeneic graft-versus-leukemia," *Science*, vol. 276, no. 5319, pp. 1719–1724, 1997.

[28] F. Ciceri, C. Bonini, M. T. L. Stanghellini et al., "Infusion of suicide-gene-engineered donor lymphocytes after family haploidentical haemopoietic stem-cell transplantation for leukaemia (the TK007 trial): a non-randomised phase I-II study," *The Lancet Oncology*, vol. 10, no. 5, pp. 489–500, 2009.

[29] A. Di Stasi, S.-K. Tey, G. Dotti et al., "Inducible apoptosis as a safety switch for adoptive cell therapy," *The New England Journal of Medicine*, vol. 365, no. 18, pp. 1673–1683, 2011.

[30] X. J. Huang, D. H. Liu, K. Y. Liu et al., "Haploidentical hematopoietic stem cell transplantation without in vitro T-cell depletion for the treatment of hematological malignances," *Bone Marrow Transplant*, vol. 38, no. 4, pp. 291–297, 2006.

[31] D. Liu, X. Huang, K. Liu et al., "Haploidentical hematopoietic stem cell transplantation without in vitro T cell depletion for treatment of hematological malignancies in children," *Biology of Blood and Marrow Transplantation*, vol. 14, no. 4, pp. 469–477, 2008.

[32] P. Di Bartolomeo, S. Santarone, G. De Angelis et al., "Haploidentical, unmanipulated, G-CSF-primed bone marrow transplantation for patients with high-risk hematologic malignancies," *Blood*, vol. 121, no. 5, pp. 849–857, 2013.

[33] L. Luznik, P. V. O'Donnell, H. J. Symons et al., "HLA-haploidentical bone marrow transplantation for hematologic

malignancies using nonmyeloablative conditioning and high-dose, posttransplantation cyclophosphamide," *Biology of Blood and Marrow Transplantation*, vol. 14, no. 6, pp. 641–650, 2008.

[34] P. V. O'Donnell, L. Luznik, R. J. Jones et al., "Nonmyeloablative bone marrow transplantation from partially HLA-mismatched related donors using posttransplantation cyclophosphamide," *Biology of Blood and Marrow Transplantation*, vol. 8, no. 7, pp. 377–386, 2002.

[35] S. R. McCurdy, J. A. Kanakry, M. M. Showel et al., "Risk-stratified outcomes of nonmyeloablative HLA-haploidentical BMT with high-dose posttransplantation cyclophosphamide," *Blood*, vol. 125, no. 19, pp. 3024–3031, 2015.

[36] D. R. Shook, B. M. Triplett, P. W. Eldridge, G. Kang, A. Srinivasan, and W. Leung, "Haploidentical stem cell transplantation augmented by CD45RA negative lymphocytes provides rapid engraftment and excellent tolerability," *Pediatric Blood and Cancer*, vol. 62, no. 4, pp. 666–673, 2015.

[37] B. M. Triplett, D. R. Shook, P. Eldridge et al., "Rapid memory T-cell reconstitution recapitulating CD45RA-depleted haploidentical transplant graft content in patients with hematologic malignancies," *Bone Marrow Transplantation*, vol. 50, pp. 968–977, 2015.

[38] Y. Kanda, S. Chiba, H. Hirai et al., "Allogeneic hematopoietic stem cell transplantation from family members other than HLA-identical siblings over the last decade (1991–2000)," *Blood*, vol. 102, no. 4, pp. 1541–1547, 2003.

[39] Y. Wang, D.-H. Liu, L.-P. Xu et al., "Superior graft-versus-leukemia effect associated with transplantation of haploidentical compared with HLA-identical sibling donor grafts for high-risk acute leukemia: an historic comparison," *Biology of Blood and Marrow Transplantation*, vol. 17, no. 6, pp. 821–830, 2011.

[40] R. Szydlo, J. M. Goldman, J. P. Klein et al., "Results of allogeneic bone marrow transplants for leukemia using donors other than HLA-identical siblings," *Journal of Clinical Oncology*, vol. 15, no. 5, pp. 1767–1777, 1997.

[41] R. C. Ash, M. M. Horowitz, R. P. Gale et al., "Bone marrow transplantation from related donors other than HLA-identical siblings: effect of T cell depletion," *Bone Marrow Transplantation*, vol. 7, no. 6, pp. 443–452, 1991.

16

Vitamin D and Nonskeletal Complications among Egyptian Sickle Cell Disease Patients

Mona Hamdy,[1] **Niveen Salama** (ID)**,**[1] **Ghada Maher,**[2] **and Amira Elrefaee**[1]

[1]*Department of Pediatrics, Faculty of Medicine, Cairo University, Cairo, Egypt*
[2]*Department of Chemical Pathology, Faculty of Medicine, Cairo University, Cairo, Egypt*

Correspondence should be addressed to Niveen Salama; niveensab@yahoo.com

Academic Editor: Estella M. Matutes

Lower levels of vitamin D have been documented in many patients with sickle cell disease (SCD), but data are still inconclusive regarding the association between vitamin D deficiency (VDD) and the occurrence or the severity of various SCD complications. Our study aimed to detect the prevalence of vitamin D deficiency among Egyptian patients with SCD and to associate it with the clinical course of the disease. We measured the level of 25-hydroxy vitamin D in 140 children (age from 4.3 to 15.5years), 80 patients with SCD and 60 controls using enzyme-linked immunosorbent assay. Vitamin D was deficient in 60% of SCD compared to 26.7% of controls. Severe VDD was significantly higher in SCD patients than controls. Patients were divided into 2 groups; Normal group (32 patients) and Deficient group (48 patients). There were statistically significant differences between the 2 groups regarding their age, height percentile, the presence of clinical jaundice, and osseous changes (P values 0.043, 0.024, 0.001, and 0.015, respectively). Hemoglobin and hematocrit values were significantly lower in Deficient group (P values 0.022 and 0.004, respectively) while the levels of aspartate aminotransferase, lactate dehydrogenase, and total and indirect bilirubin were significantly higher in the same group (P values 0.006, 0.001, 0.038, and 0.016, respectively). The frequency of blood transfusions, hospitalization, and vasoocclusive crisis previous year as well as the history of bone fracture and recurrent infections proved to be significantly higher in Deficient group. These findings suggest that VDD may play a role in the pathogenesis of hemolysis and other complication of SCD. Vitamin D monitoring and supplementation in patients with SCD should be implemented as a standard of care to potentially improve health outcomes in these affected patients.

1. Introduction

Vitamin D has been the focus of attention of many researchers concerned with general health as well as specific diseases. Though exposure of the skin to the ultraviolet (UV) sun rays is the main source of de novo vitamin D synthesis [1], North African and Middle Eastern countries, with abundant sun all over the year, reported the highest frequencies of vitamin D deficiency (VDD) in all age groups world-wide [2, 3].

Studies in patients with sickle cell disease (SCD) revealed high prevalence of VDD in these patients regardless of their age or ethnic background [4–7]. Predisposing factors that can contribute to such deficiency include decreased synthesis of vitamin D from sunlight due to skin pigmentation and limited outdoor activity, diminished exogenous supply as a result of poor appetite and impaired absorption by the

damaged intestinal mucosa as a complication of SCD, and increased metabolic requirements due to increased erythrocyte production to compensate for shortened lifespan of the red cells and also decreased level of vitamin D binding protein 'which is known in inflammatory conditions as SCD' resulting in decreased serum level of vitamin D. Finally impaired renal function which is known in many patients with SCD interferes with hydroxylation of vitamin D to 25-hydroxy-vitamin D (25-OHD) [4, 8].

Vitamin D deficiency has been linked to many skeletal and extraskeletal disorders including cardiovascular diseases [9], respiratory disorders, and asthma [10]. Vitamin D also has immunomodulatory and antimicrobial activities that affect both innate and acquired immunity [11]; all these disorders could have direct impact on the clinical course of SCD. In addition, suboptimal vitamin D levels have been detected in many pathological conditions associated with SCD such as vasoocclusive crises (VOC) [8], chronic pain [12], bone fragility [13], renal impairment [14], and autoimmune and inflammatory disorders [15]. Whether VDD initiates or exacerbates these disorders and the effect of its supplementation on their clinical courses remains to be determined.

Few studies are available regarding the nutritional status of SCD patients, including their vitamin D levels, and even fewer correlate specific nutritional deficiencies to the clinical profile of these patients.

Aim of Work. Our study was conducted to determine vitamin D status in Egyptian children and adolescents with sickle cell disease and to detect the effect of its deficiency on the clinical course of the disease as regards VOC, hemolysis, and other complications of the disease.

2. Materials and Methods

This is a case control cross-sectional study conducted on the Hematology Clinic, New Children Hospital, Cairo University. Eighty SCD patients and 60 age and sex frequency matched healthy control were enrolled. Informed consent was obtained from all patients, controls, and/or their legal guardians. Our study was conducted in accordance with the Declaration of Helsinki and was approved by the ethical committee of the New Children Hospital, Cairo University. All cases were in steady state indicated by the absence of any painful episodes in last 4 weeks prior to enrollment [17]. Patients older than 20 years and those with renal impairment, chronic malabsorption, osteoporosis, osteopenia, intercurrent infection or inflammation, and ongoing steroid therapy were excluded from the study. Clinical data were obtained from the patients' interviewing and medical records including anthropometric measures, number of blood transfusions, VOC, and hospital admissions in the last year.

VOC were classified as mild, moderate, and severe where mild and moderate VOC were managed at home (with non-steroidal anti-inflammatory drugs and weak opioid, respectively) while severe VOC required hospitalization and the use of strong opioid [18].

The cross-sectional nature of the study and the limited financial resources due to self-funding of the study hinder our ability to monitor vitamin D level all over the year, so blood sampling was performed during the summer months 'from June to August', taking into consideration the seasonal variation of vitamin D level with expected higher level of the vitamin during summer, assuming that deficient patients during summer are deficient in the other seasons.

Blood was withdrawn from all study populations in the outpatient clinic. Laboratory investigations included complete blood count, reticulocyte count, aspartate transaminase (AST), alanine transaminase (ALT), lactate dehydrogenase (LDH), and total and indirect serum bilirubin.

2.1. 25-Hyroxyvitamin D. 25-OHD was measured for case and control groups as it is the major circulating form of

TABLE 1: The ranges for the classification of 25-hydrxyvitamin D status [16].

Vitamin D status	25-OH Vitamin D (ng/ml)
Severe deficiency	<10
Deficiency	10-20
Sufficiency	20-30.
Toxicity	>100

vitamin D and is considered the most accurate marker for vitamin D status [19].

2.2. Sample Collection, Storage, and Preparation. Blood samples were collected by venipuncture, allowed to clot, and then centrifuged at room temperature for 1 hour. Specimens were stored at 8 Celsius degrees for 3 days and or -20 Celsius longer duration.

2.3. Assay Procedures. Enzyme-linked immunosorbent assay (ELISA) was based on competitive binding using the DRY-HYBRID-XL 25-OH Vitamin D kits. The walls of the reagents cartridge are coated with vitamin D binding protein (VDBP). Endogenous 25-OHD of the samples competes with a 25-OHD-biotin for binding to the coated VDBP. After incubation the unbound conjugate is washed off, thereafter, bound 25-OHD-biotin conjugate is detected by streptavidin-conjugated peroxidase (Enzyme complex). The amount of bound peroxidase conjugate is inversely proportional to the concentration of 25-OHD in the sample [20].

2.4. Expected Normal Values. Each laboratory should determine its own normal and pathological values. Our laboratory suggests the ranges in Table 1 for the classification of 25-OHD status [16].

The dynamic range of the assay is defined by the limit of detection and the maximum values of the Master curves. Values found below the measuring range are indicated as < 4.6 ng/mL and values above the measuring ranges are indicated as > 130 ng/ml.

2.5. Statistical Analysis. The data were analyzed using the S-plus Statistics Software *(SPSS version 21)*. Descriptive statistical calculations (mean ± standard deviation) were done to quantitative values. Statistical analyses were performed using the independent *t*-test as applicable for quantitative variables. *Fisher exact test* and *Pearson Chi-Square test* were used for qualitative variables. *Two-tailed P-values* of less than 0.05 were considered to be significant. *The Pearson correlation coefficient* (r) was used to express the relationship between quantitative variables in different groups.

3. Results

The study populations were composed of 80 Egyptian cases with SCD, compared to 60 age and sex frequency matched healthy controls with male-to-female ratios 1.4: 1 and 1.3:1, respectively. Case group consisted of 59 (73.8%) patients with

TABLE 2: Demographic and laboratory data of the case and control groups.

Variable	Case(n=80)	Control(n=60)	P-value
Age: in years:median (IQR)	9 (7.5)	9.5 (8)	0.753
Sex: n (%)			0.522
Male (%)	47 (58.8%)	34 (56.6%)	
Female (%)	33 (41.2%)	26 (43.3%)	
Hemoglobin (g/dl): mean ± SD	8.3 ±1.4	13.2 ±1.8	**Less than 0.001**
Hematocrit (%): mean ± SD	25.5 ±4.8	37 ±3.9	**Less than 0.001**
MCV (FL): mean ± SD:	84.5 ±8.8	88.1 ± 6.8	**0.008**
MCH (pg): mean ± SD	25.0 ±3	32.3 ±1.7	**Less than 0.001**
WBC (10^3mm^2): mean ± SD	9.2 ±4.4	7.9 ±2.1	**0.033**
Platelets (10^3mm^2): mean ± SD	328.2 ±164.4	284.7 ±106.4	0.067
25-OHD (ng/ml): mean ± SD	22 ±10.4	22.7±8.4	0.658
No Deficiency: n (%)	32 (40%)	44(73.3%)	0.061
Deficiency: n (%)	48 (60%)	16 (26.7%)	0.058
Severe deficiency: n (%)	13 (16.2%)	5 (8.3%)	**0.021**
25-OHD in VDD groups (ng/ml): mean ± SD	9.9 ±2.1	11±1.8	**0.049**

n= number. IQR= interquartile range. SD = standard deviation. 25-OHD =25-hydroxyvitamin D. MCV = mean corpuscular volume. MCH= mean corpuscular hemoglobin. WBC= white blood cells. VDD= vitamin D deficiency. Bold values indicate statistical significance.

homozygous hemoglobin S *(HBSS)* and 21(26.2%) patients with sickle β-thalassemia *(HBSβ)*. The demographic and laboratory data of the 2 groups are shown in Table 2.

There were statistically significant differences between case and control groups regarding the level of hemoglobin (Hb), hematocrit, mean corpuscular volume (MCV), mean corpuscular hemoglobin (MCH), and white blood cell (WBC) counts.

Cases of sickle cell disease were divided into 2 groups: 'Normal group' with normal vitamin D level (32 patients) and 'Deficient group' with VDD (48 patients). Table 3 showed the demographic and laboratory data of the 2 groups.

There were statistically significant differences between the 2 groups regarding their age, height percentile, and the presence of clinical jaundice and osseous changes (P values 0.043, 0.024, 0.001 and 0.015, respectively). Regarding lab results, hemoglobin and hematocrit values were significantly lower in Deficient group (P values 0.022 and 0.004, respectively) while the levels of aspartate aminotransferase, lactate dehydrogenase, and total and indirect bilirubin were significantly higher in the same group (P values 0.006, 0.001, 0.038, and 0.016, respectively).

Data from Table 4 shows weak but statistically significant correlation between serum 25-OHD and the biomarker of hemolysis and red blood cell turnover. VDD patients had lower level of hemoglobin and hematocrit and higher level of AST, LDH, and total and indirect bilirubin.

The association between VDD and the clinical course and complications of SCD is shown in Table 5.

The frequencies of blood transfusions and hospitalization last year were significantly higher in Deficient group; also the occurrence of vasoocclusive crises last year and the presence of old fractured bone and recurrent infections proved to be statistically significant.

4. Discussion

The reported incidences of VDD range from 20 to 80% in some Middle Eastern counties [21]. Despite these high incidences, VDD often remained underdiagnosed and untreated especially in patients with SCD where chronic pain of VDD was usually credited to SCD, as the pain in both conditions is dull aching and deeply seated and involves the back and extremities [22].

In our study, we found 26.7% incidence of VDD among the healthy control group; however, further population based studies are needed to evaluate vitamin D status among the Egyptians. Forty-eight (60%) of our SCD patients and 16 (26.7%) of controls were found to have VDD, with 13 cases and 5 controls having severe deficiency with statistically significant difference between the two groups. These results are in close approximation to those obtained from Spain [23] and Turkey [24] where the prevalence of VDD among SCD patients was 56.4% and 63.1%, respectively, while the prevalence of severe VDD (25-OH D level < 10 ng/ml) was 12% in a study on sickle patients conducted in Saudi Arabia [25].

We detected a weak negative correlation between age and vitamin D level; the older the age, the lower the level. This correlation 'which is well established by other studies [1, 26]' could be weak due to the proximity in age distribution between our studied patients with VDD and those with normal vitamin D level. In older age patients, this negative correlation could be explained by prolonged course of the disease with more skin pigmentation, more intestinal mucosal damage, and renal impairment which all affect vitamin D metabolism.

We did not detect any significant correlation between sickle disease genotype and vitamin D status. This finding

TABLE 3: Demographic and laboratory data of the 2 groups.

Variable	Normal Group (n=32)	Deficient Group (n=48)	P-value
Age: in years:median (IQR)	8 (9.235)	11(5)	**0.043**
Sex: n (%)			0.732
Male (%)	17 (53.1%)	30 (62.5%)	
Female (%)	15 (46.9%)	18 (37.5%)	
Weight percentile: mean ± SD	29.7±20.2	22.1±18.2	0.072
Height percentile: mean ± SD	33.8±26.5	22.2±24.8	**0.024**
Hemoglobin genotype: n (%)			0.635
HBSS (%)	26 (81.3%)	33 (68.7%)	
HBSB+ (%)	5 (15.6%)	11 (20.8%)	
HBSB0 (%)	1 (3.1%)	4 (10.5%)	
Splenomegaly: n (%) (n= 28)	12 (37.5)	16 (33.4)	0.655
Splenectomy: n (%) (n=22)	7 (31.8)	15 (68.2)	0.156
Pallor: n (%) (n=38)	12 (31.5)	26 (68.5)	0.267
Jaundice: n (%) (n=21)	1 (4.8)	20 (95.2)	**0.001**
Osseous changes: n (%) (n=13)	3 (23)	10 (76)	**0.015**
Hemoglobin (g/dL): mean ± SD	8.6±1.1	7.9±1.6	**0.022**
Hematocrit (%): mean ± SD	26.9±4	23.9±5.1	**0.004**
Reticulocyte count (%): mean ± SD	4.8±2.9	6.5±4.1	0.063
Corrected Reticulocyte count (%): mean ± SD	2.6±1.4	3±2.1	0.401
AST (IU/L): mean ± SD	43.3±23.3	54.4±20.1	**0.006**
ALT (IU/L): mean ± SD	25.1±20.3	27.1±18.8	0.540
LDH (IU/L): mean ± SD	454.8±279.4	634.9±277.8	**0.001**
TSB (mg/dL): mean ± SD	4.2±2.4	5.9±3.5	**0.038**
Indirect bilirubin (mg/dL): mean ± SD	2±1.8	2.6±1.4	**0.016**

n = number. IQR = interquartile range. SD = standard deviation. *HBSS*= homozygous hemoglobin S; $HBS\beta^+$ = $S\beta^+$ thalassemia; $HBS\beta^0$ = $S\beta^0$ thalassemia; AST = aspartate aminotransferase; ALT = alanine aminotransferase; LDH = lactate dehydrogenase; TSB = total serum bilirubin. Bold values indicate statistical significance.

TABLE 4: Correlation between Serum 25-OHD and biomarkers of intravascular femolysis.

Variable	Correlation Coefficient(r)	P.value
Hemoglobin (g/dl)	0.27	**0.019**
Hematocrit (%)	0.29	**0.011**
Reticulocyte count (%)	-0.31	**0.007**
Corrected Reticulocyte count (%)	-0.22	0.061
AST	-0.33	**0.003**
ALT	-0.05	0.618
LDH	-0.27	**0.017**
TSB	-0.29	**0.010**
Indirect SB	-0.35	**0.002**

AST = aspartate transaminase; ALT = alanine transaminase; LDH = lactate dehydrogenase; TSB = total serum bilirubin; indirect SB = indirect serum bilirubin. Bold values indicate statistical significance.

was supported by similar study performed on SCD patients in Spanish population [23].

In our study, we found significantly lower height percentile in SCD patient with VDD than those with normal vitamin D level, while the weight percentile was lower though did not reach significance. Other studies [24, 25] showed impairment in both weight and height percentile among SCD patients with VDD compared to those with sufficient

vitamin D. Further verification studies are needed to detect the impacts of VDD on the patients' growth parameters.

A statistically significant correlation was observed between vitamin D level and biomarkers of hemolysis. Lower vitamin D levels were associated with lower hemoglobin and hematocrit but with higher reticulocyte counts, AST, LDH, and total and indirect serum bilirubin levels. Whether VDD increases hemolysis or excessive hemolysis increases

TABLE 5: Association between VDD, clinical course, and complications of SCD.

Variable	Normal Group (n=32)	Deficient Group (n=48)	P-value
Blood transfusion: n (%) (n=69)	30 (43.4)	39 (56.6)	0.475
Age at 1st blood transfusion (years)	2.3 ± 1.9	1.6 ±1.0	0.351
Frequency of blood transfusion/ Last year	3.6 ± 2.8	5.4 ± 3.5	**0.021**
Positive VOC/ Last year: n (%) (n=68)	24 (35.2)	44 (64.8)	**0.032**
Degree of VOC: n (%)			0.732
Mild (n=41)	13 (31.7)	28 (68.3)	
Moderate (n= 21)	10 (47.6)	11 (52.4)	
Severe (n= 6)	1 (16.6)	5 (83.4)	
Hospital admission/ Last year: n (%) (n=44)	14 (31.8)	30 (68.2)	**0.012**
Bone fracture: n (%) (n=8)	1 (12.5)	7 (87.5)	**0.034**
Recurrent infection: n (%) (n= 36)	7 (19.5)	29 (80.5)	**0.036**
Viral hepatitis (B&C): n (%) (n=12)	5 (41.6)	7 (58.4)	0.219
Pulmonary hypertension: n (%)(n=11)	3 (27.3)	8 (72.7)	0.068
Diabetes Mellitus: n (%) (n=4)	2 (50)	2 (50)	0.721
Abnormal TCD: n (%) (n= 2)	1 (50)	1 (50)	0.834
Gall Bladder stones: n (%) (n= 3)	1 (33.3)	2 (66.7)	0.059

n = number; SD = standard deviation; VOC = vasoocclusive crisis; TCD= transcranial Doppler. Bold values indicate statistical significance.

the demand of vitamin D is still debatable. Winters and colleagues suggested that increased hemolysis and bone marrow activity may interfere with vitamin D absorption leading to VDD [26], while other authors suggested that VDD may increase hemolysis of RBCs in patient with SCD [19].

Low "hemoglobin and hematocrit" and high "reticulocyte count and LDH" were associated with significantly lower level of vitamin D in other studies [27–29]. A recent study showed a positive correlation between hemoglobin concentration and vitamin D level where 1g/L hemoglobin increase was associated with 0.4 nmol/L increase of serum vitamin D level [30]; however, others showed nonsignificant correlation between vitamin D level and hemoglobin, hematocrit, reticulocyte count, or AST level [5, 19, 31].

We have noticed that, throughout the year prior to enrollment, SCD patients with VDD had significantly higher incidences of VOC, blood transfusions, hospital or emergency room visits, and recurrent infections as compared to those with normal vitamin D level.

Vasoocclusive crisis is the hallmark of SCD and the main cause of healthcare utilization. Our study along with other studies [8, 32] provided evidence that painful episodes in SCD correlate positively with VDD, the mechanism of which is still unclear, but a recent study associates lower vitamin D level to increased expression of SLC6A5 gene which encodes for a neuronal pain pathway protein called glycine tranporter-2 which may have a direct effect on the nervous system. Impaired bone health may also contribute to these painful episodes [32, 33]; Osunkwo and colleagues also proved that proper vitamin D therapy could reduce the number of painful days and improve quality of life [12]. Though others failed to detect any association between VDD and the number of painful episode, this could be explained by the high incidence (96.4%) of VDD among the studied sample [34].

The role of vitamin D in both innate and acquired immunity has been well established; vitamin D activated at extrarenal sites supports innate immunity by stimulating the expression of Cathelicidin, "member of a group of antimicrobial peptide called Defensins", which is usually suppressed by pathogens [11]. Vitamin D also exhibits a pivotal role in both cell mediated and humoral immune responses by modulating the proliferation of T lymphocytes and regulating cytokines production and also through downregulation of B lymphocyte proliferation, antibodies production, and cell switching to plasma or memory cell [35, 36]. In our study, we detected a significantly higher incidence of respiratory and urinary tract infections among patients with VDD. Several studies conducted in children confirmed our findings of significant association between VDD and increased risk of viral and bacterial respiratory tract infections [37–39]; Urashima and colleagues even suggest that vitamin D supplementation plays a role in prevention of seasonal influenza [40]. Other authors encounter more than 50% reduction of the respiratory illness rate on the second year of monthly vitamin D supplementation [41].

Our study has its own limitations: first, the studied sample being collected from patient attending SCD clinic at a single tertiary care hospital which may not represent all patients with SCD; second, the lack of community-based studies to detect the prevalence of VDD among the Egyptian population; lastly, the lack of proper dietary and medication history including vitamins supplementation.

5. Conclusions and Recommendations

Vitamin D deficiency is a major nutritional health problem in patients with sickle cell disease that may aggravate the disease process and increase the risk of its complications. Further prospective and interventional studies are needed to confirm the causal relationship between VDD and suspected complications and the effect and proper dose of vitamin D replacement before considering vitamin D as an adjunct therapy in SCD management; however, periodic measurement of vitamin D level should be implemented as primary care point in patients with SCD.

Disclosure

The current address of Mona Hamdy, Niveen Salama and Amira Elrefaee is New Children Hospital, Abu El Rish, Cairo University Hospital, Cairo, Egypt. The current address of Ghada Maher is Kaser El Einy Hospital, Cairo University Hospital, Cairo, Egypt. This study is self-funded by the authors.

Conflicts of Interest

The authors declare that they have no conflicts of interest.

Authors' Contributions

Mona Hamdy and Niveen Salama contributed equally in this work being joint senior authors. Ghada Maher and Amira Elrefaee also contributed equally in this work being responsible for samples collection and analysis.

Acknowledgments

The authors would like to express their sincere gratitude and respect to all the staff at the Hematology Clinic of Cairo University Children's Hospital, for their continuous efforts, support, and patience. Without their help and guidance, this study could not be conducted. They would like also to thank all the patients with sickle cell disease for their great spirits, cooperation, and commitment in providing the required data and samples.

References

[1] C. Wykes, A. Arasaretnam, S. O'Driscoll, L. Farnham, C. Moniz, and D. C. Rees, "Vitamin D deficiency and its correction in children with sickle cell anaemia," *Annals of Hematology*, vol. 93, no. 12, pp. 2051–2056, 2014.

[2] C. Palacios and L. Gonzalez, "Is vitamin D deficiency a major global public health problem?" *The Journal of Steroid Biochemistry and Molecular Biology*, vol. 144, no. Part A, pp. 138–145, 2014.

[3] D. Bassil, M. Rahme, M. Hoteit, and G. E.-H. Fuleihan, "Hypovitaminosis D in the Middle East and North Africa Prevalence, risk factors and impact on outcomes," *Dermato-Endocrinology*, vol. 5, no. 2, pp. 274–298, 2013.

[4] V. G. Nolan, K. A. Nottage, E. W. Cole, J. S. Hankins, and J. G. Gurney, "Prevalence of vitamin D deficiency in sickle cell disease: a systematic review," *PLoS ONE*, vol. 10, no. 3, Article ID e0119908, 2015.

[5] A. M. Buison, D. A. Kawchak, J. Schall, K. Ohene-Frempong, V. A. Stallings, and B. S. Zemel, "Low vitamin D status in children with sickle cell disease," *Journal of Pediatrics*, vol. 145, no. 5, pp. 622–627, 2004.

[6] P. C. Boettger, C. L. Knupp, D. K. Liles, and K. Walker, "Vitamin D Deficiency in Adult Sickle Cell Patients," *Journal of the National Medical Association*, vol. 109, no. 1, pp. 36–43, 2017.

[7] B. O. Tayo, T. S. Akingbola, B. L. Salako et al., "Vitamin D levels are low in adult patients with sickle cell disease in Jamaica and West Africa," *BMC Hematology*, vol. 14, no. 1, 2014.

[8] M. T. Lee, M. Licursi, and D. J. Mcmahon, "Vitamin D deficiency and acute vaso-occlusive complications in children with sickle cell disease," *Pediatric Blood & Cancer*, vol. 62, no. 4, pp. 643–647, 2015.

[9] T. J. Wang, M. J. Pencina, S. L. Booth et al., "Vitamin D deficiency and risk of cardiovascular disease," *Circulation*, vol. 117, no. 4, pp. 503–511, 2008.

[10] A. Gupta, A. Sjoukes, D. Richards et al., "Relationship between serum vitamin D, disease severity, and airway remodeling in children with asthma," *American Journal of Respiratory and Critical Care Medicine*, vol. 184, no. 12, pp. 1342–1349, 2011.

[11] J. S. Adams and M. Hewison, "Unexpected actions of vitamin D: new perspectives on the regulation of innate and adaptive immunity," *Nature Clinical Practice: Endocrinology & Metabolism*, vol. 4, no. 2, pp. 80–90, 2008.

[12] I. Osunkwo, E. I. Hodgman, K. Cherry et al., "Vitamin D deficiency and chronic pain in sickle cell disease," *British Journal of Haematology*, vol. 153, no. 4, pp. 538–540, 2011.

[13] J.-B. Arlet, M. Courbebaisse, G. Chatellier et al., "Relationship between vitamin D deficiency and bone fragility in sickle cell disease: a cohort study of 56 adults," *Bone*, vol. 52, no. 1, pp. 206–211, 2013.

[14] D. C. Rees and J. S. Gibson, "Biomarkers in sickle cell disease," *British Journal of Haematology*, vol. 156, no. 4, pp. 433–445, 2012.

[15] S. Unal, Y. Oztas, G. Eskandari, L. T. Gumus, and O. Nuriman, "The Association Between Vitamin D and Inflammation in Sickle Cell Disease," in *Blood*, vol. 124, 21 edition, 2014.

[16] M. F. Holick, N. C. Binkley, H. A. Bischoff-Ferrari et al., "Evaluation, treatment, and prevention of vitamin D deficiency: an endocrine society clinical practice guideline," *The Journal of Clinical Endocrinology & Metabolism*, vol. 96, no. 7, pp. 1911–1930, 2011.

[17] S. K. Ballas, "More definitions in sickle cell disease: steady state v base line data," *American Journal of Hematology*, vol. 87, no. 3, p. 338, 2012.

[18] D. S. Darbari, Z. Wang, M. Kwak, M. Hildesheim, J. Nichols, and D. Allen, "Severe Painful Vaso-Occlusive Crises and Mortality in a Contemporary Adult Sickle Cell Anemia Cohort Study. PLoS One," in *DOI*, vol. 8, pp. e79923-10, e79923, 8(11, 2013.

[19] S. A. Adegoke, J. A. P. Braga, A. D. Adekile, and M. S. Figueiredo, "The Association of Serum 25-Hydroxyvitamin D with Biomarkers of Hemolysis in Pediatric Patients with Sickle Cell Disease," *Journal of Pediatric Hematology/Oncology*, vol. 40, no. 2, pp. 159–162, 2018.

[20] B. W. Hollis, "Editorial: The determination of circulating 25-hydroxyvitamin D: No easy task," *The Journal of Clinical Endocrinology & Metabolism*, vol. 89, no. 7, pp. 3149–3151, 2004.

[21] G. El-Hajj Fuleihan, "Vitamin D deficiency in the Middle East and its health consequences for children and adults," *Clinical*

Reviews in Bone and Mineral Metabolism, vol. 7, no. 1, pp. 77–93, 2009.

[22] A. AlJama, M. AlKhalifah, I. A. Al-Dabbous, and G. Alqudaihi, "Vitamin D deficiency in sickle cell disease patients in the Eastern Province of Saudi Arabia," *Annals of Saudi Medicine*, vol. 38, no. 2, pp. 130–136, 2018.

[23] C. Garrido, E. Cela, C. Beléndez, C. Mata, and J. Huerta, "Status of vitamin D in children with sickle cell disease living in Madrid, Spain," *European Journal of Pediatrics*, vol. 171, no. 12, pp. 1793–1798, 2012.

[24] S. Özen, S. Ünal, N. Erçetin, and B. Taşdelen, "Frequency and risk factors of endocrine complications in Turkish children and adolescents with sickle cell anemia," *Turkish Journal of Hematology*, vol. 30, no. 1, pp. 25–31, 2013.

[25] S. Mohammed, S. Addae, S. Suleiman et al., "Serum calcium, parathyroid hormone, and vitamin D status in children and young adults with sickle cell disease," *Annals of Clinical Biochemistry*, vol. 30, no. 1, pp. 45–51, 1993.

[26] A. C. Winters, W. Kethman, R. Kruse-Jarres, and J. Kanter, "Vitamin D insufficiency is a frequent finding in pediatric and adult patients with sickle cell disease and correlates with markers of cell turnover," *Journal of Nutritional Disorders and Therapy*, vol. 4, no. 140, 2014.

[27] A. Lal, E. B. Fung, Z. Pakbaz, E. Hackney-Stephens, and E. P. Vichinsky, "Bone mineral density in children with sickle cell anemia," *Pediatric Blood & Cancer*, vol. 47, no. 7, pp. 901–906, 2006.

[28] T. S. Garadah, A. B. Hassan, A. A. Jaradat et al., "Predictors of abnormal bone mass density in adult patients with homozygous sickle-cell disease," *Clinical Medicine Insights: Endocrinology and Diabetes*, vol. 8, pp. 35–40, 2015.

[29] M. Sarrai, H. Duroseau, J. D'Augustine, S. Moktan, and R. Bellevue, "Bone mass density in adults with sickle cell disease," *British Journal of Haematology*, vol. 136, no. 4, pp. 666–672, 2007.

[30] K. Samson, H. McCartney, S. Vercauteren, J. Wu, and C. Karakochuk, "Prevalence of Vitamin D Deficiency Varies Widely by Season in Canadian Children and Adolescents with Sickle Cell Disease," *Journal of Clinical Medicine*, vol. 7, no. 2, p. 14, 2018.

[31] A. Ashraf, J. Alvarez, K. Saenz, B. Gower, K. McCormick, and F. Franklin, "Threshold for effects of vitamin D deficiency on glucose metabolism in obese female African-American adolescents," *The Journal of Clinical Endocrinology & Metabolism*, vol. 94, no. 9, pp. 3200–3206, 2009.

[32] I. Osunkwo, T. R. Ziegler, J. Alvarez et al., "High dose vitamin D therapy for chronic pain in children and adolescents with sickle cell disease: results of a randomized double blind pilot study," *British Journal of Haematology*, vol. 159, no. 2, pp. 211–215, 2012.

[33] J. Han, X. Zhang, S. L. Saraf et al., "Risk factors for vitamin D deficiency in sickle cell disease," *British Journal of Haematology*, vol. 181, no. 6, pp. 828–835, 2018.

[34] T. C. Jackson, M. J. Krauss, M. R. Debaun, R. C. Strunk, and A. M. Arbeláez, "Vitamin D deficiency and comorbidities in children with sickle cell anemia," *Pediatric Hematology and Oncology*, vol. 29, no. 3, pp. 261–266, 2012.

[35] S. Chen, G. P. Sims, X. C. Xiao, Y. G. Yue, and P. E. Lipsky, "Modulatory effects of 1,25-dihydroxyvitamin D_3 on human B cell differentiation," *The Journal of Immunology*, vol. 179, no. 3, pp. 1634–1647, 2007.

[36] S. Romagnani, "Regulation of the T cell response," *Clinical & Experimental Allergy*, vol. 36, no. 11, pp. 1357–1366, 2006.

[37] J. R. Sabetta, P. DePetrillo, R. J. Cipriani, J. Smardin, L. A. Burns, and M. L. Landry, "Serum 25-hydroxyvitamin D and the incidence of acute viral respiratory tract infections in healthy adults," *PLoS ONE*, vol. 5, no. 6, Article ID e11088, 2010.

[38] S. A. Quraishi, E. A. Bittner, K. B. Christopher, C. A. Camargo, and J. Salluh, "Vitamin D Status and Community-Acquired Pneumonia: Results from the Third National Health and Nutrition Examination Survey," *PLoS ONE*, vol. 8, no. 11, p. e81120, 2013.

[39] A. A. Ginde, J. M. Mansbach, and C. A. Camargo, "Vitamin D, respiratory infections, and asthma," *Current Allergy and Asthma Reports*, vol. 9, no. 1, pp. 81–87, 2009.

[40] M. Urashima, T. Segawa, M. Okazaki, M. Kurihara, Y. Wada, and H. Ida, "Randomized trial of vitamin D supplementation to prevent seasonal influenza A in schoolchildren," *American Journal of Clinical Nutrition*, vol. 91, no. 5, pp. 1255–1260, 2010.

[41] M. T. Lee, M. Kattan, I. Fennoy et al., "Randomized phase 2 trial of monthly vitamin D to prevent respiratory complications in children with sickle cell disease," *Blood Advances*, vol. 2, no. 9, pp. 969–978, 2018.

17

Choice of Unmanipulated T Cell Replete Graft for Haploidentical Stem Cell Transplant and Posttransplant Cyclophosphamide in Hematologic Malignancies in Adults: Peripheral Blood or Bone Marrow

Shatha Farhan, Edward Peres, and Nalini Janakiraman

Stem Cell Transplant Program, Henry Ford Hospital, Detroit, MI 48202, USA

Correspondence should be addressed to Shatha Farhan; sfarhan1@hfhs.org

Academic Editor: Suparno Chakrabarti

Allogeneic hematopoietic stem cell transplantation (SCT) is often the only curative option for many patients with malignant and benign hematological stem cell disorders. However, some issues are still of concern regarding finding a donor like shrinking family sizes in many societies, underrepresentation of the ethnic minorities in the registries, genetic variability for some races, and significant delays in obtaining stem cells after starting the search. So there is a considerable need to develop alternate donor stem cell sources. The rapid and near universal availability of the haploidentical donor is an advantage of the haploidentical SCT and an opportunity that is being explored currently in many centers especially using T cell replete graft and posttransplant cyclophosphamide. This is probably because it does not require expertise in graft manipulation and because of the lower costs. However, there are still lots of unanswered questions, like the effect of use of bone marrow versus peripheral blood as the source of stem cells on graft-versus-host disease, graft versus tumor, overall survival, immune reconstitution, and quality of life. Here we review the available publications on bone marrow and peripheral blood experience in the haploidentical SCT setting.

1. Introduction

Allogeneic hematopoietic stem cell transplantation (SCT) is often the only curative option for many patients with malignant and benign hematological stem cell disorders [1]. An HLA-matched related sibling/donor (MRD) is the preferred donor; however, donor availability for many patients still remains a significant challenge as only approximately one-third of patients have an MRD and the shrinking family sizes in many societies are further reducing this probability. The likelihood of identifying a volunteer unrelated donor that is suitably matched at HLA-A, HLA-B, HLA-C, and HLA-DRB1 is population specific ranging from about 79% for Caucasian patients of European descent to 30%–50% for patients of other ethnic backgrounds [2]. This is secondary to the underrepresentation of the ethnic minorities in the registries, significant genetic variability for some races, and

expansion of the number of mixed race individuals [3]. In addition, as the age cutoff for reduced intensity conditioning (RIC) and nonmyeloablative (NMA) transplant eligibility has increased, there has been a critical need for alternative donors for those who may not have a suitable HLA-MRD or matched unrelated donor (MUD). Moreover, there are significant delays in obtaining stem cells of couple of months from initiation of the donor search to transplantation [4]. Because high-risk diseases like acute leukemia are more common among the elderly, the time taken to secure a MUD [5] increases the risk of leukemia relapse in this group that needs to proceed to SCT promptly. Even if a matched unrelated donor is identified, the likelihood of proceeding to transplant is less than 50% because of disease progression during the search process [3].

Transplantation from a full haplotype mismatch family donor has been studied for several decades. Potential

HLA-haploidentical donors include biological parents or children of a patient, and each sibling has a 50% chance of sharing exactly one HLA haplotype. In most centers, it is possible to identify at least one HLA-haploidentical first-degree relative for more than 95% of patients, and the average number of HLA-haploidentical donors per patient is 2.7 [6]. This rapid and near universal availability of the donor is an advantage of haploidentical SCT and an opportunity that is being explored currently in many centers. However, there are two major historical barriers to a successful haploidentical SCT which include graft rejection and graft-versus-host disease (GVHD) arising from the intense bidirectional alloreactivity and hence a high nonrelapse mortality (NRM) after transplantation. Recently, utilization of different methods to overcome these issues, like the GIAC protocol, pioneered in China, comprising granulocyte-colony-stimulating factor (GCSF) stimulation of the donor; intensified immunosuppression through posttransplantation cyclosporine, mycophenolate mofetil (MMF), and short-course methotrexate; antithymocyte globulin and combination of peripheral blood stem cell and bone marrow allografts; and the use of posttransplantation cyclophosphamide (Cy) [7, 8], and the development of novel methods of selective depletion of T cell subsets, such as the use of $\alpha\beta$ TCD [9, 10], have improved safety of haploidentical SCT.

Because of lower rate of severe opportunistic infections and less NRM with T replete compared to T cell deplete stem cell transplantation [11, 12] and because T cell depletion is relatively inexpensive and does not require expertise in graft manipulation and the feasibility of posttransplant Cy, T cell replete unmanipulated haploidentical graft is now considered to be a viable alternative option for patients. Posttransplant Cy can induce donor-host tolerance to allografting and decrease GVHD probably by eliminating alloreactive T cell clones without myeloablation [7]. Hematopoietic stem cells are quiescent nondividing cells which express high levels of aldehyde dehydrogenase, likely responsible for cellular resistance to Cy, while T, B, and NK cells express low levels of this enzyme, rendering them sensitive to Cy cytotoxicity [13]. The use of posttransplant Cy has been based on evidence dating back to the 1960s by Berenbaum and Santos who reported that the use of high-dose posttransplant Cy can prevent skin graft rejection when administered 2-3 days after allografting [8]. Immunosuppression after transplant has been shown to promote allograft tolerance and prevent or alleviate GVHD. Storb and colleagues reported that posttransplantation immunosuppression administration with cyclosporine and MMF permits engraftment of major MHC-identical allogeneic bone marrow in dogs with only 200 cGy total body irradiation (TBI) [14]. When this strategy was applied to patients, a 20% incidence of graft failure was noted [15]; this subsequently decreased to 3% after adding a 3-day course of fludarabine to the pretransplant conditioning regimen [16]. The group of Luznik et al. was able to achieve tolerance and multilineage mixed hematopoietic chimerism across MHC barriers in mice conditioned with fludarabine and 200 cGy TBI and given cyclophosphamide 200 mg/kg intraperitoneally on day 2. This regimen was truly NMA as autologous hematopoiesis recovered in mice that were conditioned but did not receive an infusion of marrow [17]. In addition to suppressing graft rejection in sublethally conditioned mice, posttransplant Cy also inhibited GVHD in lethally irradiated mice given MHC-mismatched bone marrow plus a high dose of donor T cells. The administration of cyclosporine or corticosteroids before cyclophosphamide treatment disrupted the tolerance that should be achieved by posttransplant Cy [18, 19] but the tolerance was not affected by the administration of G-CSF starting the day after posttransplant Cy treatment [20]. It was also noted that, in contrast to the conventional GVHD prophylaxis where NRM increase with increasing genetic disparity [21, 22], when using posttransplant Cy, GVHD and NRM were not associated with the degree of HLA mismatching [23].

2. Haploidentical Stem Cell Transplantation: Bone Marrow Experience

Researchers from Johns Hopkins Hospital (JHH) reported in 2002 the result of a phase I trial of 13 patients (median age: 53 years) who received a full haplotype mismatched T cell replete bone marrow (BM) graft treated with a NMA regimen consisting of fludarabine 30 mg/m² administered daily for 4 days and 2 Gy TBI followed by posttransplant Cy administration (50 mg/m²) on day +3 [24]. The pretransplant conditioning was increased in 10 patients by adding Cy at 14 mg/kg on days −6 and −5 due to an initial higher rate of graft failure noted in the first 3 treated patients. For additional GVHD prophylaxis, MMF and tacrolimus were administered the day after patients received posttransplant Cy (day +4) and continued for at least 30 days. Engraftment was achieved in 8/10 patients in the second cohort (80%), with a median time to absolute neutrophil count >500/microL of 15 days and to unsupported platelet count >20,000/microL of 14 days. All patients with engraftment achieved ≥95% donor chimerism within 60 days of transplantation. Two patients with myelodysplastic syndrome (MDS) rejected their grafts but experienced autologous neutrophil recovery at 24 and 44 days. Grade II–IV acute GVHD developed in 6/13 patients (46%), while grade III–IV acute GVHD developed in only 3/13 patients (23%). After a median follow-up of 6.5 months, 6/10 patients were alive, with 5 remaining in complete remission after transplant [24]. Subsequently, Fred Hutchinson Cancer Center (FHCC) and JHH group published a phase I/II trial of 68 patients who received T cell replete BM haploidentical SCT using Cy 14.5 mg/kg/day on days −6 and −5, fludarabine 30 mg/m²/day on days −6 to −2, and 200 cGy TBI on day −1 followed by one or two posttransplant days of 50 mg/m² Cy (day +3 ± day +4) [25]. Twenty-eight patients received one dose and 40 received 2 doses of posttransplant Cy. Tacrolimus and MMF were also used after transplant but tacrolimus was continued until day 180. GCSF support was started on day +1. The median times to neutrophil and platelet recovery were 15 and 24 days, respectively. Graft failure occurred in 9 of 66 (13%) evaluable patients [25]. The cumulative incidence of grades II–IV and grades III–IV acute GVHD was 34% and 6%, respectively. While no significant difference was seen in the incidence of acute GVHD between the two groups, a strong trend towards less extensive chronic GVHD was seen for patients receiving 2 doses as compared with one dose of posttransplant Cy [25]. The cumulative incidence of NRM at day 100 and 1 year was 4% and 15%, respectively. Low rates of NRM, acute GVHD, and chronic GVHD were also reported in a longer follow-up in the expanded cohorts treated in line with the JHH protocol [38]. With 4.1-year median follow-up, 3-year probabilities of relapse, progression-free survival (PFS), and overall survival (OS) were 46%, 40%, and 50%, respectively. On multivariable analyses, the Disease Risk Index (DRI) was statistically significantly associated with relapse, PFS, and OS.

The Blood and Marrow Transplant Clinical Trials Network conducted multicenter phase 2 trials for individuals with leukemia or lymphoma and no suitable related donor. Cyclophosphamide, fludarabine, and 200 cGy of TBI were used with HLA-haploidentical related donor BM transplantation (n = 50). The median time to neutrophil and platelet recovery was 16 and 24 days, respectively. The 100-day cumulative incidence of grades II–IV acute GVHD was 32%. There were no reported cases of grades III-IV acute GVHD. The 1-year cumulative incidences of NRM and relapse after haploidentical BM transplantation were 7% and 45%, respectively [27]. The 1-year probabilities of OS and PFS were 62% and 48%, respectively. In this study too, the most frequent cause of death was relapse.

MD Anderson (MDACC) [28, 39], the Italian group [30, 40], and others reported their experience with BM haploidentical SCT using a potentially more ablative conditioning regimen trying to provide more antitumor activity and decrease relapse rate. MDACC used fludarabine, melphalan 100–140 mg/m^2 based regimen with thiotepa, or TBI 200 cGy. Eighty-four patients had a BM graft except 4 pts. (95%). Overall, for the entire cohort, relapse rate was 32% and PFS was 42.3%. The median OS for first transplants was 25.6 months and it was 6.5 months for second transplant patients. Of the 49 patients who had first transplant for acute myeloid leukemia (AML)/MDS, 27 (55.1%) were in complete remission prior to transplant. NRM for these patients was 9%, relapse rate was 24.3%, and PFS was 66.8% at 50 months of median follow-up [28]. When they compared 32 patients with AML/MDS who received BM haploidentical SCT with MRD and MUD who underwent matched transplantations and received melphalan-based conditioning regimen and conventional GVHD prophylaxis, results were comparable. However, the median time to neutrophil and platelet recovery for haploidentical SCT recipients was 18 and 25 days compared to 13-12 and 14–16 days in MUD and MRD. These differences were probably related to the use of bone marrow stem cells in the haploidentical SCT group [41].

Raiola et al. [30] reported the results of 50 patients with high-risk hematologic malignancies who underwent an unmanipulated haploidentical BM transplant followed by posttransplant Cy. The myeloablative conditioning consisted of thiotepa, busulfan, fludarabine (n = 35, 8/35 received reduced dose of busulfan), or TBI 9.9 Gy and fludarabine (n = 15). The median age was 42 years (range: 18–66 years); 23 patients were in remission, 27 patients had active disease, and 10 patients were receiving a second allograft. In this study, they used cyclosporine and MMF which were

started on days 0 and +1, respectively, in order to better control GVHD, and the second dose of Cy was moved from day +4 to day +5 to decrease the acute toxicity. GCSF was started on day +5. Three patients died before engraftment, and 2 patients had autologous recovery: 45 patients (90%) had full-donor chimerism on day +30. The median day for neutrophil engraftment was day +18. The cumulative incidence of grades II-III acute GVHD was 12%, and that of moderate chronic GVHD was 10%. With a median follow-up for surviving patients of 10.7 months, the cumulative incidence of transplant related mortality (TRM) was 18%, and the rate of relapse was 26%. The actuarial 22-month disease-free survival (DFS) rate was 68% for patients in remission and 37% for patients with active disease (P < 0.001). They also published a recent update on 148 patients with encouraging results in terms of engraftment; there was only one patient who developed primary graft failure (0.7%), low rates of GVHD, and transplant mortality. The rate of GVHD, both acute and chronic, was low, and 80% of patients were off cyclosporine at 1 year. Major causes of death were relapse (22%), GVHD (2%), and infections (6%) [40]. When they compared the results of haploidentical SCT to other graft sources including MRD, unrelated donors, and cord, haploidentical SCT grafts were comparable to MRD, whereas UCB had inferior survival [42].

Symons et al. also reported the results of a phase II clinical trial of T cell replete HLA-haploidentical BM transplant using a myeloablative regimen and posttransplant Cy that initially enrolled subjects with refractory hematologic malignancies only, with the later addition of high-risk leukemias in remission and chemosensitive lymphomas. The majority (67%) of patients were not in remission at the time of transplant. Conditioning consisted of IV busulfan (pharmacokinetically adjusted) on days −6 to −3, Cy (50 mg/kg/day) on days −2 and −1 in twenty-seven patients, or Cy (50 mg/kg/day) on days −5 and −4 and TBI (300 cGy/day) on days −3 to 0 in three patients. Donor engraftment at day 60 occurred in all but one evaluable patient (96%, 24/25). The median times to neutrophil and platelet recovery were 25 and 32 days, respectively. The cumulative incidences of grades II–IV and grades III-IV acute GVHD at day 100 were 14% and 7.3%, respectively. The cumulative incidence of chronic GVHD at one year was 13%. The cumulative incidence of NRM at 100 days was 12%. There were no deaths from infection. The cumulative incidence of relapse at 1 year was 66%, in this poor-risk cohort. The cumulative incidence of relapse among patients in complete remission prior to transplant was 13% at 1 year. With a median follow-up of surviving patients of 5.5 months, actuarial OS was 40% at one year. With a median follow-up of event-free patients of 4.5 months, actuarial event-free survival (EFS) was 23.5% at one year [26]. However, disease progression remained a problem in patients with refractory leukemia.

A recent report by the Center for International Blood and Marrow Transplant Research which looked at adults with AML after haploidentical donor (n = 192, 162/192 (84%) were BM) and 8/8 HLA-matched unrelated donor (MUD) (n = 1982, 1671/1982 (84%) were PB) showed data suggesting that survival for patients with AML after haploidentical transplantation with posttransplant Cy is comparable with MUD. Neutrophil recovery on day 30 after MUD was similar to haploidentical donor in the RIC transplant group, while it was higher in the myeloablative transplant group, and this is probably related to use of BM in most of the haploidentical SCT. In the myeloablative setting, 3-month acute grades II–IV GVHD (16% versus 33%, $P < 0.0001$) and 3-year chronic GVHD (30% versus 53%, $P < 0.0001$) were lower after haploidentical donor compared to MUD. Similar differences were observed after RIC transplants, 19% versus 28% ($P = 0.05$) and 34% versus 52% ($P = 0.002$). Whether the observed low rate of GVHD was solely explained by the use of BM in most of the haploidentical SCT or use of posttransplant Cy or the combination of both cannot be determined. When Ciurea et al. compared chronic GVHD rates in the subset of patients transplanted with BM, there were no differences in 3-year rates of chronic GVHD after haploidentical donor and MUD with myeloablative regimens (30%, $n = 85$ versus 36%, $n = 231$) or with reduced intensity regimens (34%, $n = 77$ versus 30%, $n = 80$), but these numbers are small and might not show the difference. In addition, 39% of patients who got reduced intensity regimen and 23% of patients who got the myeloablative regimens in the MUD group also received in vivo T cell depletion. Among recipients of reduced intensity regimens, NRM risks were lower after haploidentical compared with MUD transplantation. However, any advantage derived from lower mortality risks with the very low intensity regimen for haploidentical transplantation was negated by higher relapse risks in this group. In the myeloablative setting, an effect of donor type on NRM or relapse risks was not seen. OS was similar between the haploidentical and MUD groups [43].

3. Haploidentical Stem Cell Transplantation: Peripheral Blood Experience

Collection of BM stem cells involves the use of the operating room which can be cumbersome, presents an increased risk of complications to the donor, and can make it difficult to reach target CD34 when there is great disparity in weight between the donor and recipient. In addition, in cases of major ABO incompatibility, further time-consuming and complex processing is required. Therefore, there is considerable interest in developing peripheral blood stem cells as a graft source in haploidentical SCT. Recently, emerging data suggest that G-CSF mobilized peripheral blood stem cell (PBSC) graft can also safely be used for haploidentical SCT with posttransplant Cy.

Solomon and colleagues [29, 44] reported the use of busulfan based conditioning regimen with fludarabine and cyclophosphamide (Bu/Flu/Cy) in 20 patients of whom 11 had relapsed/refractory disease. In response to increased rates of mucositis, fludarabine and busulfan doses were decreased by 30% and 15%, respectively, in 15 patients. On day 0, patients received an unmanipulated peripheral blood T cell replete allograft. The cumulative incidence of severe acute GVHD and chronic GVHD was low at 10% and 5%, respectively, with a day 100 NRM of only 10%. For standard-risk patients, NRM was 0% at 100 days and 1 year. The 1-year OS and

relapse rates were 69% and 40%, respectively, and were better for standard-risk patients (88% and 33%, resp.). Noninfectious fever (median Tmax 103.9; 101.2–106.8) developed in 18 of 20 patients within a median of 2.5-day (range: 1–5 days) transplantation and resolved in all patients after posttransplant Cy administration. Achievement of full-donor chimerism was rapid with all evaluable patients achieving durable complete donor T cell and myeloid chimerism by day +30. However, they noticed high rates of BK-linked hemorrhagic cystitis (75% of patients) so they published recently the result of Flu/TBI (12 Gy) regimen and PBSC haploidentical SCT [34]. All patients engrafted and achieved sustained complete donor T cell and myeloid chimerism by day +30. When compared with a contemporaneously treated cohort of patients receiving myeloablative HLA-MUD transplantation at their institution, outcomes were statistically similar, with 2-year OS and DFS being 78% and 73%, respectively, after haploidentical SCT versus 71% and 64%, respectively, after MUD transplantation. In patients with DRI low/intermediate risk disease, 2-year DFS was superior after haploidentical compared with MUD transplantations (100% versus 74%, $P = 0.032$), whereas there was no difference in DFS in patients with high/very high-risk disease (39% versus 37% for haploidentical donor and MUD, resp., $P = 0.821$). Rates of grades II to IV acute GVHD were less after haploidentical compared with MUD transplantation (43% versus 63%, $P = 0.049$) as was moderate-to-severe chronic GVHD (22% versus 58%, $P = 0.003$) in spite of the use of PBSC as the stem cell source in all 30 haploidentical transplant recipients compared with 32 of 48 MUD transplant recipients (100% versus 67%, $P < 0.001$). However, GVHD prophylaxis was tacrolimus and methotrexate in all MUD patients, and no patients received in vivo T cell depletion. BK virus-associated cystitis was significantly less frequent after TBI-based myeloablative conditioning with clinically significant hemorrhagic cystitis occurring in only 2 (7%) patients.

Raj et al. published a 4-center experience of 55 patients who underwent T cell replete haploidentical PBSC transplant using RIC followed by posttransplant Cy. The 1-year cumulative incidences of grades II to III acute GVHD were 53% and 8%, respectively. There were no cases of grade IV GVHD. The 2-year cumulative incidence of chronic GVHD was 18%. With a median follow-up of 509 days, OS and EFS at 2 years were 48% and 51%, respectively. The 2-year cumulative incidences of NRM and relapse were 23% and 28%, respectively [31].

Using the same protocol of NMA conditioning regimen, GVHD prophylaxis, growth factor support, and antimicrobial prophylaxis previously reported by Luznik et al. [25], Bhamidipati et al. reported the results of 18 patients who received PBSC haploidentical SCT [32]. Despite the high CD3+ cell dose (median of 19.7×10^7/kg), the cumulative incidence of acute GVHD (all grades) was 41 and 53% on days +60 and +90, respectively. Three patients (17%) developed grades III-IV acute GVHD. The cumulative incidence of chronic GVHD at 1 and 2 years was 8% at both the time points and extensive chronic GVHD developed in only one patient. One-year OS was 62% for all patients and 70% in those patients who underwent transplant in complete remission.

TABLE 1: Platforms of conditioning regimens, GVHD prophylaxis, and graft source.

Reference	Conditioning regimen	GVHD prophylaxis	Graft source
O'Donnell et al., 2002 [24]	FluCyTBI	PTCy D +3, Tac MMF	BM
Luznik et al., 2008 [25]	FluCyTBI	PTCy D +3 ± D +4, Tac MMF	BM
Symons et al., 2011 [26]	BuCy or CyTBI	PTCy, Tac MMF	BM
Brunstein et al., 2011 [27]	FluCyTBI	PTCy, Tac MMF	BM
Pingali et al., 2014 [28]	FluMel Thiotepa or TBI	PTCy, Tac MMF	BM (94%)
Solomon et al., 2012 [29]	FluBuCy	PTCy, Tac MMF	PBSC
Raiola et al., 2013 [30]	FluBu Thiotepa ($n = 35$) FluTBI 9.9 Gy ($n = 15$)	PTCy, CsA MMF	BM
Raj et al., 2014 [31]	FluCyTBI	PTCy, Tac MMF	PBSC
Bhamidipati et al., 2014 [32]	FluCyTBI	PTCy, Tac MMF	PBSC
Castagna et al., 2014 [33]	BM FluCyTBI	PTCy, Tac MMF 74% PTCy, CsA MMF 26%	BM $n = 46$ (67%)
	PBSC FluCyTBI	PTCy, Tac MMF	PBSC $n = 23$ (33%)
Solomon et al., 2015 [34]	Flu/TBI (12 Gy)	PTCy, Tac MMF	PBSC
Bradstock et al., 2015 [35]	BM FluCyTBI	BM PTCy D +3, Tac MMF	BM $n = 13$
	PBSC FluCyTBI	PBSC PTCy D +3 D +4, Tac MMF	PBSC $n = 23$
Gayoso et al., 2013 [36]	NMA 77.5% MA 22.5%	PTCy, CNI, MMF	BM 51% PBSC 49%
Sugita et al., 2015 [37]	FluCyBuTBI	PTCy, Tac MMF	PBSC

BM, bone marrow; Bu, busulfan; CsA, cyclosporine; CNI, calcineurin inhibitor; Cy, cyclophosphamide; D, day; Flu, fludarabine; Mel, melphalan; MMF, mycophenolate; PTCy, posttransplant cyclophosphamide; Tac, tacrolimus; TBI, total body irradiation; PBSC, peripheral blood stem cells.

Hundred-day and 1-year NRM were 11 and 17%, respectively. The relapse-free survival at 1 year was 53% [32].

More recently retrospective data comparing BM with PB in haploidentical SCT have been reported. Castagna et al. [33] retrospectively looked at the outcome of 2-center haploidentical SCT comparing PBSC and BM in patients with mostly lymphoid malignancies. 46 patients had BM with a median age of 44, while 23 patients had PBSC with median age of 54. They all received FluCyTBI. The incidence of grades II to IV acute GVHD was similar in both groups, 25% and 33% after BM and PBSC infusions, respectively. In addition, chronic GVHD was also similar, 13% after both BM and PBSC infusions. This is probably related to the short term follow-up and the small number of patients which may impair the statistical power of the comparison. No major differences between the 2 cohorts were observed in terms of infectious complications. The relapse incidence was similar in the two cohorts. However, patients in complete remission had a significant lower incidence of relapse (14% versus 33%, $P = 0.04$) and superior PFS (68% versus 49%, $P = 0.05$) compared with those who were not in complete remission. The 2-year overall NRM was 18% (BM: 22%; PBSC: 12%; $P = 0.96$). OS and NRM were not statistically different between the 2 cohorts of patients. They also reported 49 patients with refractory lymphoma (most of them received BM (80%)) who received T-repleted haploidentical SCT with a nonmyeloablative regimen and posttransplant Cy; also in this group the median number of CD34+ cells infused was

3.3×10^6/kg in BM group compared to 5.1×10^6/kg in PBSC group but the median number of days to engraft was similar. Relapse rate was low (18%) [45].

Bradstock et al. [35] compared outcomes for two retrospective cohorts of patients undergoing RIC therapy transplants using haploidentical graft and posttransplant Cy. The graft used was BM in 13 patients and PBSC in 23 patients. Ten of these patients were previously reported [31]. The BM cohort received a single 60 mg/kg dose of cyclophosphamide on day +3, whereas the PBSC cohort received 2 doses on days +3 and +4 and so the 24-month cumulative rates for chronic GVHD were similar in both groups, 28.6% for BM and 32.3% for PBSCs. The 6-month cumulative incidences of acute GVHD were also similar in both groups, 55.1% for BM and 48.5% for PBSCs. Patients in the PBSC group received double the number of CD34+ cells in the stem cell graft; however, times to neutrophil and platelet recovery were not different between the 2 groups. Three patients, all receiving PBSCs, failed to engraft but survived; 2 of these had Philadelphia chromosome positive ALL in first remission, and both recovered with autologous Philadelphia chromosome negative hemopoiesis. The third patient had AML in second remission and because of morbid obesity was unable to receive TBI; he recovered with autologous hemopoiesis. None had significant titers of anti-donor HLA antibodies in their serum, and there is therefore no obvious explanation for this happening in the 2 ALL patients, both of whom had received significant prior chemotherapy. The remaining 33

TABLE 2: Patients, donors, and graft characteristics.

Reference	Pts. number	Med. age (range)	Donors	Disease	Med. CD34 ×10⁶	Med. CD3 ×10⁸
O'Donnell et al., 2002 [24]	13	53	Parent 16% Sib 38% Child 46%	AML/MDS 7 ALL 2 CML 2 MM 1 NHL 1	5.3	0.32
Luznik et al., 2008 [25]	68	46	Parent 28% Sib 48% Child 24%	AML/MDS 28 ALL 4 CML/CMML 6 CLL/NHL 13 HL 13 MM 3 PNH 1	4.8	0.42
Symons et al., 2011 [26]	30	43	NA	AML 16 3 ALL 2 CML 9 NHL	NA	NA
Brunstein et al., 2011 [27]	50	48	Parent 30% Sib 34% Child 36%	AML 22 ALL 9 NHL 12 HL 7	NA	NA
Pingali et al., 2014 [28]	84	46	Parent 15% Sib 42% Child 42% Cousin 1%	AML/MDS 49 ALL 10 CML 9 Lymphoma 13 3 others	NA	NA
Solomon et al., 2012 [29]	20	44	Parent 15% Sib 65% Child 20%	AML 20 ALL 2 NHL 2 HL 1 CML 3	5	1.73
Raiola et al., 2013 [30]	50	42	NA	AML 25 ALL 12 Lymphoma 5 MPD 5 CML 3	4	0.35
Raj et al., 2014 [31]	55	49	Parent 24% Sib 37% Child 39%	AML/MDS 21 ALL 2 NHL 12 HL 9	6.4	2
Bhamidipati et al., 2014 [32]	18	41	Parent 28% Sib 33% Child 39%	AML 12 ALL 2 NHL 2 Other 2	5	1.97
Castagna et al., 2014 [33]	BM, n = 46 (67%)	44	NA	AML/MDS 2 ALL 2 HL 23 NHL/CLL 16 MM 2	3	0.34
	PBSC, n = 23 (33%)	54	NA	AML/MDS 2 HL 6 NHL/CLL 12 MM 2	5.1	2.73
Solomon et al., 2015 [34]	30	46.5	Parent 7% Sib 40% Child 53%	AML/MDS 17 ALL 6 CML 5 NHL 2	5.01	1.55

TABLE 2: Continued.

Reference	Pts. number	Med. age (range)	Donors	Disease	Med. CD34 $\times 10^6$	Med. CD3 $\times 10^8$
Bradstock et al., 2015 [35]	BM, $n = 13$	53	Parent 7% Sib 66% Child 27%	AML 10 NHL 2 CML 1	2.5	NA
	PBSC, $n = 23$	44		AML/MDS 11 NHL 4 ALL 4 Other 4	5.8	NA
Gayoso et al., 2013 [36]	80	37	Parent 35% Sib 44% Child 21%	AML/MDS 30 NHL 5 HL 29 ALL 9 Other 6	NA	NA
Sugita et al., 2015 [37]	31	48	Parent 22.6% Sib 29% Child 45.1% Other 3.2%	AML/MDS 21 ALL 8 NHL 2	4.0	NA

ALL, acute lymphoid leukemia/lymphoma; AML, acute myeloid leukemia; CLL, chronic lymphocytic leukemia; CML, chronic myeloid leukemia; CMML, chronic myelomonocytic leukemia; HL, Hodgkin lymphoma; MDS, myelodysplastic syndrome; MM, multiple myeloma; MPD, myeloproliferative disorder; NHL, non-Hodgkin lymphoma; PNH, paroxysmal nocturnal hemoglobinuria.

patients engrafted, with complete donor chimerism documented on DNA testing of blood T cells and granulocytes. The 2-year cumulative incidences of relapse were 43.9% for BM and 23.5% for PBSCs ($P = 0.286$). For the 33 patients with hematological malignancies, the distribution of relapse-free survival did not differ significantly between BM and PBSC groups and at 2 years was 44.9% and 72.7%, respectively. OS at 2 years was significantly better for PBSC patients ($P = 0.028$), at 83.4% versus 52.7% for BM. Patients in the first cohort were slightly older and had a higher proportion of acute myeloid leukemia, but there were no differences in the distribution of DRI scores between the 2 groups. No serious episodes of opportunistic infection occurred in both cohorts and no posttransplant lymphoproliferative disorder was observed.

Another abstract from 14 centers in Spain [36] reported the results of 80 patients (16–66-year-old) who received NMA (77.5%) or myeloablative (22.5%) conditioning regimens and posttransplant Cy with MMF and calcineurin inhibitor. Almost half of the patients (51%) got BM, while the other half (49%) got PBSC. TRM was 19% at 6 months. Grades II–IV acute GVHD was 33% while grades III-IV acute GVHD was 14%. Chronic GVHD was present in 24%, being extensive in 12%. Another multicenter but prospective phase II study was conducted by the Japan Study Group for Cell Therapy and Transplantation [37]. They used a reduced intensity regimen containing busulfan (6.4 mg/kg). GVHD prophylaxis consisted of Cy (50 mg/kg/day on days 3 and 4), tacrolimus (days 5 to 180), and MMF (days 5 to 60). They included large numbers of patients who were not in remission and patients with a history of prior allogeneic SCT compared to other studies. One-year relapse rate was 45% with 1-year DFS and OS rates of 34% and 45%. Grades II–IV acute GVHD was 23%, while grades III-IV acute GVHD was 3%. Chronic GVHD was present in 15%, without any severe GVHD. Subgroup analysis showed that patients who

had a history of prior allogeneic SCT ($n = 13$) had lower engraftment (69% versus 100%).

4. Conclusions and Future Directions

The studies in Tables 1–3 and others reported over the last decade represent considerable evidence to suggest that haploidentical SCT is a safe and practical option for patients with no donors with almost comparable results to MRD or MUD transplant [38, 43, 44, 46–50] and is superior to conventional consolidation/maintenance chemotherapy as postremission therapy for high-risk diseases [51, 52]. BM has been replaced by PBSC as a stem cell source in MRD and MUD SCT because of the higher engraftment rates due to the larger number of CD34+ stem cells and because of a potential higher graft versus tumor effect linked to a larger number of T cells. In the haploidentical SCT setting, graft rejection rate appears to be similar or slightly lower in most of the studies utilizing PBSC rather than BM as in Table 3. The median days to neutrophils and platelet engraftments appear to be similar between BM and PBSC grafts in spite of higher median CD34 cells in the PBSC grafts. High fever at 4 to 5 days after transplant was observed in both studies with BM or PBSC; however, the median Tmax of patients transplanted with PBSCs was significantly higher than the Tmax of patients transplanted with BM, probably related to high number of T cells [53].

In the study reported by the Blood and Marrow Transplant Clinical Trials Network, chronic GVHD occurred more frequently after PBSC MUD where most patients did not get in vivo T cell depletion, without effect on OS [54], and, in MRD, the higher incidence and greater severity of chronic GVHD in PBSC MRD SCT had little impact on the patient's performance status or survival [55, 56]. Most of the studies that compared haploidentical SCT to MRD or MUD transplants showed less GVHD especially chronic GVHD

TABLE 3: Transplant outcomes.

Reference	Engraf. failure	Med. days to neut./PLT eng.	aGVHD II–IV/III–IV	cGVHD	NRM	Relapse	EFS/PFS	OS
O'Donnell et al., 2002 [24]	20% Cohort 2	15/14	46%/23%	1/10 limited	1/10 died of GVHD	4/10 cohort 2 relapsed	At med. f/u 6 mo. 5/10 in CR	At med. f/u 6 mo. 6/10 (cohort 2) alive
Luznik et al., 2008 [25]	13%	15/24	34%/6%	Ext. 5% in 2 doses of CY versus 25% in one dose of Cy	1y 15%	1y 51%	2y EFS 26%	2y 36%
Symons et al., 2011 [26]	4%	25/32	14%/7.3%	13%	100 D 12%	1y 66% poor risk 1y 13% in CR	1y 23.5%	1y 40%
Brunstein et al., 2011 [27]	2%	16/24	32%/0	1y 13%	1y 7%	1y 45%	1y PFS 48%	1y 62%
Pingali et al., 2014 [28]	4.7%	18/NA	32.6%/7.8%	21.3%/Ext. 10%	25%	3y 30.1%	3y PFS 42.3%	1y OS 64% Median OS for 1st SCT 25.6 mo. 2nd SCT 6.5 mo.
Solomon et al., 2012 [29]	0%	16/27	30%/10%	35%/severe 5%	1y 10%	1y 40%	1y DFS 50%	1y 69%
Raiola et al., 2013 [30]	6%	18/23	12%/6%	26%/Ext. 0	6 mo. 18%	18 mo. 22%	DFS 18 mo. 51%	18 mo. 62%
Raj et al., 2014 [31]	4%	17/21	II 35% III 8% IV 0%	18% @ 2 y 2 severe cases	1y 17%	2y 28%	2y 51%	2y 48%
Bhamidipati et al., 2014 [32]	6%	15/18	All grades 53%/17%	8% @ 2 y Ext. only in 1 patient	1y 17%	1y 38%	1y 53%	1y 62%
Castagna et al., 2014 [33]	NA NA	BM 21/29 PB 20/27	25%/3% 33%/14%	13% 13%	2y 19%	1y 22% 1y 12%	2y PFS 62%	2y 68%
Solomon et al., 2015 [34]	0	16/25	43%/23%	56%/Ext. 10%	2y 3%	2y 24%	2y DFS 73%	2y 78%
Bradstock et al., 2015 [35]	0	15/18	I–III 55.1% No IV	28.6%	6 mo. 0	2y 43.9%	2y EFS 44.9%	2y 52.7%
	13%	16/24	I–III 48.5% No IV	32.3%	6 mo. 0	2y 23.5%	2y EFS 63.6%	2y 83.4%
Gayoso et al., 2013 [36]	NA	18/27	33%/14%	24%/Ext. 12%	6 mo. 19%	NA	1y EFS 48%	1y 60%
Sugita et al., 2015 [37]	13% (0 in no h/o SCT; 31% in h/o SCT)	19/35	23%/3%	15%/none severe	1y 23%	1y 45%	1y DFS 34%	1y 45%

aGVHD, acute graft versus host disease; cGVHD, chronic graft versus host disease; CR, complete remission; Cy, cyclophosphamide; D, day; DFS, disease-free survival; Engraf, engraftment; EFS, event-free survival; Ext, extensive; mo., months; neut., neutrophils; NRM, nonrelapse mortality; OS, overall survival; PFS, progression-free survival; PLT, platelets; y, year.

[41] but it is difficult to tell if this is from the use of BM in most of haploidentical SCT studies or from the use of posttransplant Cy or from both. In the study that compared PBSC haploidentical SCT to MUD SCT [34], rates of acute and moderate-to-severe GVHD were less in haploidentical SCT which may be attributed to use of BM in some of patients in the MUD group and no in vivo T cell depletion or use of posttransplant Cy which is cytotoxic to alloreactive T cells. Interestingly, the number of CD3+ T cells reported in PBSC allografts was about 5-fold higher than the one reported in BM allografts (Table 2) and hence there were higher but acceptable rates of acute GVHD in most of them and similar rates in others (Table 3). Most PBSC studies also showed low rates of severe acute and chronic GVHD and most of them were responsive to steroids. However, most of these studies are from single centers with the small number of patients and short term follow-up especially for the PBSC grafts. The two studies that compared PB with BM [33, 35] are retrospective and small which may impair the statistical power of the comparison. In addition, it is difficult to compare across different trials because of the heterogeneity of patient population and conditioning regimens.

Regarding relapse, the high relapse rate in some of the haploidentical studies compared to other graft sources could be related to the NMA regimen used, use of the BM grafts with low graft versus tumor effect, or lower NRM in haploidentical studies, which puts more patients at risk of relapse. Also effect is probably different depending on the disease too, myeloid or lymphoid malignancies. The effects of the substitution of BM with PBSC in the haploidentical setting on graft versus tumor effect and relapse are also unclear and difficult to assess because of the lack of prospective studies and heterogeneity between the above studies regarding disease risk and regimens used. However, in most of the studies, the most relative factor contributing to outcome was disease risk prior to transplant.

Despite limitations, these studies suggest that BM or PBSC could be safely used as allograft sources for haploidentical transplantation with good outcomes and acceptable rates of GVHD and graft failure, which helps provide more options for patients and donors. However, there is need for prospective adequately powered studies to evaluate the effect of use of BM versus PBSC in haploidentical SCT setting on GVHD, graft versus tumor, OS, immune reconstitution, and quality of life. Since disease relapse or progression remains a problem in high-risk patients, novel therapies added in the conditioning regimens or posttransplant need to be evaluated.

Competing Interests

The authors declare that they have no competing interests.

References

[1] E. A. Copelan, "Hematopoietic stem-cell transplantation," *The New England Journal of Medicine*, vol. 354, no. 17, pp. 1813–1826, 2006.

[2] G. E. Switzer, J. G. Bruce, L. Myaskovsky et al., "Race and ethnicity in decisions about unrelated hematopoietic stem cell donation," *Blood*, vol. 121, no. 8, pp. 1469–1476, 2013.

[3] J. Pidala, J. Kim, M. Schell et al., "Race/ethnicity affects the probability of finding an HLA-A,-B,-C and-DRB1 allele-matched unrelated donor and likelihood of subsequent transplant utilization," *Bone Marrow Transplantation*, vol. 48, no. 3, pp. 346–350, 2013.

[4] M. A. Sanz and G. F. Sanz, "Unrelated donor umbilical cord blood transplantation in adults," *Leukemia*, vol. 16, no. 10, pp. 1984–1991, 2002.

[5] D. Confer and P. Robinett, "The US National Marrow Donor Program role in unrelated donor hematopoietic cell transplantation," *Bone Marrow Transplantation*, vol. 42, supplement 1, pp. S3–S5, 2008.

[6] G. J. Ruiz-Argüelles, G. J. Ruiz-Delgado, O. González-Llano, and D. Gómez-Almaguer, "Haploidentical bone marrow transplantation in 2015 and beyond," *Current Oncology Reports*, vol. 17, no. 12, article 57, 2015.

[7] H. Mayumi, M. Umesue, and K. Nomoto, "Cyclophosphamide-induced immunological tolerance: an overview," *Immunobiology*, vol. 195, no. 2, pp. 129–139, 1996.

[8] M. C. Berenbaum and I. N. Brown, "Prolongation of homograft survival in mice with single doses of cyclophosphamide," *Nature*, vol. 200, no. 4901, p. 84, 1963.

[9] M. Schumm, P. Lang, W. Bethge et al., "Depletion of T-cell receptor alpha/beta and CD19 positive cells from apheresis products with the CliniMACS device," *Cytotherapy*, vol. 15, no. 10, pp. 1253–1258, 2013.

[10] W. R. Drobyski, S. Vodanovic-Jankovic, and J. Klein, "Adoptively transferred γδ T cells indirectly regulate murine graft-versus-host reactivity following donor leukocyte infusion therapy in mice," *Journal of Immunology*, vol. 165, no. 3, pp. 1634–1640, 2000.

[11] S. Kato, H. Yabe, M. Yasui et al., "Allogeneic hematopoietic transplantation of CD34+ selected cells from an HLA haploidentical related donor. A long-term follow-up of 135 patients and a comparison of stem cell source between the bone marrow and the peripheral blood," *Bone Marrow Transplantation*, vol. 26, no. 12, pp. 1281–1290, 2000.

[12] R. Crocchiolo, S. Bramanti, A. Vai et al., "Infections after T-replete haploidentical transplantation and high-dose cyclophosphamide as graft-versus-host disease prophylaxis," *Transplant Infectious Disease*, vol. 17, no. 2, pp. 242–249, 2015.

[13] R. J. Jones, J. P. Barber, M. S. Vala et al., "Assessment of aldehyde dehydrogenase in viable cells," *Blood*, vol. 85, no. 10, pp. 2742–2746, 1995.

[14] R. Storb, C. Yu, J. L. Wagner et al., "Stable mixed hematopoietic chimerism in DLA-identical littermate dogs given sublethal total body irradiation before and pharmacological immunosuppression after marrow transplantation," *Blood*, vol. 89, no. 8, pp. 3048–3054, 1997.

[15] P. A. McSweeney, D. Niederwieser, J. A. Shizuru et al., "Hematopoietic cell transplantation in older patients with hematologic malignancies: replacing high-dose cytotoxic therapy with graft-versus-tumor effects," *Blood*, vol. 97, no. 11, pp. 3390–3400, 2001.

[16] M. Maris, A. Woolfrey, P. A. McSweeney et al., "Nonmyeloablative hematopoietic stem cell transplantation: transplantation for the 21st century," *Frontiers in Bioscience*, vol. 6, pp. G13–G16, 2001.

[17] L. Luznik, S. Jalla, L. W. Engstrom, R. Lannone, and E. J. Fuchs, "Durable engraftment of major histocompatibility complex-incompatible cells after nonmyeloablative conditioning with fludarabine, low-dose total body irradiation, and posttransplantation cyclophosphamide," *Blood*, vol. 98, no. 12, pp. 3456–3464, 2001.

[18] K. Nomoto, M. Eto, K. Yanaga, Y. Nishimura, T. Maeda, and K. Nomoto, "Interference with cyclophosphamide-induced skin allograft tolerance by cyclosporin A," *Journal of Immunology*, vol. 149, no. 8, pp. 2668–2674, 1992.

[19] P. Dukor and F. M. Dietrich, "Prevention of cyclophosphamide-induced tolerance to erythrocytes by pretreatment with cortisone," *Proceedings of the Society for Experimental Biology and Medicine*, vol. 133, no. 1, pp. 280–285, 1970.

[20] Y. Nishimura, H. Mayumi, Y. Tomita, M. Eto, T. Maeda, and K. Nomoto, "Recombinant human granulocyte colony-stimulating factor improves the compromised State of recipient mice without affecting the induction of specific tolerance in the cyclophosphamide-induced tolerance system," *Journal of Immunology*, vol. 146, no. 8, pp. 2639–2647, 1991.

[21] C. Anasetti, P. G. Beatty, R. Storb et al., "Effect of HLA incompatibility on graft-versus-host disease, relapse, and survival after marrow transplantation for patients with leukemia or lymphoma," *Human Immunology*, vol. 29, no. 2, pp. 79–91, 1990.

[22] T. Kawase, Y. Morishima, K. Matsuo et al., "High-risk HLA allele mismatch combinations responsible for severe acute graft-versus-host disease and implication for its molecular mechanism," *Blood*, vol. 110, no. 7, pp. 2235–2241, 2007.

[23] Y. L. Kasamon, L. Luznik, M. S. Leffell et al., "Nonmyeloablative HLA-haploidentical bone marrow transplantation with high-dose posttransplantation cyclophosphamide: effect of HLA disparity on outcome," *Biology of Blood and Marrow Transplantation*, vol. 16, no. 4, pp. 482–489, 2010.

[24] P. V. O'Donnell, L. Luznik, R. J. Jones et al., "Nonmyeloablative bone marrow transplantation from partially HLA-mismatched related donors using posttransplantation cyclophosphamide," *Biology of Blood and Marrow Transplantation*, vol. 8, no. 7, pp. 377–386, 2002.

[25] L. Luznik, P. V. O'Donnell, H. J. Symons et al., "HLA-haploidentical bone marrow transplantation for hematologic malignancies using nonmyeloablative conditioning and high-dose, posttransplantation cyclophosphamide," *Biology of Blood and Marrow Transplantation*, vol. 14, no. 6, pp. 641–650, 2008.

[26] H. Symons, A. Chen, L. Luznik et al., "Myeloablative haploidentical bone marrow transplantation with T cell replete grafts and post-transplant cyclophosphamide: results of a phase II clinical trial," *Blood*, vol. 118, no. 21, p. 4151, 2011.

[27] C. G. Brunstein, E. J. Fuchs, S. L. Carter et al., "Alternative donor transplantation after reduced intensity conditioning: Results of parallel phase 2 trials using partially HLA-mismatched related bone marrow or unrelated double umbilical cord blood grafts," *Blood*, vol. 118, no. 2, pp. 282–288, 2011.

[28] S. R. Pingali, D. Milton, A. di Stasi et al., "Haploidentical transplantation for advanced hematologic malignancies using melphalan-based conditioning—mature results from a single center," *Biology of Blood and Marrow Transplantation*, vol. 20, supplement 2, pp. S40–S41, 2014.

[29] S. R. Solomon, C. A. Sizemore, M. Sanacore et al., "Haploidentical transplantation using t cell replete peripheral blood stem cells and myeloablative conditioning in patients with high-risk hematologic malignancies who lack conventional donors is well tolerated and produces excellent relapse-free survival: results

of a prospective phase II trial," *Biology of Blood and Marrow Transplantation*, vol. 18, no. 12, pp. 1859–1866, 2012.

[30] A. M. Raiola, A. Dominietto, A. Ghiso et al., "Unmanipulated haploidentical bone marrow transplantation and posttransplantation cyclophosphamide for hematologic malignancies after myeloablative conditioning," *Biology of Blood and Marrow Transplantation*, vol. 19, no. 1, pp. 117–122, 2013.

[31] K. Raj, A. Pagliuca, K. Bradstock et al., "Peripheral blood hematopoietic stem cells for transplantation of hematological diseases from related, haploidentical donors after reduced-intensity conditioning," *Biology of Blood and Marrow Transplantation*, vol. 20, no. 6, pp. 890–895, 2014.

[32] P. K. Bhamidipati, J. F. Dipersio, K. Stokerl-Goldstein et al., "Haploidentical transplantation using G-CSF-mobilized T-cell replete PBSCs and post-transplantation CY after non-myeloablative conditioning is safe and is associated with favorable outcomes," *Bone Marrow Transplantation*, vol. 49, no. 8, pp. 1124–1126, 2014.

[33] L. Castagna, R. Crocchiolo, S. Furst et al., "Bone marrow compared with peripheral blood stem cells for haploidentical transplantation with a nonmyeloablative conditioning regimen and post-transplantation cyclophosphamide," *Biology of Blood and Marrow Transplantation*, vol. 20, no. 5, pp. 724–729, 2014.

[34] S. R. Solomon, C. A. Sizemore, M. Sanacore et al., "Total body irradiation-based myeloablative haploidentical stem cell transplantation is a safe and effective alternative to unrelated donor transplantation in patients without matched sibling donors," *Biology of Blood and Marrow Transplantation*, vol. 21, no. 7, pp. 1299–1307, 2015.

[35] K. Bradstock, I. Bilmon, J. Kwan et al., "Influence of stem cell source on outcomes of allogeneic reduced-intensity conditioning therapy transplants using haploidentical related donors," *Biology of Blood and Marrow Transplantation*, vol. 21, no. 9, pp. 1641–1645, 2015.

[36] J. Gayoso, P. Balsalobre, C. Castilla-Llorente et al., "Haploidentical stem cell transplantation (HAPLO-HSCT) with reduced intensity conditioning (RIC) regimens and high dose cylophosphamide post-transplant (HD-CY) as GVHD prophylaxis in patients with relapsed or refractory Hodgkin's disease: multicentric Spanish experience," *Blood*, vol. 122, no. 21, p. 3406, 2013.

[37] J. Sugita, N. Kawashima, T. Fujisaki et al., "HLA-haploidentical peripheral blood stem cell transplantation with post-transplant cyclophosphamide after busulfan-containing reduced-intensity conditioning," *Biology of Blood and Marrow Transplantation*, vol. 21, no. 9, pp. 1646–1652, 2015.

[38] S. R. McCurdy, J. A. Kanakry, M. M. Showel et al., "Risk-stratified outcomes of nonmyeloablative HLA-haploidentical BMT with high-dose posttransplantation cyclophosphamide," *Blood*, vol. 125, no. 19, pp. 3024–3031, 2015.

[39] C. G. Kanakry, E. J. Fuchs, and L. Luznik, "Modern approaches to HLA-haploidentical blood or marrow transplantation," *Nature Reviews Clinical Oncology*, vol. 13, no. 2, pp. 10–24, 2015.

[40] A. Bacigalupo, A. Dominietto, A. Ghiso et al., "Unmanipulated haploidentical bone marrow transplantation and post-transplant cyclophosphamide for hematologic malignanices following a myeloablative conditioning: an update," *Bone Marrow Transplantation*, vol. 50, supplement 2, pp. S37–S39, 2015.

[41] S. R. McCurdy and E. J. Fuchs, "Comparable outcomes for hematologic malignancies after HLA-haploidentical transplantation with posttransplantation cyclophosphamide and HLA-matched transplantation," *Advances in Hematology*, vol. 2015, Article ID 431923, 9 pages, 2015.

[42] C. G. Kanakry, E. J. Fuchs, and L. Luznik, "Modern approaches to HLA-haploidentical blood or marrow transplantation," *Nature Reviews Clinical Oncology*, vol. 13, no. 1, pp. 10–24, 2015.

[43] S. O. Ciurea, M.-J. Zhang, A. A. Bacigalupo et al., "Haploidentical transplant with posttransplant cyclophosphamide vs matched unrelated donor transplant for acute myeloid leukemia," *Blood*, vol. 126, no. 8, pp. 1033–1040, 2015.

[44] A. Bashey, X. Zhang, C. A. Sizemore et al., "T-cell-replete HLA-haploidentical hematopoietic transplantation for hematologic malignancies using post-transplantation cyclophosphamide results in outcomes equivalent to those of contemporaneous HLA-matched related and unrelated donor transplantation," *Journal of Clinical Oncology*, vol. 31, no. 10, pp. 1310–1316, 2013.

[45] L. Castagna, S. Bramanti, S. Furst et al., "Nonmyeloablative conditioning, unmanipulated haploidentical SCT and post-infusion CY for advanced lymphomas," *Bone Marrow Transplantation*, vol. 49, no. 12, pp. 1475–1480, 2014.

[46] D.-P. Lu, L. Dong, T. Wu et al., "Conditioning including antithymocyte globulin followed by unmanipulated HLA-mismatched/haploidentical blood and marrow transplantation can achieve comparable outcomes with HLA-identical sibling transplantation," *Blood*, vol. 107, no. 8, pp. 3065–3073, 2006.

[47] X.-H. Chen, L. Gao, X. Zhang et al., "HLA-haploidentical blood and bone marrow transplantation with anti-thymocyte globulin: long-term comparison with HLA-identical sibling transplantation," *Blood Cells, Molecules, and Diseases*, vol. 43, no. 1, pp. 98–104, 2009.

[48] Y. Luo, H. Xiao, X. Lai et al., "T-cell-replete haploidentical HSCT with low-dose anti-T-lymphocyte globulin compared with matched sibling HSCT and unrelated HSCT," *Blood*, vol. 124, no. 17, pp. 2735–2743, 2014.

[49] Y. Wang, Q.-F. Liu, L.-P. Xu et al., "Haploidentical vs identical-sibling transplant for AML in remission: a multicenter, prospective study," *Blood*, vol. 125, no. 25, pp. 3956–3962, 2015.

[50] A. Di Stasi, D. R. Milton, L. M. Poon et al., "Similar transplantation outcomes for acute myeloid leukemia and myelodysplastic syndrome patients with haploidentical versus 10/10 human leukocyte antigen-matched unrelated and related donors," *Biology of Blood and Marrow Transplantation*, vol. 20, no. 12, pp. 1975–1981, 2014.

[51] Y.-Q. Sun, J. Wang, Q. Jiang et al., "Haploidentical hematopoietic SCT may be superior to conventional consolidation/maintenance chemotherapy as post-remission therapy for high-risk adult ALL," *Bone Marrow Transplantation*, vol. 50, no. 1, pp. 20–25, 2015.

[52] X.-J. Huang, H.-H. Zhu, Y.-J. Chang et al., "The superiority of haploidentical related stem cell transplantation over chemotherapy alone as postremission treatment for patients with intermediate- or high-risk acute myeloid leukemia in first complete remission," *Blood*, vol. 119, no. 23, pp. 5584–5590, 2012.

[53] A. Bashey and S. R. Solomon, "T-cell replete haploidentical donor transplantation using post-transplant CY: an emerging standard-of-care option for patients who lack an HLA-identical sibling donor," *Bone Marrow Transplantation*, vol. 49, no. 8, pp. 999–1008, 2014.

[54] C. Anasetti, B. R. Logan, S. J. Lee et al., "Peripheral-blood stem cells versus bone marrow from unrelated donors," *The New England Journal of Medicine*, vol. 367, no. 16, pp. 1487–1496, 2012.

[55] N. Schmitz, M. Beksac, A. Bacigalupo et al., "Filgrastim-mobilized peripheral blood progenitor cells versus bone marrow transplantation for treating leukemia: 3-year results from the EBMT randomized trial," *Haematologica*, vol. 90, no. 5, pp. 643–648, 2005.

[56] D. Gallardo, R. de la Cámara, J. B. Nieto et al., "Is mobilized peripheral blood comparable with bone marrow as a source of hematopoietic stem cells for allogeneic transplantation from HLA-identical sibling donors? A case-control study," *Haematologica*, vol. 94, no. 9, pp. 1282–1288, 2009.

18

Study of Erythrocyte Indices, Erythrocyte Morphometric Indicators, and Oxygen-Binding Properties of Hemoglobin Hematoporphyrin Patients with Cardiovascular Diseases

Victor V. Revin,[1] Antonina A. Ushakova,[1] Natalia V. Gromova,[1] Larisa A. Balykova,[1] Elvira S. Revina,[1] Vera V. Stolyarova,[1] Tatiana A. Stolbova,[1] Ilya N. Solomadin,[1] Alexander Yu. Tychkov,[1] Nadezhda V. Revina,[1] and Oksana G. Imarova[2]

[1]*Federal State-Financed Academic Institution of Higher Education "National Research Ogarev Mordovia State University", Saransk 430005, Russia*
[2]*GBUZ RM "National Hospital for War Veterans", Saransk 430005, Russia*

Correspondence should be addressed to Natalia V. Gromova; nataly_grom@mail.ru

Academic Editor: Bashir A. Lwaleed

The current study investigates the functional state of erythrocytes and indices of the oxygen-binding capacity of hemoglobin in blood samples from healthy donors and from patients with coronary artery disease and myocardial infarction before and after treatment. It has been established that, in cardiovascular diseases, erythrocyte morphology and hemoglobin oxygen-transporting disorders are observed. Standard therapy does not result in the restoration of the structure and properties of erythrocytes. The authors believe that it is necessary for future therapeutic treatment to include preparations other than cardiovascular agents to enhance the capacity of hemoglobin to transport oxygen to the tissues.

1. Introduction

Currently, cardiovascular diseases are the most common diseases and are one of the leading causes of death and disability among able-bodied populations in economically developed countries [1–3]. By 2020, the World Health Organization estimates that there will be nearly 25 million deaths due to cardiovascular diseases worldwide.

More than half of deaths due to cardiovascular system diseases are caused by coronary artery disease (CAD). One in five men aged from 50 to 59 years suffers from this disease, and the incidence and mortality rates are increasing every year.

Coronary artery disease may cause myocardial infarction, apoplectic attack, or heart failure. Acute heart failure (AHF) remains one of the most actual and important problems of modern cardiology. Acute heart failure is a clinical syndrome characterised by early onset of disturbed cardiac function symptoms (reduced cardiac output and inadequate blood supply) [4, 5]. At present, the most common causes of acute heart failure are myocardial infarction (MI), decompensated chronic heart failure (CHF), and heart rhythm disorders, including atrial fibrillation [5].

Abnormalities of blood rheology are of great importance among significant factors determining hemodynamic disorders found in patients with CAD [6–8].

Among other factors underlying the pathogenesis of CAD (coronary atherosclerosis, hemodynamic findings, and coagulation system imbalances), hemorheological disorders influence CAD severity, expected treatment response, and patient treatment success [8–10].

Retrogressive changes in hemorheological indices are closely related to changes in erythrocyte morphometric indicators, which, in turn, determine their functional properties and reflect the state of both erythrocyte and cell membranes. Moreover, changes in erythrocyte morphometry may serve as an indicator of conduct therapy efficiency.

Hypoxia plays a significant role in the pathophysiology of a majority of cardiovascular diseases. Hypoxia causes disorders of blood gas transport function and very often leads to decreases in the efficiency of oxygen transport with the assistance of erythrocytes. In such cases, disorders of endothelial structure and function play a crucial role, whereas the role of erythrocytes and their oxygen-transporting capacity in the progress of peripheral vascular diseases still remains under investigated [3, 11].

One of the main reasons for disorders of the erythrocyte oxygen-transporting function is the conformational change of hemoglobin hematoporphyrin (Hb) and hemoglobin oxygen affinity (O_2). The use of Raman scattering spectroscopy makes it possible to determine changes in the conformation of hematoporphyrin in patients with severe arterial hypertension [12], patients with circulatory failure [13–15], and patients with stable effort angina under therapeutic interval hypoxia [12]. It is also important that the oxygen-binding and oxygen-transporting properties of hemoglobin depend on the morphofunctional state of erythrocyte membranes [16, 17].

A change of the conformation of hemoglobin hematoporphyrin (both cytoplasmic and membrane-bound) is may be interconnected with changes in the morphometric indicators of erythrocytes (erythrocyte surface area, phase height, phase volume, and hemoglobin distribution). Erythrocyte indices are an additional characteristic of the morphological and functional properties of erythrocytes.

The purpose of this study was to investigate erythrocyte morphology, the functional state of erythrocytes, and the conformational changes in hemoglobin in both healthy donors and patients with cardiovascular diseases.

To achieve our designated research purpose, the following aims were set:

(1) To study the functional characteristics of erythrocytes and the state of hemoglobin healthy donors and in patients suffering from CAD with various levels of severity for angina of effort and MI on their admission to hospital

(2) To evaluate the changes in the functional characteristics of erythrocytes and the state and oxygen-binding capacity of hemoglobin in patients with CAD and other cardiovascular diseases after standard medical treatment

2. Materials and Methods

2.1. Patients. This study included 40 patients from a cardiovascular care unit (Veterans Hospital of the Republic of Mordovia). Patients were males aged from 41 to 60 years (average age is 53.6 ± 4.2 years).

A clinicofunctional analysis of the condition of 20 patients suffering from CAD with stable angina (SA) of effort of the functional classes II-III was carried out.

Patients selected for subsequent examination did not smoke, had no genetically determined diseases, and had body mass indices ranging 24–29.

Twenty male patients diagnosed with "acute myocardial infarction" were also examined.

Therefore, all patients were divided into 2 groups based on a disease:

Group 1: stable angina, $n = 20$

Group 2: acute myocardial infarction, $n = 20$

Treatment included standard methods of clinical research study. All patients provided their consent to participate in the study.

The patients were randomly selected, and patients older than 60 years were excluded. The research was assessed by experts and approved by Local Ethics Committee at the Mordovia State University. The research was conducted in accordance with the Good Clinical Practice principles.

2.2. Control Group. There was also a control group consisting of 20 practically healthy donors (aged 41–60 years) who had periodic health examinations and did not have a history of cardiovascular diseases. These donors were selected in such a way that their gender and age corresponded to the parameters of patients with heart diseases from the other studied groups. Their average hematological parameters corresponded to physiologically normal parameters typical for such gender and age.

2.3. Sample Collection. Patient blood samples were taken from patients with diseases in the morning before taking medications or consuming food. Samples were taken from the ulnar vein and were collected into 5 ml vacuum tubes. The blood samples were taken from patients at their admission to hospital and after the protracted treatment based on the background therapy. The standard therapy in case of cardiac angina (CA) and MI included the following: regimen, diet, intake of statins (atorvastatin $C_{33}H_{35}FN_2O_5$), ACE inhibitors (enalapril $C_{20}H_{28}N_2O_5$) or blockers of the angiotensin receptor (valsartan $C_{24}H_{29}N_5O_3$), beta-blockers (bisoprolol $NC_{18}HNO_4$), antiaggregants (if CA, aspirin $C_9H_8O_4$; if MI, additionally, clopidogrel $C_{16}H_{16}ClNO_2S$), if MI, anticoagulants (heparin $C_{12}H_{19}NO_{20}S_3$), and nitrates (nitroglycerin) on demand. On medical indications, in case of MI, we administered analgesics (morphine), diuretics (verospiron), antiarrhythmic medication, and cardiac tonics. As for the group with MI, our study included patients who were delivered stenting (bare metal stents).

Thus, all 100% of CA patients took aspirin, and MI patients received 3-component therapy: aspirin + clopidogrel + heparin during 7–10 days under the control of APTT.

Blood was taken according to a standard procedure of blood taking [18].

For complete blood counts (CBC), vacuum systems with K3-EDTA anticoagulant were used. Roche Diagnostics (Switzerland) reagents were used in addition to dilution reagent (Cellpack), lysing solution (Stromatolyser 4DL, Sulfolyser), leucocyte differentiation reagent (Stromatolyser 4DS), and caustic cleaner (Cellclean).

2.4. Hematologic Research. Hematologic research was conducted by means of an XT-2000i automatic hematology analyser (Sysmex, Japan). For hematological indices, we determined the following indicators: erythrocyte levels (RBC count), mean corpuscular volume (MCV), mean corpuscular hemoglobin (MCH), and mean corpuscular hemoglobin concentration (MCHC).

2.5. Raman Analysis. The oxygen-binding properties of hemoglobin were evaluated by examining changes in the conformation of hemoglobin hematoporphyrin in native erythrocytes by means of Raman spectroscopy using an inVia Raman-scattering spectrometer (Renishaw, United Kingdom) with a short focal distance and high transmission monochromator with a focal distance no longer than 250 mm. A laser was used to obtain spectra (radiation wavelengths: 532 nm; peak radiated power: 100 mW; field lens: 100x). For data recording, a CCD detector (1024 × 256 pixels with a Peltier cooling module maintaining it at −70°C) with a grating of 1800 lines per mm was used. Digitised spectra are adapted using the WiRE 3.3 program. Spectral smoothing and baseline correction were also performed.

Whole blood was centrifuged during 10 min at 4000g. After removing the supernatant liquid, the sediment of erythrocytes was washed 10-fold volume of the solution for washing the erythrocytes and then again centrifuged 10 min at 4000g (at a temperature of 4°C). The above-described procedure was repeated 3 times. The obtained erythrocytic mass was stored in the washing medium at 4°C. Time of storage did not exceed 1 hour.

Smear was prepared on the slide (glass) by a standard method (slide was degreased with alcohol and dried prior to smearing), immediately after preparation measurements were taken of spectra of hemoglobin hematoporphyrin of erythrocytes (in the range 300–2000 sm^{-1}).

To evaluate the conformation of hemoglobin hematoporphyrin (Hb) and hemoglobin oxygen-binding properties, specific Raman-scattering spectral lines were used (maximum values are given): 1355, 1375, 1550, and 1580 cm^{-1}.

The nature of the Raman spectra for hemoglobin hematoporphyrin [19] allows one to identify the degree of oxidation of its iron atom, its spin state, and the existence of ligands. It also reflects changes in globin structure that lead to hematoporphyrin deformation and influencing the oxygen-binding properties of hemoglobin [14].

The intensities of the 1355 and 1375 cm^{-1} spectral lines are connected with symmetrical oscillations of pyrrole rings in molecules of deoxygenated hemoglobin and hemoglobin and with ligands, respectively [13]. The intensity of the 1375 cm^{-1} line is determined by oxygenated hemoglobin contents because the amount of oxygen in blood is 3-4 times higher than the contents of other ligands (e.g., NO or CO). Thus, the intensity ratio $I_{1375}/(I_{1355} + I_{1375})$ is proportional to the relative amount of oxygenated hemoglobin in blood. Intensities of the 1550 cm^{-1} and 1580 cm^{-1} spectral lines characterise the spin state of iron in deoxy- and oxy-forms, respectively. Therefore, they act as markers to evaluate the structural characteristics of iron in a prosthetic group, which provides the opportunity to use the spectral line intensity ratio I_{1355}/I_{1550} and I_{1375}/I_{1580} to evaluate the capacity of hemoglobin molecules in erythrocytes to bind and donate oxygen molecules, given the internal state of hemoglobin molecules. After division of one ratio by another $(I_{1355}/I_{1550})/(I_{1375}/I_{1580})$, it is possible to obtain the characteristic reflecting hemoglobin molecule oxygen affinity in native erythrocytes [20, 21].

2.6. Laser Interference Microscopy. Morphometric indices (morphology) were studied by laser interference microscopy. In contrast to the conventional methods of optical microscopy based on the registration of light intensity distribution, laser interference microscopy allows one to obtain the phase distribution in the interference image [22, 23].

For this study, an MII-4M modulation interference microscope, built by "Amphora Laboratory" (Moscow, Russia), was used. We also used a 635 nm laser with a lens with a magnification of 33.4 diameters and a numerical aperture of 0.65 [24]. A preliminary calibration of the microscope using 2 μm and 7.5 μm silicone particles was performed. Using a laser and interference microscope, the following morphological properties of erythrocytes were determined: the optical path difference (OPD), the surface area of the erythrocyte phase image (S), the physical height (Z), and phase volume of erythrocytes (V) [25].

The principle underlying the operation of this device is as follows: a laser beam L is divided into reference (control) and object beams. The reference beam reflects off the inspection mirror and goes to the detector. The object beam passes through the object, which is placed into a special chamber with the mirror bottom, reflects off the mirrored base sheet, passes through the object again, and goes to the detector, where it interferes with the first beam. Due to the difference in refractive indices of environment and the object between beams, there is optical path difference or phase height.

OPD value search point of the object forms phase image of the object [26–28]. The phase image for all the cells depends on the refractive index distribution and geometrical size of the cell. If geometrical size of the cell does not change during the experiment, then changes of phase height are determined only by changes of the refractive index. Thus, by the phase image, we can judge refractive index distribution in the cell, by the OPD change, the refractive index dynamics, and hence intracellular processes [29].

We placed 5–10 μl of erythrocytic suspension diluted with normal saline at a ratio of 1 : 200 onto special preparation glass with a smooth surface, and the sample was then covered with glass and placed under the microscope lens.

The mirrored base sheet on which the preparation with erythrocytes was placed reflected transmitted light, resulting in a double-phase shift of the coherent light source beam at every point on the object, and by means of an additional wave from the same source, the interference cell image was formed. At least 100 cells were imaged for each test [22, 25].

Interference images processing was carried out using FIJI software [30]. Using this program, the registration of the surface area volume of erythrocytes and maximum path length difference were performed. Further analysis of the results was carried out using Microsoft Office Excel 2013 and OriginPro 8.1 programs.

We calculated the erythrocyte phase volume using the following formula:

$$V = \frac{\Phi_{mean} * S}{n_{cell} - n_m}. \tag{1}$$

We calculated physical height using the following formula:

$$Z_{cell} = \frac{\Phi_{mean}}{n_{cell} - n_m}. \tag{2}$$

Φ_{mean} is mean value of measured parameter of the optical path length difference, proportional thickness.

S is surface area of the phase image of the cell.

n_{cell} is erythrocyte refractive index, which is 1.405.

n_m is refractive index of the surrounding solution (normal saline), which was 1.333 [25].

Refractive index was measured by using the Refractometer PTR46 [31–33].

Therefore, the erythrocyte phase portrait forming the phase shift distribution in various parts of the object was obtained. Phase shift values were used to create a three-dimensional (3D) image of the cell.

2.7. Statistical Analysis. At the first stage of statistical analysis, we evaluated the normality of value distribution for every sample using Geary's criterion [34]. We then evaluated the homogeneity of variance. We conducted the analysis of variance model and ANOVA for repeated measurements. In case of statistically significant differences between average values, we used ex post facto Tukey's method to compare individual means analysis [35].

The findings are presented in the form of arithmetical mean and standard deviation (mean ± SD).

3. Results

3.1. RBC Count and Erythrocyte Indices in the Blood of Apparently Healthy People and in Patients with SA and MI before and after Treatment. Erythrocyte indices are calculated values that allow for the quantification of important indicators of the erythrocyte state. These indices include the total number of erythrocytes, MCV, MCH, and MCHC. These indices are used to assess the functional activity of erythrocytes. For example, the MCHC is a sensitive indicator of hemoglobin formation violations, as it shows the degree of hemoglobin saturation in erythrocytes regardless of the amount of formed elements. The MCH indicator (mean corpuscular hemoglobin) estimates the weight of hemoglobin in an erythrocyte or the hemoglobin ratio to the cell volume.

Haemogram assessment has been based on physiological standards corresponding to the international system of units (SI) in clinical studies [36].

We found that the red blood cell count of apparently healthy people was $4.47 \pm 0.21 \times 10^{12}$ cells/L, the mean corpuscular volume was 94.51 ± 4.41 fL, and the mean corpuscular hemoglobin and the mean corpuscular hemoglobin concentrations were 31.17 ± 1.17 pg and 343.3 ± 8.23 pg, respectively. These indices that do not differ from physiological standards and literature data have been used as controls in our research (Table 1).

The data of patients with SA and MI admitted to the hospital were analysed before treatment and after the patient's hospital discharge.

At the time of hospital admission, the red blood cell counts of patients with CAD corresponded to physiological standards, although they exceeded the control group indices by 8% (Table 1).

Erythrocyte indices in patients with IHD and with MI corresponded to physiological norms. At the same time, all indices in the patient groups were significantly lower than those of the control group of donors.

Statistically significant changes in the studied indices were not observed after treatment.

Qualitative and quantitative changes, observed in the red blood cell system, are important diagnostic and prognostic indicators of various pathological processes and diseases. However, RBC indicators and erythrocyte indices provide only an indirect understanding of the processes occurring in the cytoplasmic membrane of red blood cells and can show not only the degree of erythrocyte damage (change in the morphology of each erythrocyte) but also the state (conformation and form) of hemoglobin in the erythrocyte.

Since the RBC count, MCV, MCHC, and MCH of patients with SA and MI were within normal physiological standards, we could not estimate real changes in the morphology of each erythrocyte. In addition, it was difficult to understand which hemoglobin form (oxyhemoglobin, deoxyhemoglobin, and methemoglobin) is within the erythrocyte and how the hematoporphyrin conformation and the hemoglobin oxygen-binding capacity change.

In this manner, we studied the morphometric characteristics of red blood cells using laser interference microscopy (LIM).

3.2. Morphometric Characteristics of Erythrocytes from Apparently Healthy People and from Patients with SA and MI before and after Treatment. The mean value of the optical path difference (OPD), the phase image area of erythrocytes (S), the geometric height (Z), and the erythrocyte phase volume (V) was estimated in patients with SA and MI.

Patients with CAD had erythrocyte morphometric characteristics that differed from that those of healthy people (Table 2).

The OPD and geometric height of erythrocytes exceeded the control group indices by 17%, whereas the erythrocyte phase volume was 9.8% greater than that of controls. In addition, we noted a decrease in the erythrocyte phase image area in relation to controls by 6.5%. MI patients, upon admission to hospital, had a mean OPD, erythrocyte geometric height, and erythrocyte phase volume that exceeded the indices of

TABLE 1: RBC count and erythrocyte indices in the blood of apparently healthy people and in patients with SA and MI before and after treatment, $n = 20$ (M ± SD).

Test groups	Indices			
	RBC count $(3.8–5.3) \times 10^{12}$cells/L	MCV (80–100) fL (femtolitre)	MCH in one erythrocyte (27–32) pg (picogram)	MCHC (320–360) pg (picogram)
Control	4.47 ± 0.20	94.51 ± 4.41	31.17 ± 1.18	343.3 ± 8.23
SA patients before treatment	$4.87 \pm 0.41^{**}$	$88.37 \pm 4.09^{**}$	$29.98 \pm 1.06^{*}$	$330.6 \pm 20.45^{*}$
SA patients after treatment	4.75 ± 0.34	90.35 ± 4.81	30.09 ± 1.20	332.0 ± 3.66
MI patients before treatment	$4.76 \pm 0.31^{*}$	$88.3 \pm 4.14^{**}$	$29.54 \pm 1.63^{*}$	$329.3 \pm 12.57^{*}$
MI patients after treatment	4.52 ± 0.45	$90.12 \pm 2.74^{*}$	30.22 ± 1.03	333.85 ± 12.29

$^{*}p < 0.05$; $^{**}p < 0.01$.

TABLE 2: Morphometric characteristics of erythrocytes from apparently healthy people and from patients with SA and MI before and after treatment, $n = 20$ (M ± SD).

Test groups	Indices			
	The mean value of optical path difference (OPD), Φ_{mean}, nm	Phase image area of erythrocyte, S, μm^2	Geometric mean height of the erythrocyte, Z, μm	Erythrocyte phase volume, V, μm^3
Control	151.82 ± 6.46	43.43 ± 3.79	2.02 ± 0.11	87.73 ± 4.82
SA patients before treatment	$177.39 \pm 5.39^{*}$	40.80 ± 3.30	$2.36 \pm 0.14^{*}$	$96.29 \pm 3.55^{*}$
SA patients after treatment	$115.38 \pm 4.61^{*\Delta}$	$55.99 \pm 2.93^{*\Delta}$	$1.53 \pm 0.11^{*\Delta}$	$75.59 \pm 3.99^{*\Delta}$
MI patients before treatment	$187.53 \pm 6.41^{*}$	40.66 ± 2.90	$2.50 \pm 0.15^{*}$	$101.65 \pm 2.98^{*}$
MI patients after treatment	$114.39 \pm 3.82^{*\Delta}$	$59.40 \pm 2.25^{\Delta}$	$1.52 \pm 0.14^{*\Delta}$	$74.25 \pm 4.46^{\Delta}$

$^{*}p < 0.05$, reliability in relation to donors' indicators; $^{\Delta}p < 0.05$, reliability in relation to pretreatment indicators.

the healthy donors by 23.5%, 23.7%, and 15.9% ($p < 0.05$), respectively (Table 2). We noted a decrease in the erythrocyte phase image area in relation to the control by 6.4%.

After the treatment of patients with SA, we observed a decrease in the OPD and physical height by 35% and a decrease of the erythrocyte phase volume by 21.5% compared to the primary indices ($p < 0.05$). However, none of these indices ever returned to the control group levels.

After patients with MI were treated, their mean optical path difference and geometric height values barely changed, whereas their phase volume decreased by 27% compared to their indices at admission. Additionally, the phase image area of erythrocyte increased by 8%, significantly exceeding healthy donor group indices. Erythrocyte phase volume indices did not return to those of the control group.

We have made a correlation analysis between the morphometric parameters determined by the LIM method and values of erythrocytic indexes. When studying correlations between RBC values (red blood cell count) and LIM parameters of human erythrocytes, we detected a moderate negative correlation with the value of phase image S ($r = -0.40$) and moderate positive correlation with the values of the geometric height, phase volume, and optical path difference ($r = 0.47$, $r = 0.48$, and $r = 0.48$, resp.) ($p < 0.05$).

Moderate reverse correlation between MCH (mean hemoglobin content in the erythrocyte) and such LIM

parameters like phase volume ($r = -0.34$), geometric height ($r = -0.31$), and OPD ($r = -0.31$) was discovered ($p < 0.05$).

The average correlation coefficient was also observed between MCV values and such morphometric parameters as OPD ($r = -0.34$), the phase volume ($r = -0.35$), and geometric height ($r = -0.34$) ($p < 0.05$).

Between morphometric LIM values of human erythrocytes and the average concentration of hemoglobin in erythrocytes, MCHC correlation was not found.

Most erythrocytes from healthy people are represented by discocytes (Figure 1(a)), which is also shown by our data in the control group. SA and MI patients have had many more spherocytes among erythrocytes (Figure 1(b)). This erythrocyte class refers to the irreversibly deformed or prehemolytic forms [37]. Also stomatocytes met in large quantities (Figure 1(c)). Such changes in red blood cell shape in patients with cardiovascular diseases are primarily related to the violation of erythrocyte membrane stability [24, 38]. In the future, the output of ectoglobular hemoglobin (EGH) and its degradation products into blood plasma may be possible, which contributes to serious metabolic changes, secondary activation of lipid peroxidation, and exacerbation of ischaemic myocardial injury [39].

The number of spherocytes was reduced, whereas other pathological forms of erythrocytes related to reversible forms such as stomatocytes and echinocytes were more frequent

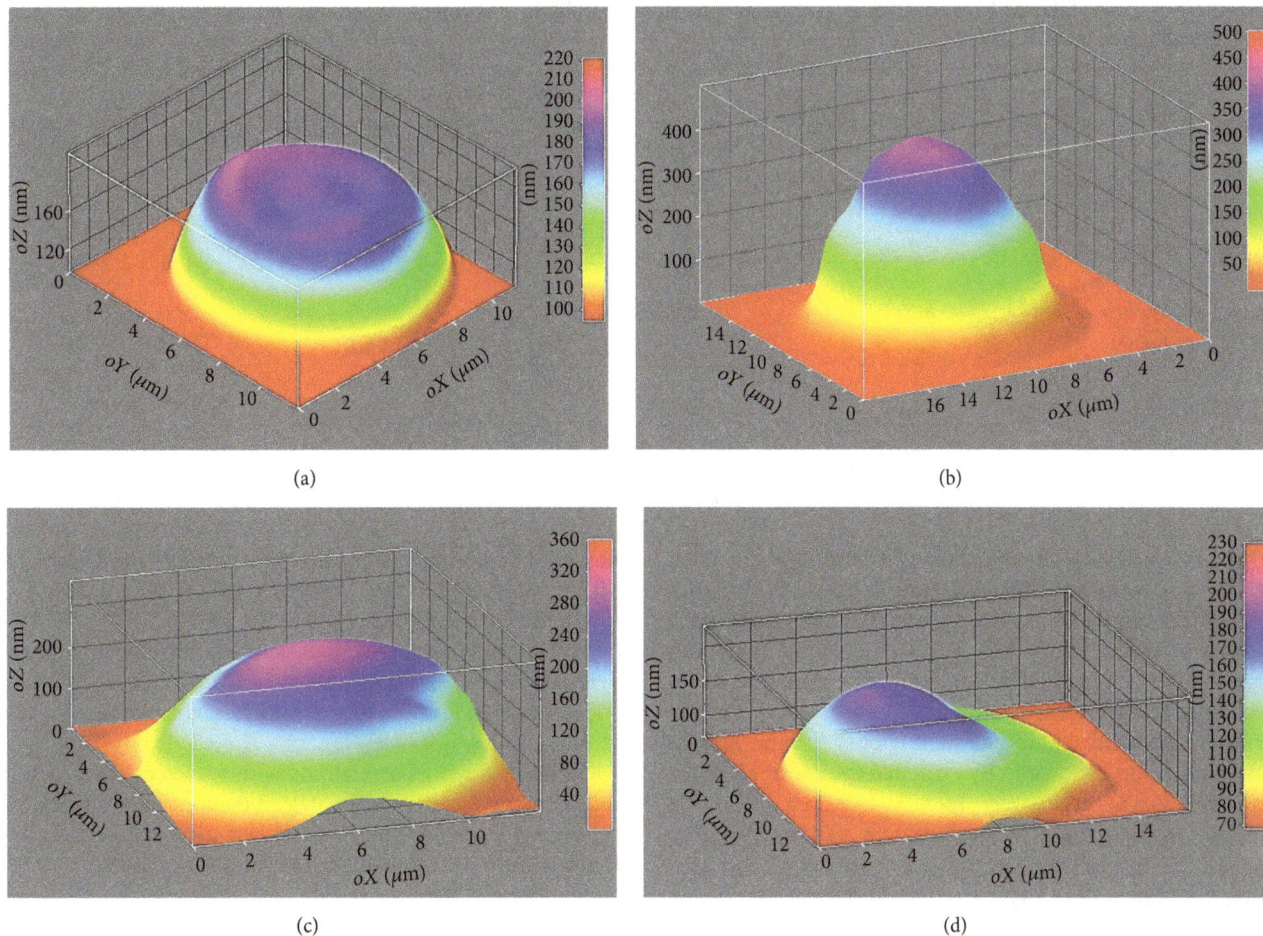

FIGURE 1: Phase images of erythrocytes, taken using LIM (oX, oY: erythrocyte sizes, μm; oZ: optical path difference (OPD), nm): (a) erythrocyte from a healthy donor (discocyte); (b) erythrocyte from a MI patient before treatment (spherocyte); (c) erythrocyte from a SA patient before treatment (stomatocyte); (d) erythrocyte from a MI patient after treatment (stomatocyte).

(Figure 1(d)) in the patient group after the treatment. Compared with discocytes, degenerative forms of red blood cells are less robust in terms of oxygen delivery function, microcirculation, and deformation capacity; therefore, their increase is an unfavourable sign [37]. Their ability to aggregate depends on their factors too. Increased erythrocyte aggregation disrupts the normal structure of the blood stream in the microcirculatory vessels and leads to increased blood viscosity, microcirculatory blocks, and tissue hypoxia [40].

3.3. Correlation of Raman Bands of Erythrocyte Hemoglobin Hematoporphyrin of Apparently Healthy People and People with SA and MI before and after Treatment.

Using the Raman method, we examined scattered intensity shifts for the relevant spectral bands of erythrocyte hemoglobin hematoporphyrin from patients with SA and MI before and after treatment in relation to the control group. The conformation of hematoporphyrin hemoglobin of red blood cells, determined by the ratio of Raman spectra, of healthy donors is shown in Figure 2.

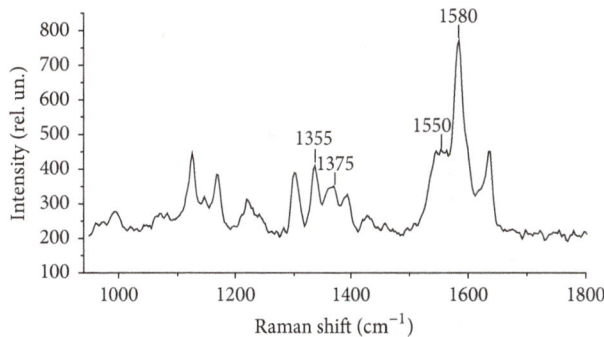

FIGURE 2: Spectrum of Raman scattering of hematoporphyrin hemoglobin. The figure shows the Raman bands with the position of the maximums of 1355, 1375, 1550, and 1580 cm^{-1}. The ordinate is the intensity of the Raman radiation, in conventional units; along the abscissa-frequency shift, cm^{-1}.

In cases of myocardial infarction and coronary artery disease, erythrocytes show changes in the correlation of band intensity.

TABLE 3: Correlation of Raman bands of erythrocyte hemoglobin hematoporphyrin of apparently healthy people and people with SA and MI before and after treatment, $n = 20$ (M ± SD).

Test groups	Indices			
	Percentage of oxyhemoglobin blood $I_{1375}/(I_{1355} + I_{1375})$	Relative ability of hemoglobin to bind ligands I_{1355}/I_{1550}	Relative ability of hemoglobin to drop off ligands I_{1375}/I_{1580}	Hemoglobin ligand affinity (O_2) $(I_{1355}/I_{1550})/(I_{1375}/I_{1580})$
Control	0.69 ± 0.03	0.61 ± 0.03	0.53 ± 0.02	1.16 ± 0.07
SA patients before treatment	$0.54 \pm 0.02^*$	$0.70 \pm 0.03^*$	$0.44 \pm 0.03^*$	$1.56 \pm 0.12^*$
SA patients after treatment	$0.61 \pm 0.03^*$	$0.67 \pm 0.04^*$	0.48 ± 0.03	$1.41 \pm 0.15^*$
MI patients before treatment	$0.52 \pm 0.03^*$	$0.76 \pm 0.03^*$	$0.40 \pm 0.02^*$	$1.90 \pm 0.11^*$
MI patients after treatment	$0.58 \pm 0.04^*$	$0.75 \pm 0.05^*$	$0.42 \pm 0.03^*$	$1.52 \pm 0.10^{*\Delta}$

$^*p < 0.05$, reliability in relation to donors' indicators; $^\Delta p < 0.05$, reliability in relation to pretreatment indicators.

The erythrocyte hemoglobin oxygen-binding ability indicators of patients with CAD at the time of hospital admission differed from those of healthy donors. Thus, the percentage of oxyhemoglobin in the blood was reduced by 21.8% and relative ability of hemoglobin to drop off ligands by 16.9% in comparison with the control group ($p < 0.05$). On the contrary, the relative ability of hemoglobin to bind ligands and hemoglobin ligand affinity exceeded the control level by 14.8% and 34.5%, respectively (Table 3).

After the treatment of patients with SA, the ability of hemoglobin to bind ligands did not reasonably change; it remained higher than that of the control group by 22.9% ($p < 0.05$) (Table 3). The ability of hemoglobin to allocate ligands has not changed. Compared to the control group, the index remained lower by 9.5% ($p < 0.05$). The hemoglobin ligand affinity was reduced by 13.5% ($p < 0.05$), although it did not reach the level of the control group. The percentage of oxyhemoglobin increased by 11.9% ($p < 0.05$), remaining lower than the control value ($p < 0.05$).

Before the treatment of patients with MI, the ability of hemoglobin to bind ligands and the hemoglobin ligand affinity increased by 24.3% and 64.8% relative to the control, and the ability of hemoglobin to shed ligands and the percentage of oxyhemoglobin decreased by 24.5% and 24.7%, respectively, compared to the control. After treatment, the ability of hemoglobin to bind ligands irrelevantly decreased, and the hemoglobin ligand affinity decreased by 9.0%; we also observed an increase of 11.4% in the percentage of oxyhemoglobin. Simultaneously, the ability of hemoglobin to allocate ligands did not change, remaining higher than the control value by 20.8%.

The studied indices still did not reach the control levels (Table 3). The changes in the study results are therefore better expressed among MI patients.

When studying correlations between the relative number oHb in the blood ($I_{1375}/(I_{1355} + I_{1505})$) and morphometric parameters of human erythrocytes, we discovered a moderate negative correlation with values of the optical path difference ($r = -0.46$), geometric altitude ($r = -0.46$), and phase volume ($r = -0.47$). High correlation coefficient was observed with values of erythrocyte indices: RBC count ($r = -0.72$), MCV ($r = 0.98$), MCH ($r = 0.95$), and MCHC ($r = 0.94$) ($p < 0.05$).

When studying correlations between the relative ability of hemoglobin to release ligands (I_{1375}/I_{1550}) and morphometric parameters of human erythrocytes, correlation was not found.

When studying correlations with values of erythrocytic indices, we detected a moderate reverse correlation with RBC count ($r = -0.44$). With MCV, MCH, and MCHC indices, we found a close direct positive correlation ($r = 0.88$, $r = 0.88$, and $r = 0.84$, resp.) ($p < 0.05$).

During the study of correlations between the relative ability of hemoglobin to bind ligands, including oxygen (I_{1355}/I_{1550}) and the morphometric parameters of human erythrocytes, correlation was also not found.

We found a moderate direct correlation with the RBC index ($r = 0.32$) and a strong reverse correlation with MCV, MCH, and MCHC indices ($r = -0.82$, $r = -0.83$, and $r = -0.78$, resp.) ($p < 0.05$).

During the study of correlations between the affinity of hemoglobin to ligands, particularly to oxygen (($I_{1355}/I_{1550})/(I_{1375}/I_{1580})$) and morphometric parameters of erythrocytes, we detected a close reverse correlation with such erythrocytic indices as MCV, MCH, and MCHC ($r = -0.87$, $r = -0.92$, and $r = -0.85$, resp.). A moderate direct correlation with OPD values, physical thickness ($r = 0.51$), and phase corpuscular volume ($r = 0.53$) was detected ($p < 0.05$).

4. Discussion

In the pathogenesis of SA and MI, the universality and severity of microcirculation disorders are highly significant [41]. The persistence of the microvasculature function is mostly determined by the rheological properties of blood [13]. Therefore, in the pathogenesis of SA and MI, rheological disorders are of great importance, and the participation of red blood cells in this process determined our interest in studying the structural and functional characteristics of red blood cells [42].

This study demonstrated that, in the case of cardiovascular diseases such as SA and MI, patient erythrocyte index values corresponded to physiological standards.

However, by using more subtle methods such as LIM and Raman spectroscopy, we discovered changes in erythrocyte morphology and the violation of the oxygen-binding ability of hemoglobin associated with conformational rearrangements of hematoporphyrin.

Therefore, cardiovascular diseases are followed by an increase in erythrocyte OPD, physical height, and phase volume. Changes in erythrocyte morphological characteristics are directly related to irregularities in the composition of the phospholipid component of erythrocyte membranes and an increase in their microviscosity [43].

It is known that CAD patients have increased erythrocyte plasma membrane viscosity [44]. At the same time, oxyhemoglobin levels reduce due to the deterioration of oxygen diffusion through the membrane and the decrease of the oxygen saturation of red blood cells, which contributes to tissue hypoxia.

An increase in hemoglobin oxygen affinity and the ability of hemoglobin to bind oxygen leads to additional increases in hypoxia processes that are already present at the development of SA and especially MI. This increase can also be caused by the deterioration of the ability of hemoglobin to shed ligands, including oxygen.

Patients with cardiovascular diseases undergo long-term drug therapy.

Among the most frequently used drugs in cardiology practice are medications containing nitrates. Currently, several medications are used: nitroglycerine (or glyceryl trinitrate), statins (Liprimar), ACE inhibitors (enalapril), beta-blockers (bisoprolol, Concor), blockers of angiotensin receptors (valsartan), and anticoagulants (heparin). Organic nitrates are donors of exogenous NO with physiological effects identical to exogenous NO. Their activity is shown after a series of metabolic transformations in which nitrogen oxide is formed, that is, a substance similar in structure and function to the endothelium-dependent relaxation factor (EDRF) [45]. The main goal of drug therapy is to decrease the venous vessel pressure. Anticoagulants prevent blood clot formation and intravascular coagulation. Statins have lipid-lowering effects and help to reduce LDL levels, which helps prevent the proliferation of atherosclerotic plaques and reduces the risk of strokes and heart attacks [46].

Unfortunately, such standard SA and MI therapies do not lead to the recovery of erythrocyte structure and the oxygen-binding ability of hemoglobin.

5. Conclusion

Cardiovascular pathology is associated not only with violations of the structure and function of the blood vessels endothelium but also with changes in the structure and oxygen-binding capacity of erythrocytes.

On the basis of our data and an analysis of the literature, we argue that, in addition to traditional drugs, which affect the status of the vessels, it is necessary to seek natural compounds that normalise the structure of red blood cells and enhance their oxygen transport function to more effectively treat patients with various cardiovascular diseases.

Conflicts of Interest

The authors declare that there are no conflicts of interest regarding the publication of this paper.

Acknowledgments

The authors are grateful for the support of the Russian Science Foundation, Grant no. 15-15-10025.

References

[1] S. Sasayama, "Heart disease in asia," *Circulation*, vol. 118, no. 25, pp. 2669–2671, 2008.

[2] P. Jeemon and K. S. Reddy, "Social determinants of cardiovascular disease outcomes in Indians," *Indian Journal of Medical Research*, vol. 132, no. 11, pp. 617–622, 2010.

[3] R. K. Upadhyay, "Emerging risk biomarkers in cardiovascular diseases and disorders," *Journal of Lipids*, vol. 2015, Article ID 971453, 50 pages, 2015.

[4] M. Gheorghiade and R. O. Bonow, "Chronic heart failure in the United States: A manifestation of coronary artery disease," *Circulation*, vol. 97, no. 3, pp. 282–289, 1998.

[5] M. Gheorghiade and P. S. Pang, "Acute heart failure syndromes," *Journal of the American College of Cardiology*, vol. 53, no. 7, pp. 557–573, 2009.

[6] L. Dintenfass, "Red cell aggregation in cardiovascular diseases and crucial role of inversion phenomenon," *Angiology*, vol. 36, no. 5, pp. 315–326, 1985.

[7] M. Mares, C. Bertolo, V. Terribile, and A. Girolami, "Hemorheological study in patients with coronary artery disease," *Cardiology*, vol. 78, no. 2, pp. 111–116, 1991.

[8] M. Bilgi, H. Güllü, and İ. Kozanoğluetal., "Evaluation of blood rheology in patients with coronary slow flow or non-obstructive coronary artery disease," *Clinical Hemorheology and Microcirculation*, vol. 53, no. 4, pp. 317–326, 2013.

[9] G. Kesmarky, K. Toth, and L. Habon, "Hemorheological parameters in coronary artery disease," *Clinical Hemorheology and Microcirculation*, vol. 18, no. 4, pp. 245–251, 1998.

[10] A. Rozanski, J. A. Blumenthal, and J. Kaplan, "Impact of psychological factors on the pathogenesis of cardiovascular disease and implications for therapy," *Circulation*, vol. 99, no. 16, pp. 2192–2217, 1999.

[11] D. J. Pierson, "Pathophysiology and clinical effects of chronic hypoxia," *Respiratory Care*, vol. 45, no. 1, pp. 39–51, 2000.

[12] G. V. Maksimov, O. V. Rodnenkov, A. A. Churin, A. B. Rubin, V. A. Tkachuk, and E. I. Chazov, "Influence of interval hypoxemic training on hemoglobin ability to bind oxygen in the blood of ischemia heart disease patient," *Cardiology*, no. 6, pp. 8–12, 2001.

[13] O. V. Rodnenkov, O. G. Luneva, N. A. Ulyanova et al., "Erythrocyte membrane fluidity and haemoglobin haemoporphyrin conformation: Features revealed in patients with heart failure," *Pathophysiology*, vol. 11, no. 4, pp. 209–213, 2005.

[14] A. I. Yusipovich, N. A. Braze, O. G. Luneva et al., "Changes in the state of hemoglobin in patients with coronary heart disease and patients with circulatory failure," *Bulletin of Experimental Biology and Medicine*, vol. 155, no. 2, pp. 233–235, 2013.

[15] V. V. Revin, N. V. Gromova, E. S. Revina et al., "Study of the structure, oxygen-transporting functions, and ionic composition of erythrocytes at vascular diseases," *BioMed Research International*, vol. 2015, Article ID 973973, 7 pages, 2015.

[16] M. Nikinmaa, "Oxygen and carbondioxide transport in vertebrate erythrocytes: an evolutionary change in the role of membrane transport," *Journal of Experimental Biology*, vol. 200, part 2, pp. 369–380, 1997.

[17] S. A. Jewell, P. G. Petrov, and C. P. Winlove, "The effect of oxidative stress on the membrane dipole potential of human red blood cells," *Biochimica et Biophysica Acta—Biomembranes*, vol. 1828, no. 4, pp. 1250–1258, 2013.

[18] R. A. McPherson and M. R. Pincus, *Clinical Diagnosis and Management by Laboratory Methods*, Elsevier, 2011.

[19] N. A. Brazhe, S. Abdali, A. R. Brazhe et al., "New insight into erythrocyte through in vivo surface-enhanced Raman spectroscopy," *Biophysical Journal*, vol. 97, no. 12, pp. 3206–3214, 2009.

[20] V. A. Mityanina, E. Y. Parshina, A. I. Yusipovich, G. V. Maksimov, and A. A. Selischeva, "Oxygen-binding characteristics of erythrocyte in children with type I diabetes mellitus of different duration," *Bulletin of Experimental Biology and Medicine*, vol. 153, no. 4, pp. 508–512, 2012.

[21] A. P. Vlasov, V. A. Trofimov, T. V. Tarasova et al., "Structural-functional state of hemoglobin in gestosis," *Modern Problems of Science and Education*, vol. 6, 8 pages, 2012.

[22] A. R. Brazhe, N. A. Brazhe, O. V. Sosnovtseva, A. N. Pavlov, E. Mosekilde, and G. V. Maksimov, "Wavelet-based analysis of cell dynamics measured by interference microscopy," *Computer Research and Modeling*, vol. 1, no. 1, pp. 77–83, 2009.

[23] V. L. Minaev and A. I. Yusipovich, "Medical and biological measurements: use of an automated interference microscope in biological research," *Measurement Techniques*, vol. 55, no. 7, pp. 839–844, 2012.

[24] V. V. Revin, S. M. Filatova, I. V. Syusin et al., "Study of correlation between state and composition of lipid phase and change in erythrocytes structure under induction of oxidative processes," *International Journal of Hematology*, vol. 101, no. 5, pp. 487–496, 2015.

[25] A. I. Yusipovich, E. Y. Parshina, N. Y. Brysgalova et al., "Laser interference microscopy in erythrocyte study," *Journal of Applied Physics*, vol. 105, no. 10, pp. 102037–102047, 2009.

[26] V. P. Tychinskiĭ, G. É. Kufal', T. V. Vyshenskaya, E. V. Perevedentseva, and S. L. Nikandrov, "Measurements of submicron structures with the Airyscan laser phase microscope," *Quantum Electronics*, vol. 27, no. 8, pp. 735–739, 1997.

[27] V. P. Tychinskiĭ, "Coherent phase microscopy of intracellular processes," *Physics-Uspekhi*, vol. 44, no. 6, pp. 617–629, 2001.

[28] N. A. Brazhe, A. R. Brazhe, A. N. Pavlov et al., "Unraveling cell processes: interference imaging interwoven with data analysis," *Journal of Biological Physics*, vol. 32, no. 3-4, pp. 191–208, 2006.

[29] A. I. Yusipovich, M. V. Zagubizhenko, G. G. Levin et al., "Laser interference microscopy of amphibian erythrocytes: impact of cell volume and refractive index," *Journal of Microscopy*, vol. 244, no. 3, pp. 223–229, 2011.

[30] J. Schindelin, I. Arganda-Carreras, E. Frise et al., "Fiji: an open-source platform for biological-image analysis," *Nature Methods*, vol. 9, no. 7, pp. 676–682, 2012.

[31] G. G. Levin, Th. V. Bulygin, and G. N. Vishnyakov, "Coherent oscillations of the molecular state of protein in live cells," *Tsitologiya*, vol. 47, no. 4, pp. 348–356, 2005.

[32] B. Rappaz, A. Barbul, F. Charrière et al., "Erythrocytes volume and refractive index measurement with a digital holographic microscope," in *Optical Diagnostics and Sensing VII, 644509*, vol. 6445 of *Proceedings of SPIE*, The International Society for Optical Engineering, February 2007.

[33] P. Mazeron, J. Didelon, S. Muller, and J.-F. Stoltz, "A theoretical approach of the measurement of osmotic fragility of erythrocytes by optical transmission," *Photochemistry and Photobiology*, vol. 72, no. 2, pp. 172–178, 2000.

[34] R. C. Geary, "Testing for normality," *Biometrika*, vol. 34, pp. 209–242, 1947.

[35] J. W. Tukey, "Comparing individual means in the analysis of variance," *Biometrics. Journal of the Biometric Society*, vol. 5, pp. 99–114, 1949.

[36] H. K. Walker, W. D. Hall, and J. W. Hurst, *Clinical Methods: The History, Physical, and Laboratory Examinations*, Butterworths, Boston, Mass, USA, 3rd edition, 1990.

[37] N. Mohandas, M. R. Clark, M. S. Jacobs, and S. B. Shohet, "Analysis of factors regulating erythrocyte deformability," *Journal of Clinical Investigation*, vol. 66, no. 3, pp. 563–573, 1980.

[38] V. V. Revin, N. V. Gromova, E. S. Revina et al., "Role of membrane lipids in the regulation of erythrocytic oxygen-transport function in cardiovascular diseases," *BioMed Research International*, vol. 2016, Article ID 3429604, 11 pages, 2016.

[39] A. Boveris and B. Chance, "The mitochondrial generation of hydrogen peroxide: general properties and effect of hyperbaric oxygen," *Biochemical Journal*, vol. 134, no. 3, pp. 707–716, 1973.

[40] V. Toschi, R. Gallo, M. Lettino et al., "Tissue factor modulates the thrombogenicity of human atherosclerotic plaques," *Circulation*, vol. 95, no. 3, pp. 594–599, 1997.

[41] F. Perticone, R. Ceravolo, A. Pujia et al., "Prognostic significance of endothelial dysfunction in hypertensive patients," *Circulation*, vol. 104, no. 2, pp. 191–196, 2001.

[42] M. Fornal, R. A. Korbut, M. Lekka et al., "Rheological properties of erythrocytes in patients with high risk of cardiovascular disease," *Clinical Hemorheology and Microcirculation*, vol. 39, no. 1-4, pp. 213–219, 2008.

[43] J. A. Jiménez, N. Loango, A. M. Giraldo, P. Landázuri, and H. Castaño, "Sphingomyelin of erythrocytes membranes is related to total cholesterol and LDL-cholesterol in patients with significant coronary arterial disease," *The Open Clinical Chemistry Journal*, vol. 5, no. 1, pp. 27–32, 2012.

[44] C. Saldanha, L. Sargenter, J. Monteiro, C. Perdigão, C. Ribeiro, and J. Martins-Silva, "Impairment of the erythrocyte membrane fluidity in survivors of acute myocardial infarction. A prospective study," *Clinical Hemorheology and Microcirculation*, vol. 20, no. 2, pp. 111–116, 1999.

[45] A. B. Levine, D. Punihaole, and T. B. Levine, "Characterization of the role of nitric oxide and its clinical applications," *Cardiology*, vol. 122, no. 1, pp. 55–68, 2012.

[46] R. Hille, J. S. Olson, and G. Palmer, "Spectral transitions of nitrosylhemes during ligand binding to hemoglobin," *The Journal of Biological Chemistry*, vol. 254, no. 23, pp. 11953–11957, 1979.

19

Prognostic Factors for Immune Thrombocytopenia Outcome in Greek Children: A Retrospective Single-Centered Analysis

Alexandros Makis,[1] Athanasios Gkoutsias,[1]
Theodoros Palianopoulos,[1] Eleni Pappa,[2] Evangelia Papapetrou,[3] Christina Tsaousi,[3]
Eleftheria Hatzimichael,[4] and Nikolaos Chaliasos[1]

[1] Department of Pediatrics, University Hospital of Ioannina, Ioannina, Greece
[2] Department of Internal Medicine, University Hospital of Ioannina, Ioannina, Greece
[3] Hematology Laboratory, University Hospital of Ioannina, Ioannina, Greece
[4] Hematology Department, University Hospital of Ioannina, Ioannina, Greece

Correspondence should be addressed to Alexandros Makis; amakis@cc.uoi.gr

Academic Editor: Michelle Baccarani

Immune thrombocytopenia (ITP) in children has a varied course and according to duration is distinguished as newly diagnosed (<3 months), persistent (3–12), and chronic (>12) types. Several studies have evaluated the prognostic factors for the progression of the disease, but similar works have yet to be performed in Greece. We aimed to identify prognostic markers for the three forms of the disease in 57 Greek children during a 13-year period. Information regarding age, gender, preceding infection, bleeding type, duration of symptoms and platelets at diagnosis, treatment, disease course, and immunological markers was recorded. 39 children had newly diagnosed, 4 persistent, and 14 chronic disease. Chronic ITP children were more likely to be of age > 10 years ($p = 0.015$) and have gradual initiation of the disease ($p = 0.001$), platelets > 10×10^9/L ($p = 0.01$), and impaired immunological markers ($p < 0.003$) compared to newly diagnosed/persistent groups. Recent history of infection was found mainly in the newly diagnosed/persistent group ($p = 0.013$). None of the children exhibited severe spontaneous bleeding. *Conclusion.* Even though ITP in children usually has a self-limited course, with rare serious bleeding complications, the chronic form of the disease is characterized by different predictive parameters, which can be used in clinical practice.

1. Introduction

Primary immune thrombocytopenia (ITP) is an autoimmune disorder characterized by low platelet count (<100 × 10^9/L) in the absence of other secondary causes. The disease is caused by increased platelet destruction by humoral or cellular immune mechanisms as well as inappropriate platelet production in the bone marrow [1]. In children, it mainly occurs between 2 and 7 years of age and usually a viral infection of the respiratory or gastrointestinal tract precedes 2–4 weeks earlier. At older ages, the precipitating factor of immune deregulation remains unknown [2].

ITP is characterized by a variety of skin and mucous membrane bleeding manifestations such as petechiae, purpura, bruising, epistaxis, gingival bleeding, and menorrhagia.

Severe intracranial bleeding is extremely rare, occurring in 0.5–1% of children when the platelet count drops below 10×10^9/L [3]. According to the standardization of terminology, definitions and outcome criteria in ITP of adults and children published by Rodeghiero et al., ITP in children is divided into newly diagnosed (duration < 3 months, 50% of the cases), persistent (3–12 months, 25% of the cases) and chronic (>12 months, 25% of the cases) type. The older time limit of 6 months to define chronicity is no longer in use [4].

Children who have no or mild bleeding can be managed with observation alone, regardless of platelet count. In cases requiring treatment, intravenous immunoglobulin (IVIG), anti-D immunoglobulin, or corticosteroids can be administered [5]. When, despite repeated doses of first-line treatment, the disease becomes resistant and chronic lasting more than twelve months, other treatments should be applied. Recently, the use of the thrombopoietin receptor agonist eltrombopag has been approved in children older than one year with chronic ITP who have not responded to the administration of first-line drugs [6]. In refractory cases, other options are the use of rituximab, a monoclonal anti-CD20 chimeric antibody, or immunosuppressant drugs (e.g., cyclosporine, azathioprine, and mycophenolate mofetil) [7]. Splenectomy is an alternative choice with a significant risk of complications and is applied only in a few, very serious chronic cases [8].

Reliable prediction of the course of the disease at time of diagnosis could be a useful tool regarding the planning of treatment, in order to minimize the risk of bleeding while avoiding drug complications. Also, it helps the patients and their parents to know what to except in the future and to cope with the changes that inevitably arise in the life of the child and the family.

The predictors of the progression of the disease have been investigated in large, international studies with focus on the distinction between acute and chronic form using the time limit of 6 months from diagnosis [9–11]. In recent studies, an effort has been made to determine the predictive parameters based on the new classification in which the time limit for chronic ITP is 12 months [12–14]. A recent meta-analysis included all studies and showed that chronic ITP is mainly correlated with the female gender, older age at diagnosis, absence of recent infection, slow onset of symptoms, higher platelet count at diagnosis, the presence of antinuclear antibodies (ANA), and treatment with corticosteroids and IVIG [15].

Since ITP is a heterogeneous disease, it is of great importance to confirm these ITP predictors at national level. In Greece, one retrospective work has been published with a large number of children from Crete and it was mainly focused on the treatment and the response to it [16]. The purpose of our study was to analyze all the ITP cases from an academic reference center in Northwestern Greece during a 13-year period and to point out the specific predictive characteristics related to the three categories of ITP (newly diagnosed, persistent, and chronic).

2. Patient and Methods

The medical records of all children with ITP hospitalized in the Pediatric Department of the University Hospital of Ioannina in Greece, from November 2002 to March 2015, were retrospectively studied. The Pediatric Department is the referral center for pediatric diseases in Northwestern Greece, with a mean number of 3.450 admissions per year. The demographic, clinical, and laboratory data of patients were recorded. The study was approved by the local ethics committee. The diagnosis of primary ITP was set in children with isolated thrombocytopenia ($<100 \times 10^9$/L) in the absence of other causes that may be associated with thrombocytopenia. Children with secondary thrombocytopenia due to systemic disease or medications, patients with incomplete clinical data, or patients that discontinued monitoring in our department were excluded from the study. All children had a minimum of 1 year of follow-up.

Demographic data were collected such as name, date of birth, age, sex, and place of residence. Medical and family history were recorded. The following information was documented at diagnosis: date of diagnosis, platelet count, type and severity of bleeding, and immunological markers (i.e., ANA, antiphospholipid antibodies, immunoglobulin levels, C3 and C4 levels, and direct antiglobulin test). We also recorded the type of treatment and the response.

Newly diagnosed ITP was defined as the presence of thrombocytopenia for <3 months after diagnosis, persistent for 3–12 months, and chronic ITP for >12 months. The onset of symptoms was defined as abrupt when bleeding symptoms lasted for less than two weeks before seeking assistance or as gradual when they lasted more than two weeks before the medical assessment. Platelet number at diagnosis was classified into $<10 \times 10^9$/L and $>10 \times 10^9$/L. This value was chosen because below this threshold spontaneous and serious bleeding manifestations can occur. A history of recent infection was defined as a recorded infection of the upper respiratory or gastrointestinal tract over four weeks before the diagnosis of ITP.

The statistical analysis was done using the SPSS 16.0 statistical program. Numerical data and categorical variables were analyzed by the Mann–Whitney U or t-tests and the chi-square test, respectively. The odds ratio (OR) and 95% confidence interval (CI) were used to determine the increased relative risk. p values less than 0.05 were considered statistically significant.

3. Results

A total of 57 children diagnosed with ITP were recorded during the study period. 39 (68%) children had newly diagnosed, 4 (7%) persistent, and 14 (25%) chronic form (Figure 1(a)). Due to the small number of children with persistent form, we decided to incorporate them to the group of children with newly diagnosed ITP. The characteristics of the newly diagnosed/persistent group were compared with the chronic ITP group. The findings are summarized in Table 1.

The age range of the patients varied from 1 from 16 years with a median value of 5.2 years. 42 of 57 children (74%) were aged <10 years. Regarding the children with newly diagnosed/persistent disease, the median age was 4.8 (range 1–12) and 34 of 43 (79%) were aged <10 years. In the chronic disease group, the median age was 11.3 (range 8–16) and 6 of 14 (43%) were below 10 years. The comparison between the two groups revealed a statistically significant result ($p = 0.015$), meaning that children <10 years of age were more likely to have newly diagnosed/persistent form (Figure 1(b)).

Of the 57 children, 27 were girls (47%) and 30 boys (53%). In the newly diagnosed/persistent disease group, 23 (53%) children were boys, while 7 (50%) children were boys in the chronic disease group, a nonstatistically significant difference ($p = 0.72$).

Recent infection history was recorded in 34 (79%) children with newly diagnosed/persistent disease and in 3 (21%) from the chronic ITP group, which was a statistically significant result ($p = 0.013$). This means that children with

TABLE 1: Characteristics between different types of pediatric immune thrombocytopenia.

Parameters	Newly diagnosed/persistent ITP (number 43)	Chronic ITP (number 14)	p
Boys	23	7	0.72
Age, years (median, range)	4.8 (1–12)	11.3 (8–16)	0.015
Recent infection	34	3	0.013
Platelet count at diagnosis, $\times 10^3/\mu L$ (median, range)	14.6 (0–52)	26.3 (0–92)	0.01
Mucosal bleeding	30	7	0.81
Abrupt onset	39	3	0.001
Abnormal immunological markers	5	9	0.003
Treatment with IVIG and/or corticosteroids	40	12	0.78

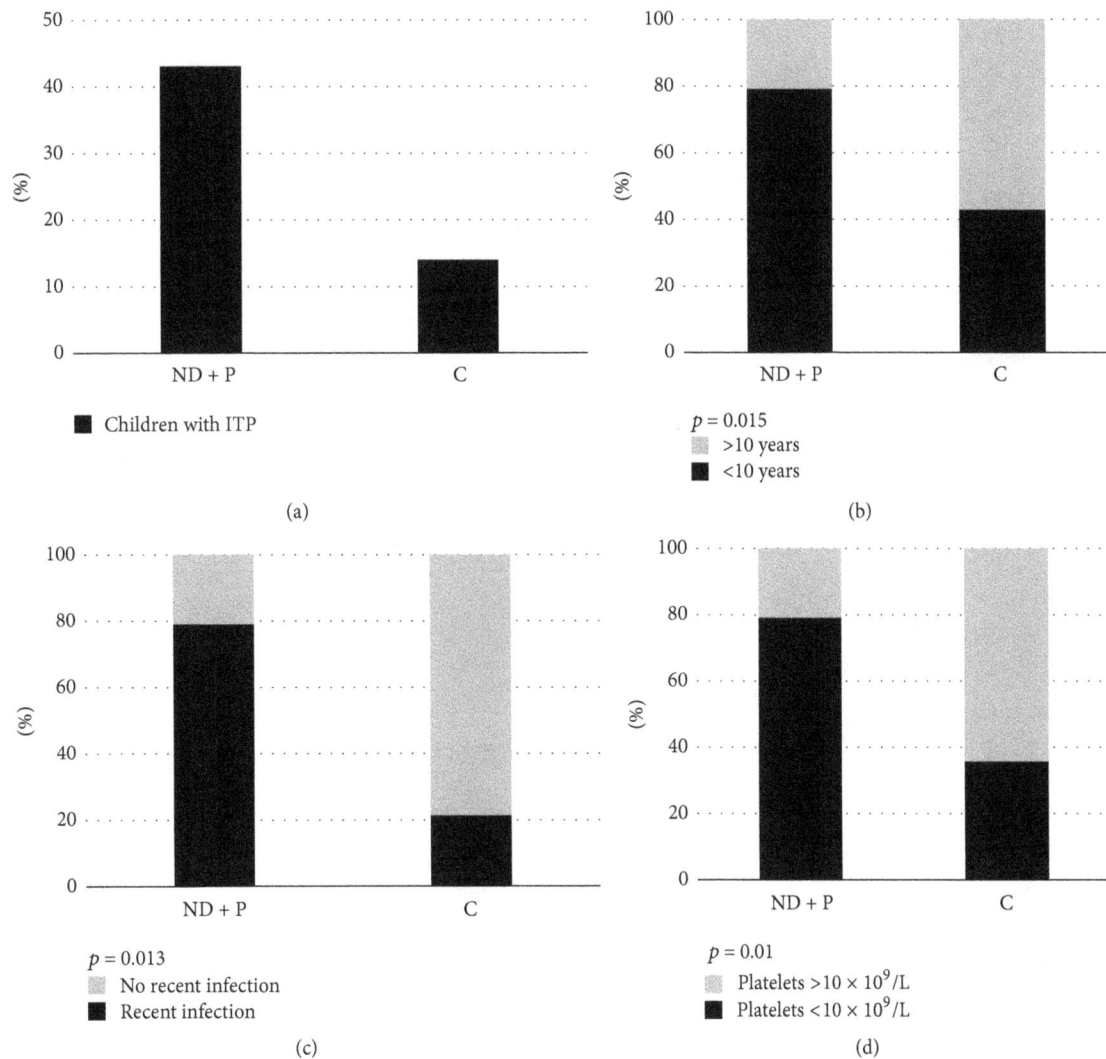

FIGURE 1: (a) Number of children with newly diagnosed/persistent (ND + P) and chronic (C) ITP, (b) percentage of children < 10 years or >10 years of age, (c) percentage of children with a history of recent infection or not, and (d) percentage of children with platelets less or more than $10 \times 10^9/L$, at diagnosis.

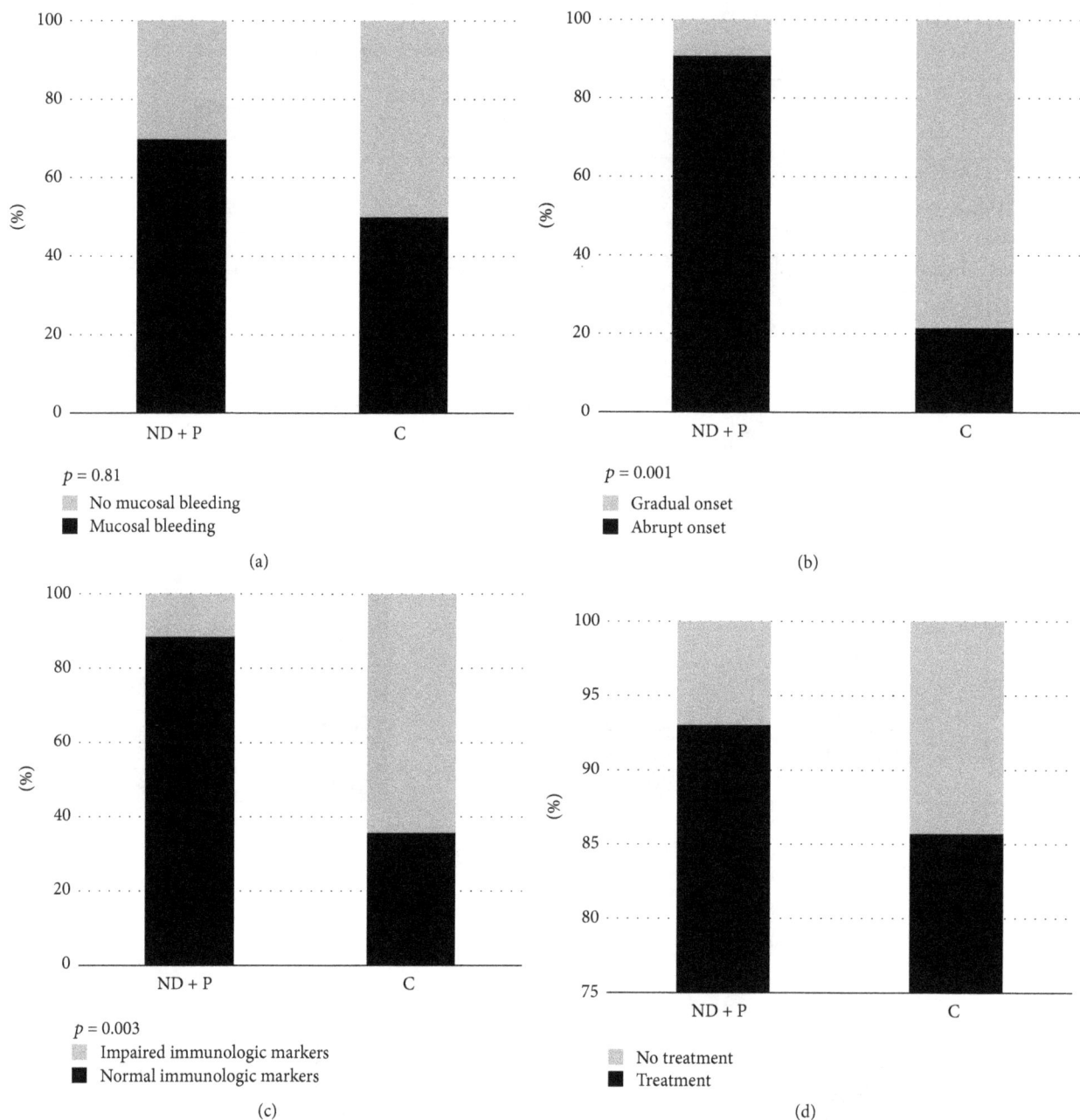

FIGURE 2: (a) Percentage of children with newly diagnosed/persistent (ND + P) and chronic (C) ITP with mucosal bleeding at diagnosis or not, (b) percentage of children with abrupt (<2 weeks) or gradual (>2 weeks) symptomatology before diagnosis, (c) percentage of children with normal or impaired immunological markers, and (d) percentage of children who received or did not receive treatment with intravenous immunoglobulin and/or corticosteroids.

newly diagnosed/persistent disease had more often a history of preceding infection (Figure 1(c)).

The median platelet count at diagnosis was 14.6×10^9/L (range 0–52) in newly diagnosed/persistent type and 26.3×10^9/L (range 0–92) in chronic ITP. Platelets below 10×10^9/L were observed in 34 of 43 children with newly diagnosed/persistent type (79%), while the same percentage was lower in children with chronic ITP (5/14, 36%) ($p = 0.01$) (Figure 1(d)).

Mucosal bleeding was observed in 37 of 57 patients (65%). In the newly diagnosed/persistent group, 30 of 43 children (70%) had mucosal bleeding, while the same number in chronic ITP group was 7/14 (50%), a nonsignificant result ($p = 0.81$) (Figure 2(a)). Only one 5-year-old boy (1 of 57, 1.75%) with newly diagnosed ITP had severe bleeding, namely, subdural hematoma. However, it was not a spontaneous bleeding, but occurred after an accidental fall and head injury. The outcome was excellent.

Concerning the onset of symptoms, the disease occurred abruptly in 39 of 43 (91%) of the cases with newly diagnosed/persistent form. In contrast, 3 of 14 (21%) children with chronic disease had abrupt onset, a statistically significant difference ($p = 0.001$) (Figure 2(b)).

Regarding immunological markers, 5 of 43 children (12%) with newly diagnosed/persistent disease had pathological results. On the contrary, chronic ITP children had more often (9 of 14 children, 65%) impaired immunological markers ($p < 0.003$) (Figure 2(c)). One 11-year-old boy with chronic disease was finally diagnosed as Evans syndrome, with positive direct antiglobulin test and markers of hemolysis, two years after diagnosis.

In total, 52 of 57 children (91%) received treatment with IVIG and/or corticosteroids sometime during the course of the disease. The percentage of children with newly diagnosed/persistent disease that required treatment was greater than those with chronic disease [40/43 (93%) versus 12/14 (86%)], but the difference was not statistically significant ($p = 0.78$) (Figure 2(d)).

Among the potential predicting factors for developing chronic ITP at diagnosis, the most significant predictors were found to be gradual onset (OR = 3.8, CI = 1.6–5.7), negative history of recent infection (OR = 3.1, CI = 1.8–4.9), age of more than 10 years (OR = 2.8, CI = 1.5–4.6), platelet count $> 10 \times 10^9$/L (OR = 2.1, CI = 1.2–4.1), and abnormal immunological markers (OR = 1.7, CI = 1.1–3.2).

4. Discussion

The present study investigated the parameters at diagnosis that distinguish the newly diagnosed/persistent from chronic ITP. According to the results, chronic ITP children are more likely to be of age older than 10 years and have negative history of recent infection, longer duration of symptoms, platelet count above 10×10^9/L, and impaired immunological markers.

The age of the patients at diagnosis has been investigated as a predictor factor in several studies with large number of patients. The investigators of the Intercontinental Childhood ITP Study Group observed that chronic ITP was more frequently found in children above 10 years of age (47.3%) rather than infants (23.1%) [9]. In another large, multicenter study, it was noticed that children at the age of 10 years were at higher risk for developing chronic ITP than at the age of 2 years [10]. In our study, we observed that children with newly diagnosed/persistent ITP were mainly under 10 years and in children with chronic disease the same proportion was significantly lower. Therefore, increased age, especially adolescence, seems to be associated with chronicity. Also, in our study, all forms of the disease showed a similar incidence in both genders, a finding that is in accordance with previous studies [17]. Of notice, the age range of our patients did not include infants.

Preceding infection has been reported as a frequent finding in childhood ITP. In a large single center study, history of recent infection at diagnosis was reported in 56% of newly diagnosed/persistent disease cases. In contrast, 77% of patients with chronic disease had no history of preceding infection [18]. In a population-based, cohort study of the predictors of chronic ITP, it was found that patients with a history of recent infection at diagnosis were less likely to develop chronic ITP than patients without a relevant history (relative risk 0.44) [10]. In our patient analysis, the findings were similar. The most common viral agents that cause infectious diseases in childhood can potentially cause a transient immunological deregulation that leads to the production of antiplatelet antibodies and ITP with acute and self-limiting characteristics. A possible explanation for this causative linkage is the theory of molecular mimicry, which suggests that similarities between pathogen antigens and platelets act as a mechanism for the transient production of antiplatelet antibodies from the patient's lymphocytes [19]. Exceptions are other infectious agents, such as cytomegalovirus, which may have more chronic and persistent influence on the immune system [20].

The duration of the bleeding symptoms before diagnosis has been reported to determine the course of the disease. Large, retrospective studies emphasized that the most important prognostic factor of chronic ITP is the slow onset of bleeding symptoms [18, 21]. In our study, the results were similar and highlight the importance of the duration of symptoms before diagnosis as an important prognostic indicator for disease progression.

Due to the immunological background of ITP, testing and monitoring for secondary autoimmune diseases are mandatory, especially in chronic and refractory cases. Lowe and Buchanan, in a sample of 126 children aged 10–18 years with ITP, found that 27% of the patients had positive ANA at diagnosis. Of these, 31% had chronic disease and 20% had the acute form [22]. Similar findings were observed in an earlier study in 87 patients with ITP. In this study, 25 children had positive ANA and most of them had chronic ITP [23]. These two studies showed that a significant proportion of patients with positive ANA had also other impaired immunological markers (e.g., anti-double stranded DNA, antiphospholipid antibodies, and anticardiolipin antibodies) and autoimmune-related symptoms. In our study, we found that children with newly diagnosed/persistent form had less frequently pathological immunological markers in contrast to the chronic form, a finding consistent with the previous studies. It must be emphasized that the presence of pathological immunological markers poses a high index of suspicion for secondary causes of ITP, including systemic lupus erythematosus, antiphospholipid syndrome, and Evans syndrome, and these children should be monitored on the basis of this risk. In our study population, a child with chronic ITP was finally diagnosed as Evans syndrome two years after diagnosis.

Platelet count at diagnosis is an important laboratory predictor of the course of ITP. In the study of Lowe and Buchanan, the mean platelet count at diagnosis was 21×10^9/L in chronic cases and 5.5×10^9/L in newly diagnosed ITP [22]. Additionally, Glanz et al. reported that a high number of platelets at diagnosis ($>20 \times 10^9$/L) combined with the age above 10 years increased the risk of chronic disease fourfold, compared to younger patients with low platelets. Moreover, at the platelet threshold above 30×10^9/L, the same risk was eleven times greater [10]. In agreement with these data, our study showed that most of patients with chronic disease had platelets above 10×10^9/L at diagnosis.

Mucosal bleeding is an important complication of ITP and when it is serious, treatment is required to increase the platelet number. However, several studies as well as ours suggest that, despite its increased incidence and severity, mucosal bleeding is associated with a short disease duration. Elalfy et al. showed that a history of mucosal bleeding at diagnosis is most often associated with acute disease. Specifically, from 224 children with acute disease, 31% had bleeding from mucous membranes, while in the group of 120 children with chronic disease the same proportion was only 6.5% [18]. Similar results were published in earlier studies [10].

The administration of IVIG or corticosteroids, when needed, is a well-documented treatment option in ITP. Data from the Intercontinental Childhood ITP Study Group showed that children with the acute type of the disease had received more often IVIG than the chronic ITP children (32.3% versus 23.8%) [24]. A recent meta-analysis provided similar findings regarding the use of IVIG and corticosteroids and concluded that they may prevent the chronic progression of the disease [15]. Likewise, in our study the percentage of children with newly diagnosed/persistent disease that received IVIG was slightly higher than in chronic disease. Although the immunomodulatory action of IVIG is not fully elucidated, it has been shown to affect both humoral and cellular immune pathways. In ITP patients, IVIG blocks the activation of Fc-receptors in macrophages of the reticuloendothelial system [25, 26]. Since ITP is considered a heterogeneous disease, IVIG may have various effects in different patients, thus explaining why not all patients respond the same way to the treatment.

In conclusion, this retrospective study determined the prognostic characteristics of ITP in children from a large area of Greece. It is confirmed that primary ITP in children is a nonthreatening and self-limited disease, usually lasting less than one year, and chronic form has different prognostic parameters. The use of these parameters can early distinguish children who are expected to have short and uneventful disease duration, in order to minimize their exposure to pharmaceutical interventions. In different case, physicians should be prepared for different diagnostic evaluation and treatment decision options for chronic disease.

Conflicts of Interest

All the authors declare no conflicts of interest.

Authors' Contributions

Alexandros Makis wrote the manuscript, provided the clinical data, performed the analysis, and cared for the studied patients; Athanasios Gkoutsias and Theodoros Palianopoulos contributed to the preparation of the manuscript; Eleni Pappa contributed to data collection and analysis; Evangelia Papapetrou and Christina Tsaousi performed the hematological analysis and contributed to the follow-up of the patients; Eleftheria Hatzimichael performed the statistical analysis and

the critical review of the manuscript; and Nikolaos Chaliasos contributed to the preparation of the manuscript and to the care of the patients. All authors discussed the results and implications and commented on the manuscript at all stages.

References

[1] U. Abadi, O. Y. Dolberg, and M. H. Ellis, "Immune thrombocytopenia: recent progress in pathophysiology and treatment," *Clinical and Applied Thrombosis/Hemostasis*, vol. 21, no. 5, pp. 397–404, 2015.

[2] P. F. Fogarty and J. B. Segal, "The epidemiology of immune thrombocytopenic purpura," *Current Opinion in Hematology*, vol. 14, no. 5, pp. 515–519, 2007.

[3] D. M. Arnold, "Bleeding complications in immune thrombocytopenia," *International Journal of Hematology*, vol. 2015, no. 1, pp. 237–242, 2015.

[4] F. Rodeghiero, R. Stasi, T. Gernsheimer et al., "Standardization of terminology, definitions and outcome criteria in immune thrombocytopenic purpura of adults and children: report from an international working group," *Blood*, vol. 113, no. 11, pp. 2386–2393, 2009.

[5] D. Provan, R. Stasi, A. C. Newland et al., "International consensus report on the investigation and management of primary immune thrombocytopenia," *Blood*, vol. 115, no. 2, pp. 168–186, 2010.

[6] C. B. Burness, G. M. Keating, and K. P. Garnock-Jones, "Eltrombopag: A Review in Paediatric Chronic Immune Thrombocytopenia," *Drugs*, vol. 76, no. 8, pp. 869–878, 2016.

[7] Y. Liang, L. Zhang, J. Gao, D. Hu, and Y. Ai, "Rituximab for children with immune thrombocytopenia: A systematic review," *PLoS ONE*, vol. 7, no. 5, Article ID e36698, 2012.

[8] P. Imbach, "Refractory Idiopathic Immune Thrombocytopenic Purpura in Children: Current and Future Treatment Options," *Pediatric Drugs*, vol. 5, no. 12, pp. 795–801, 2003.

[9] T. Kühne, G. R. Buchanan, S. Zimmerman et al., "A prospective comparative study of 2540 infants and children with newly diagnosed idiopathic thrombocytopenic purpura (ITP) from the intercontinental childhood ITP study group," *Journal of Pediatrics*, vol. 143, no. 5, pp. 605–608, 2003.

[10] J. Glanz, E. France, S. Xu, T. Hayes, and S. Hambidge, "A population-based, multisite cohort study of the predictors of chronic idiopathic thrombocytopenic purpura in children," *Pediatrics*, vol. 121, no. 3, pp. e506–e512, 2008.

[11] L. G. Robb and K. Tiedeman, "Idiopathic thrombocytopenic purpura: Predictors of chronic disease," *Archives of Disease in Childhood*, vol. 65, no. 5, pp. 502–506, 1990.

[12] S. Revel-Vilk, J. Yacobovich, S. Frank et al., "Age and duration of bleeding symptoms at diagnosis best predict resolution of childhood immune thrombocytopenia at 3, 6, and 12 months," *Journal of Pediatrics*, vol. 163, no. 5, pp. 1335–e2, 2013.

[13] P. W. Edslev, S. Rosthøj, I. Treutiger, J. Rajantie, B. Zeller, and O. G. Jonsson, "A clinical score predicting a brief and uneventful course of newly diagnosed idiopathic trombocytopenic purpura in children," *British Journal of Haematology*, vol. 138, no. 4, pp. 513–516, 2007.

[14] C. M. Bennett, C. Neunert, R. F. Grace et al., "Predictors of remission in children with newly diagnosed immune thrombocytopenia: data from the intercontinental cooperative itp study group registry ii participants," *Pediatric Blood & Cancer*, 2017.

[15] K. M. J. Heitink-Pollé, J. Nijsten, C. W. B. Boonacker, M. De Haas, and M. C. A. Bruin, "Clinical and laboratory predictors of chronic immune thrombocytopenia in children: A systematic review and meta-analysis," *Blood*, vol. 124, no. 22, pp. 3295–3307, 2014.

[16] E. Stiakaki, C. Perdikogianni, C. Thomou et al., "Idiopathic thrombocytopenic purpura in childhood: Twenty years of experience in a single center," *Pediatrics International*, vol. 54, no. 4, pp. 524–527, 2012.

[17] P. Imbach, T. Kühne, D. Müller et al., "Childhood ITP: 12 Months follow-up data from the prospective registry I of the Intercontinental Childhood ITP Study Group (ICIS)," *Pediatric Blood & Cancer*, vol. 46, no. 3, pp. 351–356, 2006.

[18] M. Elalfy, S. Farid, and A. A. Maksoud, "Predictors of chronic idiopathic thrombocytopenic purpura," *Pediatric Blood & Cancer*, vol. 54, no. 7, pp. 959–962, 2010.

[19] M. L. Rand and J. F. Wright, "Virus-associated Idiopathic Thrombocytopenic Purpura," *Transfusion Science*, vol. 19, no. 3, pp. 253–259, 1998.

[20] A. Shimanovsky, D. Patel, and J. Wasser, "Refractory immune thrombocytopenic purpura and cytomegalovirus infection: A call for a change in the current guidelines," *Mediterranean Journal of Hematology and Infectious Diseases*, vol. 8, no. 1, Article ID e2016010, 2016.

[21] B. Zeller, J. Rajantie, I. Hedlund-Treutiger et al., "Childhood idiopathic thrombocytopenic purpura in the Nordic countries: Epidemiology and predictors of chronic disease," *Acta Paediatrica*, vol. 94, no. 2, pp. 178–184, 2005.

[22] E. J. Lowe and G. R. Buchanan, "Idiopathic thrombocytopenic purpura diagnosed during the second decade of life," *Journal of Pediatrics*, vol. 141, no. 2, pp. 253–258, 2002.

[23] S. A. Zimmerman and R. E. Ware, "Clinical significance of the antinuclear antibody test in selected children with idiopathic thrombocytopenic purpura," *Journal of Pediatric Hematology/Oncology*, vol. 19, no. 4, pp. 297–303, 1997.

[24] R. Tamminga, W. Berchtold, M. Bruin, G. R. Buchanan, and T. Kühne, "Possible lower rate of chronic ITP after IVIG for acute childhood ITP an analysis from registry i of the Intercontinental Cooperative ITP Study Group (ICIS)," *British Journal of Haematology*, vol. 146, no. 2, pp. 180–184, 2009.

[25] A. Samuelsson, T. L. Towers, and J. V. Ravetch, "Anti-inflammatory activity of IVIG mediated through the inhibitory Fc receptor," *Science*, vol. 291, no. 5503, pp. 484–486, 2001.

[26] A. R. Crow, S. Song, J. Freedman et al., "IVIG-mediated amelioration of murine ITP via FcγRIIB is independent of SHIP1, SHP-1, and Btk activity," *Blood*, vol. 102, no. 2, pp. 558–560, 2003.

20

Traceability of Blood Transfusions and Reporting of Adverse Reactions in Developing Countries: A Six-Year Postpilot Phase Experience in Burkina Faso

Salam Sawadogo [ID],[1,2] Koumpingnin Nebie,[1,2] Tieba Millogo,[3] Sonia Sontie,[2] Ashmed Nana,[2] Honorine Dahourou,[2] Dieudonné Yentema Yonli,[2] Jean-Baptiste Tapko,[4] Jean-Claude Faber,[5] Eléonore Kafando,[1] and Véronique Deneys[6]

[1] University Ouaga I Professor Joseph KI-ZERBO, 03 BP 7021 Ouagadougou 03, Burkina Faso
[2] National Blood Transfusion Centre, 01 BP 5372 Ouagadougou, Burkina Faso
[3] African Institute of Public Health, 12 BP 199 Ouagadougou, Burkina Faso
[4] African Society for Blood Transfusion, Cameroon
[5] Association Luxembourgeoise des Hémophiles, 33 rue Albert Ier, 1117, Luxembourg
[6] CHU UCL Namur asbl, 15 place L. Godin, 5000 Namur, Belgium

Correspondence should be addressed to Salam Sawadogo; salemserein@hotmail.com

Academic Editor: Paolo Rebulla

Traceability is an essential tool for haemovigilance and transfusion safety. In Burkina Faso, the implementation of haemovigilance has been achieved as part of a pilot project from 2005 to 2009. Our study aims to evaluate the traceability of blood transfusions and reporting of adverse reactions over the 6-year postpilot phase. A cross-sectional study including all blood units ordered between 2010 and 2015 has been conducted in public and private health care facilities supplied with blood products by the transfusion center of Bobo-Dioulasso. The complete traceability was possible for 83.5% of blood units delivered. Adverse reactions were reported in 107 cases representing 2.1/1,000 blood units per annum. Transfusions of wrong blood to wrong patient were reported in 13 cases. Our study shows that the haemovigilance system in Burkina Faso must be improved. Healthcare workers have to be sensitized on how traceability and haemovigilance could impact the quality of care provided to patients.

1. Introduction

Blood transfusion is a life-saving treatment, generally used to replace blood lost in surgery and obstetric or to treat life-threatening anemia and inherited blood disorders. However, it is an event which carries potential risks of acute and/or delayed transfusion reactions and transfusion-transmitted infections for the recipient [1]. Therefore, it is necessary for blood services and clinical services to control the entire process through an effective Quality Management System (QMS) in order to reduce these risks.

Blood transfusion process comprises a series of steps including among others ordering of blood or blood products, administration of blood, monitoring of the transfused patient, managing of adverse reactions, and documentation of transfusion adverse events and outcomes [2].

In transfusion practices, the traceability of blood products means that, at any time, blood transfusion services must know "*who donated or who received which blood or blood product?*" Therefore, their QMS must have documentation systems for information allowing following a blood product or the procedure from the donor to the recipient (vein-to-vein) and vice versa. This implies a close collaboration between blood services and clinical services. The principle was gradually established since the scandal of HIV-infected blood in the late 1980s. The basis for this implementation is the possibility of ascending and descending surveys or look-back studies, which form undoubtedly the basis for improvement and optimization of transfusion safety [3]. Thus, traceability of blood products is an essential tool for haemovigilance and transfusion safety. Its objective is to retrieve from a donation number, the history of the donor and the recipients of the blood products processed from the donated blood [4].

This is possible if a system of information shared between blood transfusion services and health care units is in place and well functioning. In Europe, haemovigilance systems are well-defined, in which the responsibilities of each institution and every stakeholder are well described [5]. The annual report 2015 of the Haemovigilance Authority in France indicates that the average national traceability rate was 99.2% [6]. In Morocco, the traceability rates were around 51% in Casablanca [7] and 15.5% in Rabat [8].

In Burkina Faso, the National Blood Transfusion Center (CNTS) has put in place a QMS according to the ISO 9001 standards. In documents including a blood policy, quality manual and standard operating procedures (SOPs) on blood collection, blood products processing, blood products storage, and distribution, haemovigilance has been put in place. On the other hand, in many hospitals in the country, the QMS is very embryonic. There are almost no SOPs for clinical use of blood. The implementation of the haemovigilance system has been conducted as part of a pilot project from 2005 to 2009. The first data published in 2012 showed that the traceability rate was around 91% [9]. This project, supported by the World Health Organization (WHO), comprised (1°) health staff training and supervision (around 200 employees trained), (2°) design and dissemination of materials for transfusion traceability and adverse reaction reporting, and (3°) implementation of hospital transfusion committees [9].

It is well known that, in sub-Saharan African countries, one of the major challenges during the postproject phase is the sustainability of the achievements. Therefore it was important to raise the question of what happened after the end of the project of haemovigilance was implemented in Bobo-Dioulasso. Our study aimed at evaluating the traceability of blood transfusion and reporting of adverse reactions/events related to blood transfusion in public and private health care facilities supplied with blood product by the Regional Blood Transfusion Center of Bobo-Dioulasso.

2. Material and Methods

2.1. Study Setting and Design. A 6-year (2010-2015) retrospective evaluative study on haemovigilance in clinical transfusion was conducted in some health care facilities dependent on Regional Blood Transfusion Center of Bobo-Dioulasso (CRTS-B), one of the four regional blood centers in Burkina Faso. These facilities are comprised of the teaching hospital SANOU Souro of Bobo-Dioulasso, the 3 district hospitals of Dafra, Do, and Dandé, and a dozen relatively small private health care facilities located in Bobo-Dioulasso which are supplied with blood products by the CRTS-B. Clinicians from these care facilities receive the needed transfusion advice from the CRTS-B and report to this center the adverse events they observe during blood transfusion.

CRTS-B is one of the operational structures of the CNTS located in the western part of the country. The QMS implemented takes the CRTS-B into account. Indeed the entire system (organization and documentation) is harmonized at the national level for all the blood services affiliated to CNTS.

Blood is collected from voluntary and nonremunerated donors at fixed site and mobile collection. It is systematically screened for the following transfusion transmissible infections (TTIs): HIV, hepatitis B and C, and syphilis. The blood transfusion system policy is to process whole blood into blood products. Whole blood is stored in controlled cold rooms and processed, within 96 hours, into packed red blood cells (RBCs) mainly, over 90-95%, with regard to epidemiological profile and clinicians' needs. Being given the demand of therapeutic plasma and platelets is very low, as previously stated [9], a few number of whole blood units (5-10%), mainly from fixed collect sites, is processed into frozen fresh plasma (FFP) and platelet concentrates (PCs), within 6 hours after collection. Nontherapeutic plasma produced from RBCs processing is discarded.

Blood products are ordered by physicians on a standardized blood ordering form and delivered free of charge to patient. Delivered blood units are packed in cool-boxes and transported within 30 minutes to the clinical wards by employees of these services. The most distant service is located 20 minutes from blood delivery point. Each product delivered is accompanied with a posttransfusion and haemovigilance form (FPTH) on which the clinician has to record summarized information on administration of the blood unit and occurrence of adverse reactions. This form must be sent back without delay (as soon as possible) after blood transfusion, to the CRTS-B as transfusion confirmation and adverse reaction report, if applicable. The adverse reactions/events reporting system in place is a nonmandatory one.

2.2. Patients and Methods. Patients of both sexes and all ages admitted in private and public (teaching and district) hospitals, for whom blood was ordered between 2010 and 2015, were included in the study. Both medical and transfusion process information of each patient were recorded on medical software (CTS server). We extracted from this software the following information: age and gender of the recipient, hospital and ward of admission, date of blood delivery, type and number of blood products requested and delivered, confirmation that blood product was transfused, adverse events, and reactions reported where applicable.

2.3. Statistical Analysis. Excel (Microsoft Office 2007) and STATA 13 software were used for data management and data analysis. We used proportion and mean ± 2 SD to describe, respectively, qualitative and continuous variables. We used median and interquartiles 25 and 75% to describe the age of patients. The number of adverse reactions is divided by the number of traceable blood units and multiplied by

1,000 to have the incidence of adverse reaction per 1,000 blood units. The Chi-square ($\chi2$) test was used to test the differences in frequencies between groups. Groups were assumed to differ significantly when the p-values were less than 0.05.

2.4. Ethical Considerations. The study was conducted with the approval of the directorate in charge of scientific and medical activities of the National Blood Transfusion Center (CNTS). Data were collected anonymously. Patient and donor confidentiality were preserved.

3. Results

From 2010 to 2015, 61,678 blood units including 59,934 RBC units were delivered to 42,269 patients (i.e., 1.5 blood units per patient and 10,280 units per annum). The median age of the patients was 13 years (IQR [2 - 30]). The majority of patients (59.5%) were female (the sex ratio M/F was 0.68). The female patients received 62.9% of blood units delivered (Chi2=78.5; p < 0.001). Table 1 describes the distribution of patients, blood units ordered, blood units delivered and satisfaction rate per year, and type of hospital, of clinical ward, and of blood products.

Out of the 61,678 blood units delivered, the complete traceability of blood unit ("who received the blood, when, where, and from whom?") was possible in 51,533 cases (83.5% of blood units delivered). A total of 50,033 FPTH were received (i.e., 97.1%) concerning the RBC units delivered. In private health facilities, feedback was sent for only about 29% of blood units delivered. This situation concerned 16% of the products delivered in public hospitals. Figure 1 summarizes the number of blood units plotted compared to untraceable blood units according to (a) year of delivery, (b) type of hospitals, (c) clinical ward, and (d) type of blood products.

A total of 107 adverse reactions were reported over the six years. This represented 2.1 reactions per 1,000 blood units per annum, taking into account the fact that the feedback rate (proportion of FPTH returned) was 83.6%. Figure 2 shows the incidence of adverse reactions from 2010 to 2015. The reactions were nonspecific in 40 cases (i.e., 37%). They include symptoms such as sweating, dizziness, nausea, vomiting, and headache occurring during the transfusion. Figure 3 gives the frequency and type of the adverse reactions reported. Incorrect blood component transfusions (IBCT) were reported in 13 cases (i.e., 0.3 cases per 1,000 units). In 2 cases, the blood unit was transfused to a patient different from whom it has been issued for. The other cases were due to errors in blood sample labelling (9 cases) and blood group typing (2 cases).

Besides these adverse reactions, death of the patient occurred during the blood transfusion in 65 cases (1.3 per 1,000 units). But since no investigation was conducted on these deaths, it was not possible to incriminate or not blood products. In addition, 53 units of RBCs (1.06/1,000) delivered to clinical services were returned to the blood transfusion service due to blood clots present in the unit.

4. Discussion

Haemovigilance is an important tool for improving blood transfusion safety. Indeed, the WHO global strategy for safe blood transfusion defined haemovigilance as one of its important pillars [10, 11]. It is recommended to each country to build an effective haemovigilance system. The objective of such a system is to report and analyze the adverse events and reactions related to blood use in order to implement measures to correct and prevent them.

This study is one of the few studies in sub-Saharan Africa, although the need of science-based evidence to improve transfusion safety in Africa is crucial. This is the second of its kind that was carried out in our country. It revealed that the system implemented at the Regional Blood Transfusion Center of Bobo-Dioulasso allowed the traceability of 83.5% of blood units delivered and reported 2.1 adverse reactions per 1,000 units per annum.

The implementation of the haemovigilance system at the CRTS of Bobo-Dioulasso and later throughout the country has been a long and inclusive process that had combined information, training and regulation as described by Dahourou et al. in a previous study [9]. The system is theoretically well-structured with a national committee, regional committees linked to regional health directions, and hospital transfusion committees [12]. It is a variant of the French model that was implemented in Burkina Faso. Nevertheless, the blood units' traceability rate in our study was 8% lower than in the pilot phase (83% versus 91%). These findings show that the habits and good practices acquired by healthcare workers during this pilot phase tend to be lost less than a year after, even if the results remain better than those in other African countries. This suggests the need of more regulation, continuous awareness-raising action and training, effective supervision, and control of stakeholders and health facilities through regular audits and effective communication system. As described by Dahourou et al., the pilot phase of the implementation of the haemovigilance system was marked by proactive attitude of the Regional Blood Transfusion Center which organized regular training and awareness sessions for clinicians and feedback on haemovigilance indicators for each hospital [9]. It is necessary to motivate the healthcare workers, for whom transfusing blood is far from being the only concern. Indeed, traceability of blood transfusions is sometimes perceived as an administrative constraint, more than a tool to improve transfusion safety [8]. Thus, the national and regional vigilance committees and the hospital transfusion committees are invited to fully assume their role. The nonmandatory and passive reporting system could also be questioned. Despite the existence of national guidelines for good practice in blood transfusion [13], there is no legal way to oblige clinical teams to comply with all the rules. As a result, CNTS, on its own initiative, has put in place measures to require from clinicians, feedback of the first units issued for the patients in their ward before receiving additional ones, while ensuring no occurrence of any delay in blood issuing procedure that might be harmful to critical patients. These "coercive measures" are coupled with an active approach such as information, training and

TABLE 1: Distribution of patients, blood units ordered, blood units delivered and satisfaction rate per to year, type of hospital, clinical ward, and type of blood products at the Regional Blood Transfusion Center of Bobo-Dioulasso from 2010 to 2015.

	Patients (%)	Blood units ordered (%)	Blood units delivered (%)	% satisfaction of blood demand
Overall	42,269 (100)	68,381 (100)	61,678 (100)	90.2%
Years				
2010	6,430 (15.2)	12,384 (18.1)	11,271 (18.3)	91.0%
2011	6,317 (14.9)	11,297 (16.5)	10,395 (16.8)	92.0%
2012	6,984 (16.5)	11,079 (16.2)	10,156 (16.5)	91.7%
2013	5,950 (14.1)	9,252 (13.5)	8,160 (13.2)	88.2%
2014	8,508 (20.1)	12,545 (18.3)	11,569 (18.7)	92.2%
2015	8,080 (19.1)	11,824 (17.3)	10,127 (16.4)	85.6%
Hospitals				
Teaching hospital	33,678 (79.7)	52,548 (76.8)	49,520 (80.3)	94.2%
District hospitals	8,017 (19.0)	14,687 (21.5)	11,286 (18.3)	76.8%
Private health facilities	533 (1.3)	1,091 (1.6)	825 (1.3)	75.6%
Not recorded	41 (0.1)	55 (0.1)	47 (0.1)	85.5%
Clinical department				
Gynaecology-obstetric	11,472 (27.1)	23,157 (33.9)	20,741 (33.6)	89.6%
Surgical	4,983 (11.8)	11,285 (16.5)	8,739 (14.2)	77.4%
Paediatric	16,552 (39.2)	19,042 (27.8)	18,435 (29.9)	96.8%
Medical	9,221 (21.8)	14,842 (21.7)	13,716 (22.2)	92.4%
Not recorded	41 (0.1)	55 (0.1)	47 (0.1)	85.5%
Blood products				
Red blood cells	41,651 (98.5)	66,109 (96.7)	59,934 (97.2)	90.7%
Frozen fresh plasma	578 (1.4)	1,715 (2.5)	1,618 (2.6)	94.3%
Platelet concentrates	40 (0.1)	557 (0.8)	126 (0.2)	22.6%

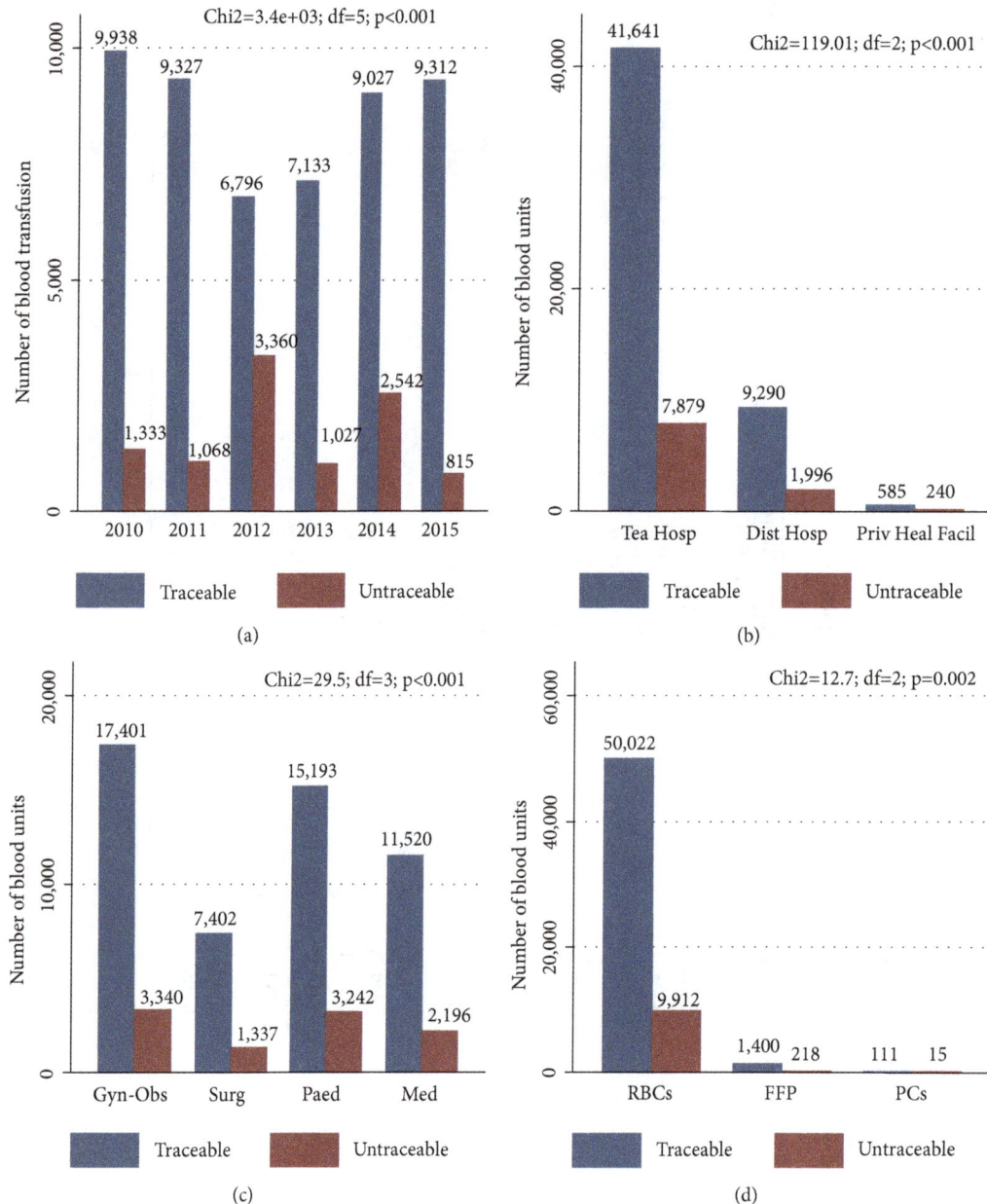

FIGURE 1: Number of blood units plotted compared to number of untraceable blood units per (a) year of delivery, (b) type of hospital, (c) clinical ward, and (d) type of blood products at the Regional Blood Transfusion Center of Bobo-Dioulasso from 2010 to 2015. Tea Hosp = Teaching Hospital; Dist Hospt = District Hospital; Priv Heal Facil = Private Health Facilities; Gyn-Obs = Gynaecology-Obstetrics; Surg = Surgery; Paed = Paediatrics; Med = Medicine; RBCs = Red blood cells; FFP = Frozen fresh plasma; PCs = Platelet concentrates.

supervision of hospital staff involved in transfusion activities [14]. This allowed substantial progress in haemovigilance in our country [15]. But most of the time, FPTH are returned only when another blood unit is requested, often several days or weeks after the last transfusion. In such cases, it was often impossible to investigate and to determine the relation with blood transfusion. So, this shows clearly that the measures implemented by the CNTS cannot replace a strong oversight by a regulatory authority (independently of blood services and care units). The regulatory authority, planned in the national blood policy, has yet to be put in place [12, 16]. For

few years by now, the CNTS is advocating the Ministry of Health to implement this independent regulatory authority.

Traceability rates in our study were higher as compared to those found in Morocco (15.5% in Rabat in 2010 and 51% in Casablanca in 2003) [7, 8]. But it was lower than in developed countries like France [6]. Haemovigilance systems in developed countries have been established since a long time (often 1994-1996), as a reaction to the human immunodeficiency virus scandal in the late 1980s/early 1990s [17]. In Africa, implementation of the first haemovigilance systems started later [9, 18].

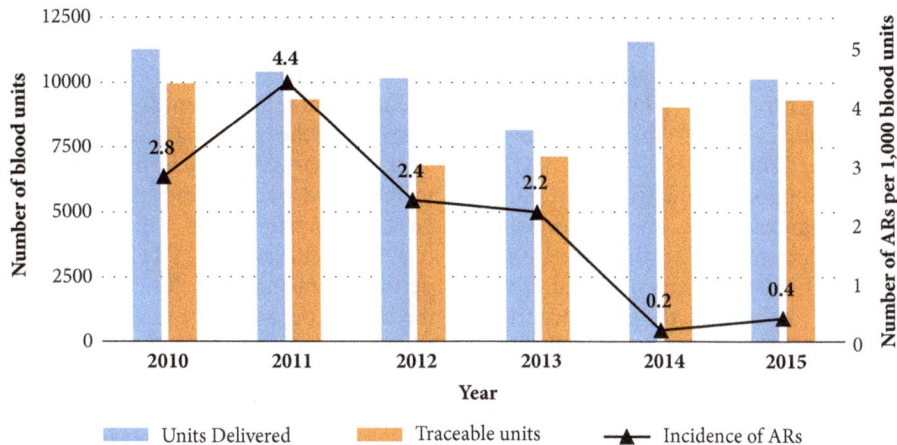

ARs = Adverse reactions

FIGURE 2: Incidence of adverse reactions reported to the Regional Blood Transfusion Center of Bobo-Dioulasso from 2010 to 2015, Burkina Faso.

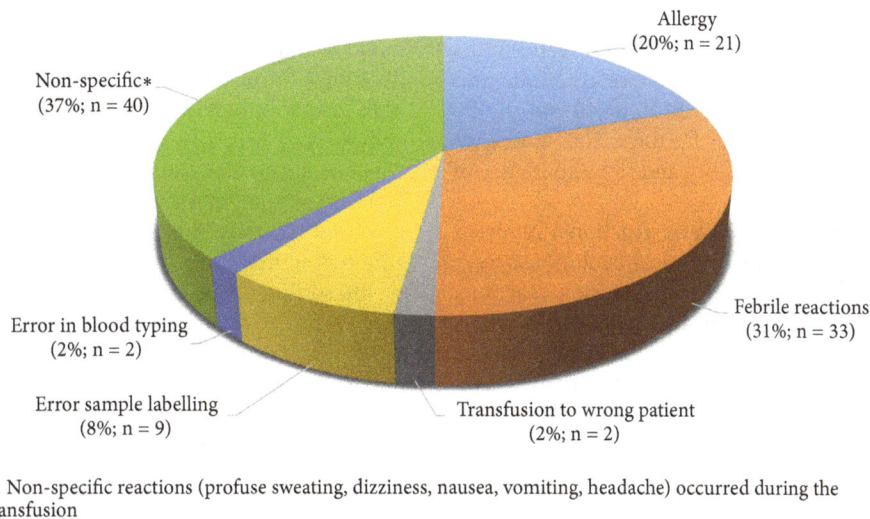

*: Non-specific reactions (profuse sweating, dizziness, nausea, vomiting, headache) occurred during the transfusion

FIGURE 3: Types of adverse reactions reported to the Regional Blood Transfusion Center of Bobo-Dioulasso from 2010 to 2015, Burkina Faso.

Adverse reactions ratio was 7 times lower in our study than in the pilot phase (2.1 versus 16.1 cases per 1,000 units). In Morocco and Tunisia, the ratio varied from 0.5 to 1.6/1,000 [7, 19] and from 0.59 to 2.19/1,000 blood units [20], respectively. In Namibian, Zimbabwean, and South African systems, these ratios were, respectively, 0.8, 0.46, and 0.82 per 1,000 blood units [18, 21, 22]. In a randomised controlled trial and prospective observational studies, JP Allain et al. [23] and AK Owusu-Ofori et al. [24] reported an adverse reactions ratio 5 to 10 times higher than our findings. The main differences with findings in these different countries could be explained by the system of adverse reactions' monitoring. In Ghana the adverse events have been noted during observational studies, while in other countries they were routine notifications; the context of the study probably affected the reporting of adverse events in Ghana.

In our study, the reported adverse reactions showed clinical symptoms that occurred during the blood transfusion or immediately after. Indeed, operational procedures and guidelines for clinical blood transfusion recommend monitoring of patients during and after blood administration, through the measurement of vital signs such as temperature, pulse, and blood pressure. But this is not well-codified and well-respected because of the insufficiency in staff number and more likely the lack of knowledge in importance of this monitoring on the quality of care and safety for patient. Adverse reactions documented on FPTH included mainly febrile reactions, chills, pruritus, profuse sweating, dizziness, etc. But many cases were reported to blood services several days or weeks posttransfusion, making any further rigorous investigation impossible. So, the severity of most of these reactions and the imputability on the transfused blood products could not be assessed. Only a few cases resulted in investigations leading to the detection of incorrect blood products transfused (wrong blood transfusions) due to patient misidentification, sample labelling and blood group typing errors. The incidence of IBCT was 0.3 cases per 1,000 units. These data are 1.5 times lower than previously observed in our country [9] and 10 to 100 times higher than those reported in Morocco (0.0025 to 0.02 per 1,000 units) and South Africa (0.03/1,000 units) [7, 19, 22]. The incidence was approximately the same as in Tunisia (0.24/1,000 units) [20].

The incorrect blood component transfusions (IBCT) represent a universally recognized cause of posttransfusion morbidity and mortality. Data in the literature show that, in around half of the cases, multiple errors occurred in the process and in more than 2/3 of the cases, the errors occurred in clinical wards. The most frequent errors are failure to perform correctly the pretransfusion controls (e.g., patient bedside test to ensure that the right blood is given to the right patient) [25, 26]. Indeed, the verification of identity concordance between the patient, the transfusion documents, and the blood product intended for transfusion at the patient's bedside are tainted by bad practice and misinterpretation [27]. In 11 cases out of 13 (i.e., 85%) in our study, errors in sample labelling and documentary verification were incriminated.

In France [6], with around 3.2 million blood units delivered in 2015, the incidence of adverse reactions was 2.4/1,000 units and the incidence of IBCT was 0.004 / 1,000 units, i.e., 100 times lower than our findings. This difference could be explained by the long culture and rich experience of haemovigilance in France.

Febrile reactions (33% of all adverse reactions) reported in this study, with regard to their clinical evolutions, were concordant with febrile nonhemolytic transfusion reactions (FNHTR). The FNHTR is a common adverse reaction occurring during blood transfusion. It could be related to the presence of cytokines in blood products, but in many cases, the mechanism remains uncertain [1, 28]. The other adverse reactions (37% of all cases) that were found in our study were nonspecific and included anxiety, vomiting, nausea, headache, and profuse sweating. These were benign symptoms presented by patients during the blood transfusion. In 65 cases (i.e., 1.3/1,000 blood units), only the mention "death during transfusion" was reported on FPTH. But there was no evidence for imputability on the transfusion of the patients' death, since no investigation was conducted. This kind of adverse reaction seems to be rather frequent and we need to put in more effort to investigate them. According to the literature, the transfusion-related acute lung injury (TRALI) and the acute haemolytic transfusion reactions are the main causes of transfusion-related deaths [27]. In our context, many patients arrive to health facilities very late and in very poor condition. This could explain our findings.

The blood clots detected in each one thousandth blood unit issued (1.06/1,000 units) could certainly be considered as grade 0 adverse events, but they constitute a serious concern. It reflects either deterioration in the quality of anticoagulant contained in collection bag or abnormalities during the collection (poor mixing of the blood with the anticoagulant). Anyway, the lack of or the poor implementation of visual inspection procedures of blood units during the processing process and mainly the delivery process is obvious.

Our study reported only data about acute adverse reactions. The FPTH, the notification materials in our system, were designed specifically for this purpose. Indeed, the primary goals of this form are the traceability of blood transfusions and the reporting of acute reactions. This means that, after the transfusion, the form must be returned immediately to the blood transfusion services. The primary aim was to create a reporting habit with the clinicians. If any adverse reaction occurs and the FPTH is returned within a reasonable period of time, the transfusion service in collaboration with the clinical department can investigate, grade the severity of reactions, and assess the imputability of blood products. In this case, a second form named "transfusion incident form (FIT)" is used. But, it is obvious that this process in not complete for all reported incidents. Only a few cases have been investigated.

Our findings show that the Regional Blood Transfusion Center of Bobo-Dioulasso does not cover the needs in blood products of the health facilities. The average satisfaction rate of blood demands was 90.2% between 2010 and 2015. This is due to insufficient blood collection, despite the many efforts made to improve the availability of blood over the last two decades (7 units donated per 1,000 inhabitants) [29]. The high rate of unmet blood demands for patients in obstetric and surgical wards (respectively, 10.5% and 22.6%) is a big concern, given that sometimes, they are in hemorrhaging and severely anemia situations that can compromise their survival. In 2012, the unmet blood requests for patients admitted in maternity were 15.6% in Ouagadougou [30].

In addition, the satisfaction rate for PCs requests was very low (22.6% compared to 90.7% and 94.3%, respectively, for RBCs and FFP). This indicates that the organization put in place for processing PCs seems to be ineffective. The platelet-rich plasma's method is used to process platelet concentrates. In a previous paper [31], we mentioned the poor setting of blood transfusion services in Burkina Faso (limited financial and material resources, shortage of trained staff, etc.), obliging them to use alternative techniques and strategies in order to make available, with a certain level of quality, the most requested blood products in hospitals. In our context, the main indications for blood transfusion are obstetrical hemorrhage and anemia caused by malaria, malnutrition, and other genetic diseases (sickle cells disease, thalassemia, etc.). This could explain the high proportion of RBCs units ordered.

Limitations to our study were that we did not report data on delayed adverse reactions and near-miss events, being given they are known to be the occult part of the errors occurring in blood transfusion. Besides that, the high number of undefined adverse reactions and patients dead during transfusion hides many abnormalities and nonconformities for which our system must put in more efforts to investigate and identify in order to improve transfusion safety.

5. Conclusion

The analysis of our haemovigilance system shows that our results, while being better than those in some other African countries, remain insufficient and decline from one year to the next, since the end of the pilot phase. This finding calls for the implementation of a quality system and management integrating haemovigilance in hospitals and indicates the need to strengthen the system in transfusion services.

Feedback and adverse reactions reporting in our system still use paper documents. Without any effective active approach, filling these papers is perceived as additional work by health staff. Implementing an electronic system could improve traceability and reporting rates, secure collection of data, and facilitate their exploitation. Anyway, corrective actions through training and regular awareness-raising of healthcare workers on how a strong traceability and haemovigilance system integrated to a quality assurance programme can improve the safety and effectiveness of care provided to patients have to be implemented.

Disclosure

The data was collected and analyzed as part of the work of the authors employed by the National Blood Transfusion Center. Data presented in this manuscript have been presented during the 18th International Haemovigilance Seminar held in Manchester on July 2018.

Conflicts of Interest

The authors declare that they have no conflicts of interest.

Acknowledgments

The authors thank all the staff of the Regional Blood Transfusion Center of Bobo-Dioulasso.

References

[1] D. R. Somagari, C. S. Sriram, C. K. Rachamalla et al., "Haemovigilance study at a tertiary care hospital in the northeast of India," *ISBT Science Series*, vol. 10, no. 2, pp. 61–64, 2015.

[2] B. Natukunda, H. Schonewille, and C. T. Smit Sibinga, "Assessment of the clinical transfusion practice at a regional referral hospital in Uganda," *Transfusion Medicine*, vol. 20, no. 3, pp. 134–139, 2010.

[3] E. Pélissier and L. Nguyen, "Traçabilité des produits sanguins labiles: définition, réglementation, bilan et perspectives," *Transfusion Clinique et Biologique*, vol. 7, suppl 1, pp. 72–74, 2000.

[4] Ministère de la santé et de l'action humanitaire, "Loi no 93-5 du 4 janvier 1993 relative à la sécurité en matière de transfusion sanguine et de médicament," *Journal officiel français*, pp. 237–245, 1993.

[5] P. Ingrand, L. Salmi, E. Benz-Lemoine, and M. Dupuis, "Évaluation de la traçabilité effective des produits sanguins labiles à partir des dossiers médicaux," *Transfusion Clinique et Biologique*, vol. 5, no. 6, pp. 397–407, 1998.

[6] Agence Nationale de Sécurité des Médicaments et des produits de santé. Rapport d'activité hémovigilance 2015. ANSM, 2016.

[7] I. Tazi, L. Loukhmas, and N. Benchemsi, "Hémovigilance : bilan 1995–2003 Casablanca," *Transfusion Clinique et Biologique*, vol. 12, no. 3, pp. 257–274, 2005.

[8] S. Ouadghiri, O. Atouf, C. Brick, N. Benseffaj, and M. Essakalli, "Traçabilité des produits sanguins labiles au Maroc : expérience de l'hôpital Ibn-Sina de Rabat entre 1999 et 2010," *Transfusion Clinique et Biologique*, vol. 19, no. 1, pp. 1–4, 2012.

[9] H. Dahourou, J. Tapko, Y. Nébié et al., "Mise en place de l'hémovigilance en Afrique subsaharienne," *Transfusion Clinique et Biologique*, vol. 19, no. 1, pp. 39–45, 2012.

[10] N. Dhingra, Making safe blood available in Africa. 2006. http://wwwlive.who.int/entity/bloodsafety/makingsafebloodavailableinafricastatement.pdf, Accessed 5 March, 2017.

[11] N. Dhingra, V. Hafner, and S. Xueref, "Hemovigilance in Countries with Scarce Resources –A WHO Perspective," *Transfusion Alternatives in Transfusion Medicine*, vol. 5, no. 1, pp. 277–284, 2003.

[12] Ministère de la santé, Burkina Faso. Décret no 2012-1033/PRES/PM/MS/ du 28 décembre 2012 portant création, attribution et organisation d'un système national de vigilance des produits de santé à usage humain.

[13] Ministère de la santé, Burkina Faso. Arrêté No2014-589/MS du 9 juin 2014, portant directives nationales de Bonnes pratiques transfusionnelles au Burkina Faso.

[14] K. Nébié, S. Ouattara, M. Sanou et al., "Poor procedures and quality control among nonaffiliated blood centers in Burkina Faso: An argument for expanding the reach of the national blood transfusion center," *Transfusion*, vol. 51, no. 7pt2, pp. 1613–1618, 2011.

[15] S. Sawadogo, E. Kafando, Y. K. Nebie et al., "Where are we with haemovigilance in Burkina Faso?" in *Proceedings of the 17th International Haemovigilance Seminar*, Blood Transfus 2016; 14 (Suppl 1): P-1-17.

[16] Décret No2015-826/PRES-TRANS/PM du 13 juillet 2015 portant adoption du document de Stratégie Nationale de transfusion sanguine. JO Burkinabè No41 du 08 OCTOBRE 2015.

[17] R. R. de Vries, "Haemovigilance: recent achievements and developments in the near future," *ISBT Science Series*, vol. 4, no. 1, pp. 60–62, 2009.

[18] B. P. L. Meza, B. Lohrke, R. Wilkinson et al., "Estimation of the prevalence and rate of acute transfusion reactions occurring in Windhoek, Namibia," *Blood Transfusion*, vol. 12, no. 3, pp. 352–361, 2014.

[19] S. Ouadghiri, C. Brick, N. Benseffaj, O. Atouf, and M. Essakalli, "Effets indésirables receveurs à l'hôpital Ibn Sina de Rabat : bilan 1999–2013," *Transfusion Clinique et Biologique*, vol. 24, no. 1, pp. 23–27, 2017.

[20] S. Mahjoub, H. Baccouche, A. Raissi, L. Ben Hamed, and N. Ben Romdhane, "Hémovigilance à Tunis (hôpital La Rabta) : bilan 2007–2013," *Transfusion Clinique et Biologique*, vol. 24, no. 1, pp. 15–22, 2017.

[21] N. Mafirakureva, S. Khoza, D. A. Mvere, M. E. Chitiyo, M. J. Postma, and M. Van Hulst, "Incidence and pattern of 12 years of reported transfusion adverse events in Zimbabwe: A retrospective analysis," *Blood Transfusion*, vol. 12, no. 3, pp. 362–367, 2014.

[22] South Africa National Blood Service. Haemovigilance Report 2012: South Africa National Blood Service; 2012.

[23] J.-P. Allain, A. K. Owusu-Ofori, S. M. Assennato, S. Marschner, R. P. Goodrich, and S. Owusu-Ofori, "Effect of Plasmodium inactivation in whole blood on the incidence of blood

transfusion-transmitted malaria in endemic regions: the African Investigation of the Mirasol System (AIMS) randomised controlled trial," *The Lancet*, vol. 387, no. 10029, pp. 1753–1761, 2016.

[24] A. K. Owusu-Ofori, S. P. Owusu-Ofori, and I. Bates, "Detection of adverse events of transfusion in a teaching hospital in Ghana," *Transfusion Medicine*, vol. 27, no. 3, pp. 175–180, 2017.

[25] P. Rouger, P. Le Pennec, and F. Noizat-Pirenne, "Analyse des risques immunologiques en transfusion sanguine: Période 1991–1998," *Transfusion Clinique et Biologique*, vol. 7, no. 1, pp. 9–14, 2000.

[26] D. Stainsby, "ABO incompatible transfusions—experience from the UK Serious Hazards of Transfusion (SHOT) scheme," *Transfusion Clinique et Biologique*, vol. 12, no. 5, pp. 385–388, 2005.

[27] E. C. Vamvakas and M. A. Blajchman, "Transfusion-related mortality: the ongoing risks of allogeneic blood transfusion and the available strategies for their prevention," *Blood*, vol. 113, no. 15, pp. 3406–3417, 2009.

[28] P.-P. Dujardin, L. R. Salmi, and P. Ingrand, "Errors in interpreting the pretransfusion bedside compatibility test. An experimental study," *Vox Sanguinis*, vol. 78, no. 1, pp. 37–43, 2000.

[29] H. Dahourou, J.-B. Tapko, K. Kienou, K. Nebie, and M. Sanou, "Recruitment of blood donors in Burkina Faso: how to avoid donations from family members?" *Biologicals*, vol. 38, no. 1, pp. 39–42, 2010.

[30] C. M. R. Ouédraogo, A. Ouédraogo, R. A. F. Kaboré et al., "Analysis of blood transfusion requirements during the gravido-puerperal period in a hospital in Ouagadougou," *Field Actions Science Report*, vol. 7, 2012.

[31] S. Sawadogo, K. Nebie, E. Kafando et al., "Preparation of red cell concentrates in low-income countries: Efficacy of whole blood settling method by simple gravity in Burkina Faso," *International Journal of Blood Transfusion and Immunohematology*, vol. 6, p. 10, 2016.

21

Chimerism in Myeloid Malignancies following Stem Cell Transplantation Using FluBu4 with and without Busulfan Pharmacokinetics versus BuCy

Shatha Farhan,[1] **Michael Bazydlo,**[2] **Klodiana Neme,**[3] **Nancy Mikulandric,**[3] **Edward Peres,**[1] **and Nalini Janakiraman**[1]

[1]*Stem Cell Transplant Program, Henry Ford Hospital, 2799 W. Grand Blvd, Detroit, MI 48202, USA*
[2]*Division of Biostatistics, Henry Ford Hospital, 2799 W. Grand Blvd, Detroit, MI 48202, USA*
[3]*Division of Pharmacy, Henry Ford Hospital, 2799 W. Grand Blvd, Detroit, MI 48202, USA*

Correspondence should be addressed to Shatha Farhan; sfarhan1@hfhs.org

Academic Editor: Suparno Chakrabarti

In the era of precision medicine, the impact of personalized dosing of busulfan is not clear. We undertook a retrospective analysis of 78 patients with myeloid malignancies who received fludarabine and busulfan (FluBu4) with or without measuring Bu pharmacokinetics (Bu PK) and those who received busulfan with cyclophosphamide (BuCy). Fifty-five patients received FluBu4, of whom 21 had Bu PK measured, and 23 patients received BuCy. Total donor cell chimerism showed that the percentage of patients maintaining 100% donor chimerism on day 100 was 66.7%, 38.2%, and 73.9% in the FluBu4 with PK, FluBu4 with no PK, and BuCy, respectively ($P = .001$). Patients who had decreasing donor chimerism by day 100 were 23.8%, 52.9%, and 26.1% in the FluBu4 with PK, FluBu4 with no PK, and BuCy, respectively ($P = .04$). Bu PK group had fewer patients with less than 95% donor chimerism on day 30, which was not statistically significant, 5% (FluBu4 PK), 31% (FluBu4 with no PK), and 21% (BuCy) ($P = .18$). Survival distributions were not statistically significant ($P = .11$). Thus, personalized drug dosing can impact donor chimerism in myeloid malignancies. This will need to be examined in larger retrospective multicenter studies and prospective clinical trials.

1. Introduction

Allogeneic stem cell transplant (SCT) which depends on chemotherapy and immunotherapy (graft versus leukemia effect) is the only potential curative treatment for most patients with acute myeloid leukemia (AML), myelodysplastic syndrome (MDS), and other myeloid malignancies. However, despite the advances in allogeneic SCT, disease relapse is still a major cause of death [1–4].

Chimerism analysis is an important tool to assess the origin of hematopoietic cells after SCT. Discrimination between donor and recipient cells allows evaluation for engraftment as well as detection of imminent graft rejection but its use as prognostic indicator for relapse is controversial [5]. Many methods have been used over the years to assess chimerism including cytogenetics, fluorescein in situ hybridization,

and variable number of tandem repeats. However a major limitation of most of these techniques is that they are time consuming and without quantification. Most recently, the use of short tandem repeats with the use of fluorescent labeling of the primers and PCR resolution products allowed accurate quantification of the degree of mixed chimerism [6].

Reduced toxicity ablative conditioning regimens are increasingly used in SCT. Busulfan (Bu) has been used for many years as a component of conditioning before SCT and now is being used more and more especially with the intravenous formulation which leads to more predictable delivery and probably improved clinical outcomes compared with oral Bu [7–9]. However, even with intravenous administration, the exposure may vary 3- to 4-fold. Recently, personalized dosing of Bu using the patient-specific Bu clearance has been used by some transplant centers. Target exposure is reflected in the measurement area under the plasma concentration-time curve (AUC) or concentration at steady state [10]. However, its impact on early and late transplant outcomes is not clear.

To explore the impact of measuring busulfan pharmacokinetics (Bu PK) in conditioning regimens on early donor chimerism in myeloid malignancies, we undertook a retrospective analysis of patients with myeloid disorders who received 4 days of fludarabine and busulfan (FluBu4) with or without measuring Bu PK and busulfan and cyclophosphamide (BuCy) at our center in the last 10 years.

2. Materials and Methods

2.1. Patients. Patients who underwent their first allogeneic SCT for AML, MDS, or myeloproliferative neoplasms involving myeloablative conditioning with FluBu4 or BuCy at our center between 2005 and 2016 were included in this retrospective analysis. Informed consent was obtained from each patient per institutional guidelines. The institutional review board also reviewed and approved this retrospective analysis.

2.2. SCT Conditioning Regimen. All patients received 1 of 3 myeloablative conditioning regimens consisting of fludarabine 40 mg/m2 with Bu 3.2 mg/kg daily for 4 days with or without Bu PK dose adjustment or Bu 3.2 mg/kg for 4 days with cyclophosphamide 60 mg/kg for 2 days. The choice of regimen was at the discretion of treating physician.

2.3. Graft versus Host Disease (GVHD) Prophylaxis. Post-transplantation graft versus host disease (GVHD) prophylaxis consisted of methotrexate on days 1, 3, 6, and 11 and tacrolimus. Patients receiving unrelated donor transplants received antithymocyte globulin 4.5 mg/kg pretransplantation in divided doses.

2.4. Chimerism Analysis. Bone marrow donor-recipient total cell chimerism analysis was performed on day 30 and day 100 using a quantitative fluorescence-based short tandem repeat polymerase chain reaction with capillary electrophoresis for polymerase chain reaction product resolution. Data are presented as peaks, and the AUC represents the percentage of host-versus-donor hematopoiesis.

2.5. Supportive Care. All supportive care measures including prophylactic antibiotics and antifungals were utilized according to institutional protocols. Ursodeoxycholic acid was started with the initiation of conditioning regimen.

2.6. Statistical Methods. Baseline characteristics were summarized by transplant group. Continuous variables were summarized as the mean, standard deviation, and range. Categorical variables were summarized as frequency counts and percentages. Patient and transplantation characteristics were compared using Fisher's exact and chi-squared test for categorical variables and Mann-Whitney's test for continuous variables. For overall tests, $P < .05$ was used to indicate statistical significance. Engraftment was defined as achieving

an absolute neutrophil count of 500/μl for 3 consecutive days. Time of platelet engraftment was defined as the first of 3 consecutive days with a platelet count 20,000/μl without transfusion support. Criteria for complete remission (CR) after transplant included absence of circulating blasts, less than 5% marrow blasts, lack of chromosomal abnormalities, and documented donor cell engraftment. Overall survival was defined as the time from SCT to the time of death or last contact. It was calculated using the Kaplan-Meier estimate.

3. Results

3.1. Patient and Transplant Characteristics. In this study, 78 patients were identified and included. Characteristics of the patients are summarized in Table 1. There were 50 males and 28 females with a median age of 59 years. Diagnoses included AML ($n = 49$), MDS ($n = 19$), and myeloproliferative neoplasms ($n = 10$). Thirty-four patients had a matched related donor, 32 had a matched unrelated donor, and 12 had a mismatched unrelated donor SCT. Peripheral blood stem cells were used in all patients. Fifty-five patients received FluBu4, of whom 21 had Bu PK measured. BuCy was given in 23 patients. Bu dose was adjusted to more than 10% change based on PK in 81% of patients in the FluBu4 PK group. The change was more than 15% and more than 20% of the dose in 71% and 62% of patients in the FluBu4 PK group, respectively, median AUC targeted was 6000 uMolxMin, and median of actual target given was 5354 uMolxMin.

Gender, donor type, cytogenetics risk group, disease risk index, median blasts at time of SCT, CD34 dose, and antithymocyte globulin use were comparable ($P > .30$) between the 3 groups. The median CD34 dose was 3.9, 4.1, and 4.4×10^6/kg of recipient in the FluBu4 with PK, FluBu4 with no PK, and BuCy, respectively. The median CD3 dose was 1.2, 1.2, and 1.1×10^8/kg of recipient in the FluBu4 with PK, FluBu4 with no PK, and BuCy, respectively. Antithymocyte globulin was used in 57%, 62%, and 44% in the FluBu4 with PK, FluBu4 with no PK, and BuCy, respectively. Disease risk index was high or very high in 57%, 53%, and 60% of patients in the FluBu4 with PK, FluBu4 with no PK, and BuCy, respectively. Median blasts at time of transplant were 4% in all 3 groups. However, patients who received BuCy were younger with a median age of 45 years compared to patients who received FluBu4 with or without PK, 59 and 63 years, respectively ($P < .001$). In addition, patients who received FluBu4 with no PK had equal cases of MDS (44%) and AML (44%) as a diagnosis compared to FluBu4 with PK and BuCy who had more AML in those groups, 71% and 82%, respectively ($P = .006$).

3.2. Engraftment and Chimerism. Median time to neutrophil engraftment was 15, 12, and 14 days in the FluBu4 with PK, FluBu4 with no PK, and BuCy, respectively. Median time to platelet engraftment was 15, 13, and 14 days in the FluBu4 with PK, FluBu4 with no PK, and BuCy, respectively.

We evaluated total donor cell chimerism values on days 30 and 100 after allogeneic SCT as a boxplot (Figure 1). The percentages of total donor chimerism which were grouped as 100%, 86%–99%, and less than 85% on day 30 and day 100 are summarized in Tables 2 and 3. Total donor cell chimerism

TABLE 1: Summary of patient characteristics by treatment group.

	FluBu4 with PK N = 21 (% or range)	FluBu4 without PK N = 34 (% or range)	BuCy N = 23 (% or range)	P value
Gender	M 14 (67%)	M 24 (70%)	M 12 (52%)	.349
	F 7 (33%)	F 10 (30%)	F 11 (48%)	
Median age at time of SCT	59 (41–70)	63 (48–72)	45 (22–63)	<.001
Disease				.006
Acute myeloid leukemia	15 (71%)	15 (44%)	19 (82%)	
MPN/MDS	6 (29%)	19 (56%)	4 (18%)	
Median blasts in bone marrow at time of SCT	4% (1–40%)	4% (1–20%)	4% (1–90%)	.910
Cytogenetic risk				.521
High	14 (67%)	17 (50%)	14 (61%)	
Intermediate	6 (29%)	16 (47%)	9 (39%)	
Low	1 (4%)	1 (3%)	0 (0%)	
Disease risk index				.372
Intermediate	9 (43%)	16 (47%)	7 (30%)	
High	5 (24%)	13 (38%)	9 (39%)	
Very high	7 (33%)	5 (15%)	7 (30%)	
Antithymocyte globulin use	12 (57%)	21 (62%)	10 (44%)	.38
CD34 dose × 10^6	3.9 ± 1.5	4.1 ± 1.3	4.4 ± 2	.534
Donor type				.401
Matched related donor	9 (43%)	13 (38%)	12 (52%)	
Matched unrelated donor	7 (33%)	15 (44%)	10 (43%)	
Mismatched unrelated donor	5 (24%)	6 (18%)	1 (5%)	

Bu, busulfan; Cy, cyclophosphamide; F, female; Flu, fludarabine; M, male; MDS, myelodysplastic syndrome; MPN; myeloproliferative neoplasm; SCT, stem cell transplant.

TABLE 2: Total donor chimerism on day 30.

	Chimerism results at day 30 FluBu4 with PK	FluBu4 with no PK	BuCy	P value
100% donor	14	17	16	
86%–99%	7	15	5	.311
<85%	0	2	2	

Bu, busulfan; Cy, cyclophosphamide; Flu, fludarabine; PK, pharmacokinetics.

TABLE 3: Total donor chimerism on day 100.

	Chimerism results at day 100 FluBu4 with PK	FluBu4 with no PK	BuCy	P value
100% donor	14	13	17	
86%–99%	3	12	0	.006
<85%	4	9	6	

Bu, busulfan; Cy, cyclophosphamide; Flu, fludarabine; PK, pharmacokinetics.

analysis showed that the percentage of patients maintaining 100% donor chimerism on day 100 was 66.7 %, 38.2%, and 73.9% in the FluBu4 with PK, FluBu4 with no PK, and BuCy, respectively (P = .001). In addition, the percentage of patients who had decreasing total donor chimerism by day 100 was 23.8 %, 52.9%, and 26.1% in the FluBu4 with PK, FluBu4

with no PK, and BuCy, respectively (P = .04) (Table 4). The Bu PK group had fewer patients with less than 95% donor chimerism by day 30 compared to the other 2 groups (no PK and BuCy) although it was not statistically significant, 5% (FluBu4 PK), 31% (FluBu4 with no PK), and 21% (BuCy) (P = .18). Since patients who received BuCy were younger and the groups who got FluBu4 with PK and BuCy had more AML as above, we looked at multivariable analysis, which suggested that patients treated with FluBu4 without PK had higher odds of experiencing a decrease in chimerism from day 30 to day 100 than patients treated with BuCy or FluBu4 with PK after adjusting for age at transplant and disease. In addition, when we looked at the effect the treatment group has on being in the 100% chimerism at day 100 group versus being in the 86%–99% or less than 86% chimerism at day 100 group, adjusting for age and disease type as in Table 5, we found that the group of FluBu4 with no PK had a higher risk of not having 100% chimerism on day 100 with P = .066 (95% CI 0.06–1.09).

3.3. GVHD and Hepatic Venoocclusive Disease. None of the patients in the 3 groups developed hepatic venoocclusive disease. Grade II and grades III-IV acute GVHD were not different between the 3 groups (P = .13). The incidence of grade II acute GVHD was 19%, 17.6%, and 21.7% in the FluBu4 with PK, FluBu4 with no PK, and BuCy, respectively. Grades III-IV acute GVHD were 4.7%, 29%, and 17.4% in FluBu4

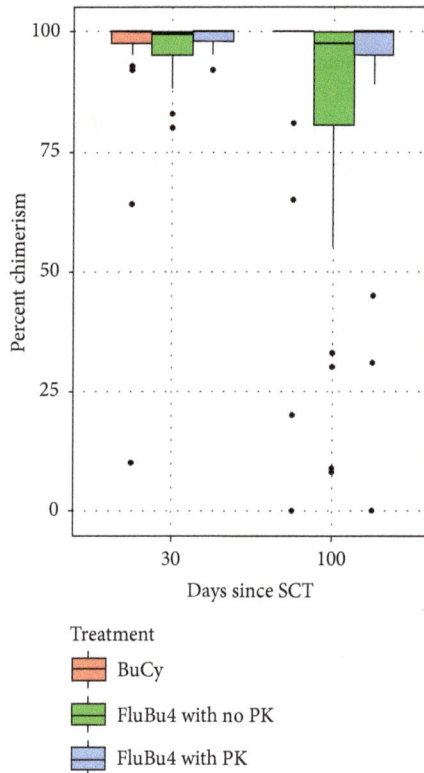

FIGURE 1: Boxplot for day 30 and day 100 chimerism for each of the 3 conditioning regimens. Bu, busulfan; Cy, cyclophosphamide; Flu, fludarabine; PK, pharmacokinetics; SCT, stem cell transplant.

TABLE 4: Decreasing and nondecreasing total chimerism between day 30 and day 100.

	Decreasing N (%)	Nondecreasing N (%)	P value
FluBu4 with no PK	18 (52.9)	16 (47.1)	
FluBu4 with PK	5 (23.8)	16 (76.2)	.04
BuCy	6 (26.1)	17 (73.9)	

Bu, busulfan; Cy, cyclophosphamide; Flu, fludarabine; PK, pharmacokinetics.

TABLE 5: Effect on the treatment group on being in the 100% chimerism on day 100 group versus being in the 86%–99% or <86% chimerism on day 100, adjusting for age and disease type.

Variable	OR	95% CI	P value
Treatment (versus BuCy)			
FluBu4 with kinetics	0.73	0.17–3.11	.672
FluBu4 without Kinetics	0.25	0.06–1.09	.066
Age at transplant	1.01	0.96–1.06	.790
Disease	1.53	0.57–4.13	.403

Bu, busulfan; Cy, cyclophosphamide; Flu, fludarabine; OR, odds ratio.

with PK, FluBu4 with no PK, and BuCy, respectively. Also looking at patients who had total donor chimerism more than 95% or less than 95% on day 100, rates of grade II and grades III-IV acute GVHD were not different between the 2 groups

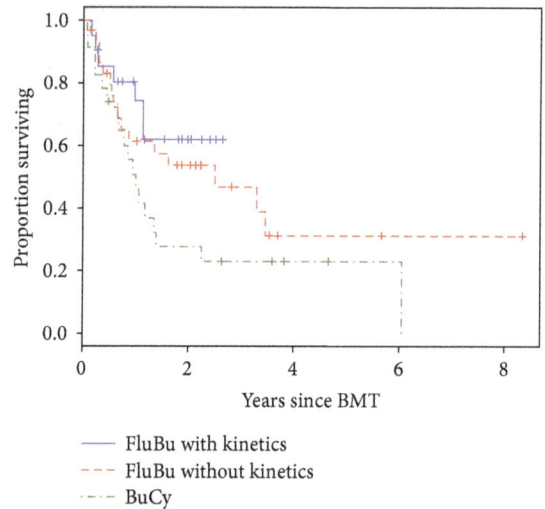

FIGURE 2: Kaplan-Meier curve for overall survival for allogeneic hematopoietic cell transplantation by conditioning regimen (P = .11). BMT, bone marrow transplant; Bu, busulfan; Cy, cyclophosphamide; Flu, fludarabine.

(P = .43). The incidence of grade II acute GVHD was 20% and 23% in the patients who had total donor chimerism more than 95% and less than 95% on day 100, respectively.

3.4. Relapse, Overall Survival, and Causes of Death. The median survival time for all patients was 1.40 years. Relapse rate was 24%, 47%, and 57% for FluBu4 with PK, FluBu4 with no PK, and BuCy, respectively (P = .085). When comparing the FluBu4 with no PK and BuCy groups, the odds ratio of relapse within the first 3 months was 2.23 (P = .194) for the no PK group. For the comparison of the FluBu4 with PK and BuCy groups, the odds ratio of relapse within the first 3 months was 1.12 (P = .87) for the FluBu4 with PK group. Survival distributions of the 3 treatment groups were not statistically significant (P = .11) (Figure 2). The cause of death was relapse in 28.5%, 35.3%, and 60% of patients in the FluBu4 with PK, FluBu4 with no PK, and BuCy groups, respectively, while the cause of death was GVHD in in 4.7%, 5.9%, and 8.7% patients in the FluBu4 with PK, FluBu4 with no PK, and BuCy, respectively. Sepsis and liver failure were cause of death in 8.7% of patients in the BuCy group. Cytomegalovirus antigenemia was documented in 35%, 34%, and 30% in the FluBu4 with PK, FluBu4 with no PK, and BuCy, respectively.

4. Discussion

Myeloablative regimens, BuCy and FluBu4, remain the standard of care for patients undergoing SCT for AML or MDS if they can tolerate it as recently shown by the Blood and Marrow Transplant Clinical Trials Network (BMT CTN 0901) [11] phase III randomized trial comparing reduced intensity and myeloablative regimens in patients with AML or MDS. This shows that intensity of chemotherapy does matter in controlling aggressive myeloid disorders. However, not all myeloablative conditioning regimens are the same and they differ in toxicity and nonrelapse mortality.

Although the intravenous form of Bu bypasses the influence of gastrointestinal enzymes that affects the oral form, there is still a lot of inter- and intraindividual variability in Bu PK [12]. The practice guidelines committee of the American Society of Blood or Marrow Transplantation (ASBMT) sought to develop an evidence-based review of personalized dosing of Bu. However that was not feasible because of the lack of the necessary controlled studies and the published literature was too heterogeneous regarding patient population, conditioning regimen, Bu dosing, and Bu PK data [10]. Several studies provided recommendation of a maximally tolerated daily exposure of Bu of less than 6,000 mMxmin for 4 days [13], while others evaluated the maximally tolerated systemic exposure of intravenous Bu in combination with fludarabine and they showed that Bu can be safely escalated to an AUC of 7000 mMxmin or more without an appreciable difference in nonrelapse mortality [14, 15] although with need of more patients and longer follow-up in those studies. In our patients, the median AUC targeted was 6000 uMolxMin and the median actual target given was 5354 uMolxMin. Bu dose had to be adjusted based on PK in 81% of patients in the FluBu4 PK group, which is similar to the percentage reported by the Center for International Blood and Marrow Transplant Research (CIBMTR) where Bu dose was adjusted based on PK in 75% of patients who got FluBu4 [16].

Many studies were published trying to compare BuCy to FluBu4 [8, 16–19]. Most of these studies included heterogeneous group of patients with myeloid and lymphoid malignancies [17, 19]; not all of them used Bu PK [17–19] nor did they all look at chimerism kinetics [8, 16, 19]. Therefore, not a lot of the studies were looking at the early effect on chimerism especially in a homogeneous group of patients. In this study we looked at the effect of these 3 regimens, BuCy, FluBu4 with PK, and FluBu4 with no PK, on early donor chimerism in a homogenous group of patients with myeloid malignancies. We found that FluBu4 with PK and BuCy have a similar effect on early donor chimerism while in the FluBu4 with no PK group more patients had decreasing donor chimerism by day 100, which was statistically significant. Even when adjusted for disease and age at transplant, FluBu4 without PK had a higher risk of decreasing donor chimerism and more patients with less than 100% donor chimerism on day 100. On day 30, patients who had PK performed had lower rates of less than 95% donor chimerism compared to others, although not statistically significant. In a randomized trial done by Lee et al. [17], the BuFlu arm had a higher degree of recipient chimerism and a lower probability of complete chimerism at 4 weeks after SCT than the BuCy arm. In addition, they had worse survival in the BuFlu group, owing mainly to excessive disease relapse, which could be related to the lack of targeted dosing by PK. In another study by Liu et al. [18], patients were randomized to get BuCy or BuFlu; fludarabine was given after busulfan. All 106 evaluable patients achieved complete donor chimerism, defined in their study by more than 95% donor, by day +30 after transplantation. They also looked at chimerism on

day +15 which was not statistically significant between the 2 groups but there was no mention of kinetic of chimerism after day 30. However, their patient population included only AML-CR1 with ages between 12 and 60 years, while our patient population has a group of higher risk diseases.

The MD Anderson Cancer Center group looked retrospectively at the effect of chimerism around day 100 (days +90 to +120) on the risk of relapse after SCT in patients with AML (81%) or MDS (19%) who got FluBu4 [20]. All patients received Bu 130 mg/m^2 daily for 4 days or Bu given with PK dose adjustment, targeting a drug concentration AUC of 6000 mMxmin. Because of the high rates of full donor myeloid chimerism by days +90 to +120 in all patients they focused solely on the impact of T lymphocyte chimerism and concluded that early T lymphocyte chimerism testing is a useful approach for predicting AML/MDS disease recurrence in patients in CR1/CR2 at the time of transplantation. However, this study excluded patients who had disease progression before day +120. In addition, they looked at chimerism at one point of time without looking at changes in chimerism over time and without comparison of groups with and without PK. In our study we did not have data about lineage-specific chimerism because it is not done routinely for all the patients in our center; in addition that will create multiple small groups of patients which would not have the power to reflect and determine differences among those small groups. Koreth et al. [21] looked at 688 patients with hematologic malignancies who received FluBu to assess the impact of early donor chimerism on long-term outcomes. They showed that total donor chimerism independently predicts long-term relapse and survival and also concluded that total donor cell chimerism is sufficient and assessing T-subset chimerism is of no additional value to predicting these endpoints. Other studies that have suggested that such analyses cannot be used reliably [22–25] had either different diseases, smaller numbers of patients, or different condition regimens.

Regarding relapse, although there was high early 100% chimerism in the BuCy group, there was also high percentage of relapse in the same group. This is probably because that group had the longest follow-up. We started sending busulfan kinetics in our center in 2013. In the BuCy group some patients had follow-up (up to 3432 days) compared to FluBu4 with no PK (up to 2945 days) and the shortest follow-up was for FluBu4 with PK (up to 1373 days) which might explain more reported relapse in the BuCy group. In addition, mechanisms of early relapse are different than those of late relapse, as early relapse can be prevented by modifying the chemotherapy regimen or preemptive therapy with immunotherapy while late relapse might be related to other mechanisms like escape from the powerful cytotoxic effect of human leukocyte antigen-mismatched donor T cells [26, 27]. So when we looked at relapse in the first 3 months, there was a tendency for higher relapse in the FluBu4 with no PK compared to the other 2 groups, which was not statistically significant.

Regarding GVHD, there was no difference between the 3 groups in our study, similar to what was found by a meta-analysis by Ben-Barouch et al. In that analysis when they looked at the randomized trials only, the risk grade II–IV acute GVHD was similar between the 2 groups FluBu4 and BuCy [28].

Our study has limitations since it is a retrospective analysis, including potential selection bias and the presence of other confounding factors that were not measured like fludarabine kinetics and prior therapies. In addition because it is retrospective, we were unable to determine any causation, only association if any. Other limitations include the small number of patients, the short follow-up, and the absence of data on lineage-specific chimerism. The strengths of this study include looking at the kinetics of chimerism and not at just one point of time chimerism and a cohort of adult patients with only myeloid malignancies treated at a single center by the same physicians with uniform peripheral blood stem cell grafts and the widely used Bu based myeloablative preparative regimens with the standard-of-care methotrexate/tacrolimus-based with or without antithymocyte globulin GVHD prophylaxis.

5. Conclusion

Currently, there are no guidelines on how and when to perform personalized dosing of Bu as part of the conditioning regimen prior to SCT. Chimerism is one of the methods used to monitor disease after SCT. However, interpretation of the results and techniques is not yet standardized. In this small cohort, we found that patients with myeloid disorders who received FluBu4 with Bu PK had a trend for higher donor chimerism similar to BuCy on day 100, while FluBu4 with no PK had a tendency to lose donor chimerism by day 100 and had more patients with less than 95% donor chimerism by day 30. Thus, in the era of precision medicine, the conditioning regimens and personalized dosing may impact early donor chimerism. This is especially important in myeloid disorders. This will need to be examined in larger retrospective multicenter studies like CIBMTR and prospective clinical trials.

Conflicts of Interest

The authors declare that there are no conflicts of interest regarding the publication of this article.

References

[1] C. Schmid, M. Labopin, A. Nagler et al., "Treatment, risk factors, and outcome of adults with relapsed AML after reduced intensity conditioning for allogeneic stem cell transplantation," *Blood*, vol. 119, no. 6, pp. 1599–1606, 2012.

[2] M. Mielcarek, B. E. Storer, M. E. D. Flowers, R. Storb, B. M. Sandmaier, and P. J. Martin, "Outcomes among patients with recurrent high-risk hematologic malignancies after allogeneic hematopoietic cell transplantation," *Biology of Blood and Marrow Transplantation*, vol. 13, no. 10, pp. 1160–1168, 2007.

[3] M. M. Bortin, M. M. Horowitz, R. P. Gale et al., "Changing trends in allogeneic bone marrow transplantation for leukemia in the 1980s," *Journal of the American Medical Association*, vol. 268, no. 5, pp. 607–612, 1992.

[4] M. M. Horowitz et al., "Transplant registries: guiding clinical decisions and improving outcomes," *Oncology (Williston Park)*, vol. 15, discussion 663-4, 666, no. 5, pp. 649–659, 2001.

[5] C. Huisman, R. A. de Weger, L. de Vries, M. G. J. Tilanus, and L. F. Verdonck, "Chimerism analysis within 6 months of allogeneic stem cell transplantation predicts relapse in acute myeloid leukemia," *Bone Marrow Transplantation*, vol. 39, no. 5, pp. 285–291, 2007.

[6] N. Kröger, U. Bacher, P. Bader et al., "NCI first international workshop on the biology, prevention, and treatment of relapse after allogeneic hematopoietic stem cell transplantation: Report from the committee on disease-specific methods and strategies for monitoring relapse following allogeneic stem cell transplantation. Part II: Chronic leukemias, myeloproliferative neoplasms, and lymphoid malignancies," *Biology of Blood and Marrow Transplantation*, vol. 16, no. 10, pp. 1325–1346, 2010.

[7] J. A. Russell and S. B. Kangarloo, "Therapeutic drug monitoring of busulfan in transplantation," *Current Pharmaceutical Design*, vol. 14, no. 20, pp. 1936–1949, 2008.

[8] B. S. Andersson, M. de Lima, P. F. Thall et al., "Once daily i.v. busulfan and fludarabine (i.v. Bu-Flu) compares favorably with i.v. busulfan and cyclophosphamide (i.v. BuCy2) as pretransplant conditioning therapy in AML/MDS," *Biology of Blood & Marrow Transplantation*, vol. 14, no. 6, pp. 672–684, 2008.

[9] I. H. Bartelink, R. G. M. Bredius, T. T. Ververs et al., "Once-daily intravenous busulfan with therapeutic drug monitoring compared to conventional oral busulfan improves survival and engraftment in children undergoing allogeneic stem cell transplantation," *Biology of Blood and Marrow Transplantation*, vol. 14, no. 1, pp. 88–98, 2008.

[10] J. Palmer, J. S. McCune, M.-A. Perales et al., "Personalizing busulfan-based conditioning: considerations from the american society for blood and marrow transplantation practice guidelines committee," *Biology of Blood and Marrow Transplantation*, vol. 22, no. 11, pp. 1915–1925, 2016.

[11] B. Scott et al., "Results of a phase III randomized, multi-center study of allogeneic stem cell transplantation after high versus reduced intensity conditioning in patients with myelodysplastic syndrome (MDS) or acute myeloid leukemia (AML): blood and marrow transplant clinical trials network (BMT CTN) 0901," *Blood*, vol. 23, no. 126, 2015.

[12] J. S. McCune, J. P. Gibbs, and J. T. Slattery, "Plasma concentration monitoring of busulfan: Does it improve clinical outcome?" *Clinical Pharmacokinetics*, vol. 39, no. 2, pp. 155–165, 2000.

[13] B. S. Andersson, P. F. Thall, T. Madden et al., "Busulfan systemic exposure relative to regimen-related toxicity and acute graft-versus-host disease: Defining a therapeutic window for IV BuCy2 in chronic myelogenous leukemia," *Biology of Blood and Marrow Transplantation*, vol. 8, no. 9, pp. 477–485, 2002.

[14] J. B. Perkins, J. Kim, C. Anasetti et al., "Maximally tolerated busulfan systemic exposure in combination with fludarabine as conditioning before allogeneic hematopoietic cell transplantation," *Biology of Blood and Marrow Transplantation*, vol. 18, no. 7, pp. 1099–1107, 2012.

[15] T. C. Shea, C. Walko, Y. Chung et al., "Phase I/II trial of dose-escalated busulfan delivered by prolonged continuous infusion in allogeneic transplant patients," *Biology of Blood and Marrow Transplantation*, vol. 21, no. 12, pp. 2129–2135, 2015.

[16] M. C. Pasquini et al., "Intravenous Busulfan-Based Myeloablative Conditioning Regimens Prior to Hematopoietic Cell Transplantation for Hematologic Malignancies," *Biol Blood Marrow Transplant*, vol. 22, no. 8, pp. 1424-30, 2016.

[17] J. H. Lee et al., "Randomized trial of myeloablative conditioning regimens: busulfan plus cyclophosphamide versus busulfan plus fludarabine," *Journal of Clinical Oncology*, vol. 31, no. 6, pp. 701–709, 2013.

[18] H. Liu, X. Zhai, Z. Song et al., "Busulfan plus fludarabine as a myeloablative conditioning regimen compared with busulfan plus cyclophosphamide for acute myeloid leukemia in first complete remission undergoing allogeneic hematopoietic stem cell transplantation: A prospective and multicenter study," *Journal of Hematology & Oncology*, vol. 6, 15 pages, 2013.

[19] Y. S. Chae, S. K. Sohn, J. G. Kim et al., "New myeloablative conditioning regimen with fludarabine and busulfan for allogeneic stem cell transplantation: Comparison with BuCy2," *Bone Marrow Transplantation*, vol. 40, no. 6, pp. 541–547, 2007.

[20] H. C. Lee, R. M. Saliba, G. Rondon et al., "Mixed T lymphocyte chimerism after allogeneic hematopoietic transplantation is predictive for relapse of acute myeloid leukemia and myelodysplastic syndromes," *Biology of Blood and Marrow Transplantation*, vol. 21, no. 11, pp. 1948–1954, 2015.

[21] J. Koreth, H. T. Kim, S. Nikiforow et al., "Donor chimerism early after reduced-intensity conditioning hematopoietic stem cell transplantation predicts relapse and survival," *Biology of Blood and Marrow Transplantation*, vol. 20, no. 10, pp. 1516–1521, 2014.

[22] Z. Y. Lim, L. Pearce, W. Ingram, A. Y. L. Ho, G. J. Mufti, and A. Pagliuca, "Chimerism does not predict for outcome after alemtuzumab-based conditioning: Lineage-specific analysis of chimerism of specific diseases may be more informative," *Bone Marrow Transplantation*, vol. 41, no. 6, pp. 587-588, 2008.

[23] K. C. Doney, M. R. Loken, E. M. Bryant, A. G. Smith, and F. R. Appelbaum, "Lack of utility of chimerism studies obtained 2-3 months after myeloablative hematopoietic cell transplantation for ALL," *Bone Marrow Transplantation*, vol. 42, no. 4, pp. 271–274, 2008.

[24] N. Schaap, A. Schattenberg, E. Mensink et al., "Long-term follow-up of persisting mixed chimerism after partially T cell-depleted allogeneic stem cell transplantation," *Leukemia*, vol. 16, no. 1, pp. 13–21, 2002.

[25] S.-J. Choi, K.-H. Lee, J.-H. Lee et al., "Prognostic value of hematopoietic chimerism in patients with acute leukemia after allogeneic bone marrow transplantation: a prospective study," *Bone Marrow Transplantation*, vol. 26, no. 3, pp. 327–332, 2000.

[26] L. Vago, C. Toffalori, F. Ciceri, and K. Fleischhauer, "Genomic loss of mismatched human leukocyte antigen and leukemia immune escape from haploidentical graft-versus-leukemia," *Seminars in Oncology*, vol. 39, no. 6, pp. 707–715, 2012.

[27] A. J. Barrett and M. Battiwalla, "Relapse after allogeneic stem cell transplantation," *Expert Review of Hematology*, vol. 3, no. 4, pp. 429–441, 2010.

[28] S. Ben-Barouch, O. Cohen, L. Vidal, I. Avivi, and R. Ram, "Busulfan fludarabine vs busulfan cyclophosphamide as a preparative regimen before allogeneic hematopoietic cell transplantation: Systematic review and meta-analysis," *Bone Marrow Transplantation*, vol. 51, no. 2, pp. 232–240, 2016.

22

Glucose-6-Phosphate Dehydrogenase Deficiency and Sickle Cell Trait among Prospective Blood Donors

Patrick Adu,[1] **David Larbi Simpong,**[1] **Godfred Takyi,**[2] **and Richard K. D. Ephraim**[1]

[1]*Department of Medical Laboratory Technology, School of Allied Health Sciences, University of Cape Coast, Cape Coast, Ghana*
[2]*Holy Family Hospital, Berekum, Brong-Ahafo Region, Ghana*

Correspondence should be addressed to Patrick Adu; patrick.adu@ucc.edu.gh

Academic Editor: Emili Montserrat

Background. Blood transfusion is a therapeutic procedure usually undertaken in patients with severe anaemia. In Ghana, severe anaemia is mostly due to malaria caused by severe *Plasmodium falciparum* infection, road traffic accidents, and haemoglobinopathy-induced acute haemolysis. *Method.* This cross-sectional study evaluated coinheritance of sickle cell haemoglobin variant and G6PD enzymopathy among individuals that donated blood at the Holy Trinity Hospital, Berekum, in the Brong-Ahafo Region, Ghana. Demographic data and other pertinent information were captured using questionnaire. Sickle cell haemoglobin variants were determined using cellulose acetate electrophoresis (pH 8.6). Qualitative G6PD status and quantitative G6PD enzyme activity were determined using methaemoglobin reduction and Trinity Biotech G6PD test kit, respectively. *Results.* Prevalence of sickle cell trait (SCT) and G6PD enzymopathy coinheritance was 7%. In addition, 19.5% of the donors had 10%–60% of normal G6PD enzyme activity suggesting that these donor units are prone to stressor-induced acute haemolysis when given to recipients. Mild G6PD activity ($p = 0.03$, OR: 2.410 (CI: 1.049–5.534)), commercial ($p = 0.020$, OR: 5.609 (CI: 1.309–24.035)), and voluntary ($p = 0.034$, OR: 2.404 (CI: 1.071–5.397)) donors were significantly associated with SCT. *Conclusion.* Screening for red cell pathologies must be incorporated into existing protocols for populations with high incidence of haemoglobinopathies to protect high-risk recipients.

1. Introduction

Blood transfusion is a therapeutic procedure usually undertaken in patients with severe anaemia. In Ghana, severe anaemia is mostly due to malaria caused by severe *Plasmodium falciparum* infection, road traffic accidents, and haemolytic episodes in individuals with haemoglobinopathies such as sickle cell anaemia and/or thalassaemia [1, 2]. It is estimated that most of the transfusions are undertaken in children under 5 years in response to severe *falciparum* infection [1]. In addition to the transfusion, such children may also be receiving antimalarial drugs (e.g., quinine and primaquine) with potential to cause oxidant stress. In these individuals, the optimal survival of the transfused red cells is of paramount importance so as to prevent adverse transfusion outcomes [3]. To ensure the safety of blood and blood products for prospective recipients, screening protocols for

transfusion-transmitted infections such as human immunodeficiency virus (HIV), hepatitis B and C, and syphilis are mandatory [4]. It has been postulated that selective pressure caused by the endemicity of *Plasmodium falciparum* infection in Ghana, and Sub-Saharan Africa in general, has led to high prevalence of certain haemoglobin variants (e.g., HbS) and/or red cell enzymopathies (e.g., G6PD deficiency) as these have been shown to offer survival advantages [5–7]. The high prevalence of these inherited red cell pathologies suggest that measures should be taken prior to donation and subsequent transfusion of such units to other individuals who might have also inherited these red cell pathologies. Some have argued that donor blood from those heterozygous for haemoglobin S or haemoglobin C should not be used for either exchange transfusion or neonatal transfusion [8, 9]. Others have also argued that those who have had previous oxidant stress-induced haemolysis as a result of G6PD enzyme deficiency

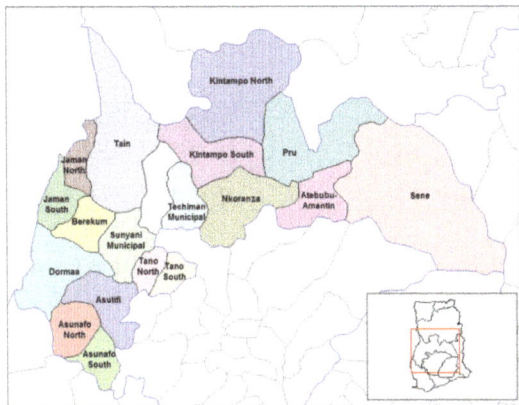

FIGURE 1: Map of Brong-Ahafo Region of Ghana (source: Google map).

must be permanently deferred for the safety of both the donor and prospective recipient [8]. Thus, knowledge of the red cell pathologies inherent in a given donor unit may be important for ensuring maximal benefit to the potential recipient.

Howes et al. estimated that the prevalence of G6PD deficiency could be as high as 32.5% across sub-Saharan Africa [10]. The WHO also estimates the prevalence of G6PD deficiency in Ghana to be 15–26% [11]. Moreover, the prevalence of sickle cell trait (SCT) in Ghana has been estimated to be between 20% and 40% [12]. However, previous studies carried out in Ghana and the subregion did not measure the G6PD enzyme activity in the donors [13, 14] and could not therefore categorize the classes of the G6PD enzymopathy in the studied donors as per the WHO recommendations [11]. In addition, the existing predonation screening protocols in Ghana do not assess for either red cell enzymopathies or haemoglobinopathies in spite of the high prevalence of these pathologies. In this study, we sought to screen for haemoglobin variants and G6PD status/enzyme activity in donor blood that had been declared fit for transfusion as per the existing predonation screening protocols. The aim was to assess whether recipients with certain medical conditions such as severe falciparum malaria or vulnerable groups like neonates requiring exchange transfusions of blood products are adequately protected from products that have the potential to complicate clinical outcomes.

2. Materials and Methods

2.1. Study Site/Study Design.
This was a hospital based cross-sectional study carried out from August 2015 to January 2016 at the Holy Family Hospital at Berekum in the Brong-Ahafo Region (Figure 1). Holy Family Hospital (HFH) is a Catholic health institution which serves as the Municipal Hospital for Berekum with Level C rating, for medical care in the PHC strategy.

2.2. Study Population.
All blood donors ≥18 years who tested negative for all the transfusion-transmitted disease screening assays were enrolled. A total of 200 donor samples

were collected for the study using a convenience sampling technique. All samples were obtained from donor blood collected in citrate phosphate dextrose adenine 1 (CPDA-1) and assayed within 24 hours of collection. Questionnaires were used to capture demographic data, medication history, donor type and history, and other pertinent information. All prospective donors on medications (Such as cotrimoxazole, aspirin, fansidar, and nitrofurantoin.) known to affect G6PD enzyme activity were excluded [15].

2.3. Ethical Considerations.
Experimental protocols were approved by the institutional review board of University of Cape Coast and Holy Trinity Hospital ethical review board (UCCIRB/CHAS/2015/61). The qualitative and quantitative G6PD assays were performed independently and were blinded to remove potential operator bias.

2.4. Qualitative G6PD Assay.
The methaemoglobin reduction test assay previously described [1] was used to qualitatively assay for G6PD status. For each sample, three tubes were set as test (T), normal (N), and deficient (D) as internal quality controls to validate the results.

2.5. Quantitative G6PD Assay.
Quantitative G6PD activity was measured in duplicate per sample using the quantitative G6PD kit from Trinity Biotech (catalog number 345-B; Trinity Biotech PLC, Bray, Ireland) according to the manufacturer's instructions. As per the manufacturer specifications, normal, intermediate, and deficient Trinity controls (catalog numbers G6888, G5029, and G5888, resp.) were run using the same method on each day of testing. 10 μL whole blood collected in CPDA-1 was added to 1 mL G6PD reagent solution and incubated at room temperature for 5 minutes. Two milliliters (2 mL) of substrate was added to the solution and mixed by inversion. The initial absorbance and final absorbance of all samples were measured using Junior Selectra chemical analyser and G6PD enzyme activity calculated in accordance with manufacturer's protocol. G6PD activity values were expressed in units per gram haemoglobin (Hb). Haemoglobin concentration was determined using Sysmex-XS haematology analyser (Sysmex Corporation, USA).

2.6. Haemoglobin Electrophoresis.
The cellulose acetate method of electrophoresis was employed to determine the haemoglobin variants of all blood samples in accordance with protocols previously described [16]. Each sample was washed four times in physiological saline and subsequently lysed in carbon tetrachloride (CCL4). The lysates were applied to the cellulose acetate paper and run for 30 minutes at 250 V and current 50 mA. For each electrophoretic run, combination of hemolysate from a sickle cell trait (AS) and HbC trait samples (ASC) served as the control.

2.7. Data Analysis.
Data were analysed using GraphPad prism 5.01 for Windows (GraphPad Software Inc., USA). Data were analysed for normality using D'Agostino and Pearson omnibus normality test and appropriate test selected for parametric and nonparametric data accordingly. For

TABLE 1: Age and gender distribution of blood donors.

Hb variant + G6PD status	Male	Female	Total
A + PD	—	4	4 (2%)
AS only	22	3	25 (12.5%)
AS + FD	14	—	14 (7%)
A + FD	19	2	21 (10.5%)
A + N	133	3	136 (68%)
Total	188 (94%)	12 (6%)	200

A and S represent haemoglobin A and haemoglobin S, respectively; N: no qualitative red cell G6PD enzyme defect; PD: partial qualitative red cell G6PD enzyme defect; FD: full qualitative red cell G6PD enzyme defect.

TABLE 2: Knowledge of blood donors on G6PD deficiency and/HbS status.

	Status		Previous donation		Total
	Yes	No	Yes	No	
G6PD	—	200	48 (24%)	152	200
Sickling	6 (3%)	194 (97%)	72 (37%)	122 (63%)	200

TABLE 3: Types of blood donors with G6PD and haemoglobin variants distribution.

Donors	G6PD-N	G6PD-D	A	AS
Commercial (n = 8)	3	5 (62.5%)	4	4 (50%)
Replacement (n = 152)	124	28 (18.4%)	128	24 (15.8%)
Voluntary (n = 40)	34	6 (15%)	28	12 (30%)
Total	161	39	160	40

G6PD-N: normal qualitative G6PD activity; G6PD-D: defective red cell G6PD activity; A: haemoglobin A; S: haemoglobin S.

TABLE 4: Number of donors as stratified by age (years).

Age (yrs)	Number of donors (%)
18–29	101 (50.5%)
30–39	81 (40.5%)
40–49	17 (8.5%)
50–59	1 (0.5%)
Total	200 (100%)

nonparametric data, multiple comparisons were undertaken using Kruskal-Wallis test with Dunn's posttest to determine statistical significant differences between groups. However, logistic regression analyses were undertaken using IBM SPSS version 16 (IBM Corporation, USA).

3. Results

As demonstrated by cellulose acetate electrophoretic mobility assay, 68% of the donors had neither the sickling haemoglobin (HbS) variant nor any qualitative G6PD defect. However, whereas 7% of the donors had both full qualitative red cell G6PD enzyme defect and haemoglobin AS phenotype, 12.5% of the donors had haemoglobin phenotype AS only, while 10.5% of the donors had full qualitative G6PD enzyme defect only (Table 1).

Whereas none of the donors had any knowledge about their G6PD status, only 3% of the study participants knew about their sickle cell haemoglobin status. However, 24% and 37% of the donors who had no knowledge about their G6PD and sickling haemoglobin status, respectively, had had previous blood donations. Overall, 19.5% of the blood donors had either HbS variant or G6PD enzymopathy (Table 2).

Of the 200 donors, 4% were commercial donors, that is, those donating for financial rewards (50% of which had HbAS phenotype), 76% were replacement (i.e., donation to a relative) donors (15.8% of which had HbAS phenotype), and 20% were voluntary blood donors (30% of which had HbAS phenotype) (Table 3).

50.5% of the study participants belonged to the 18–29 age group, whereas 40.5%, 8.5%, and 0.5%, respectively, belonged to the 30–39, 40–49, and 50–59 age groups, respectively (Table 4).

The red blood cell G6PD enzyme activities were significantly reduced in donors who demonstrated either partial

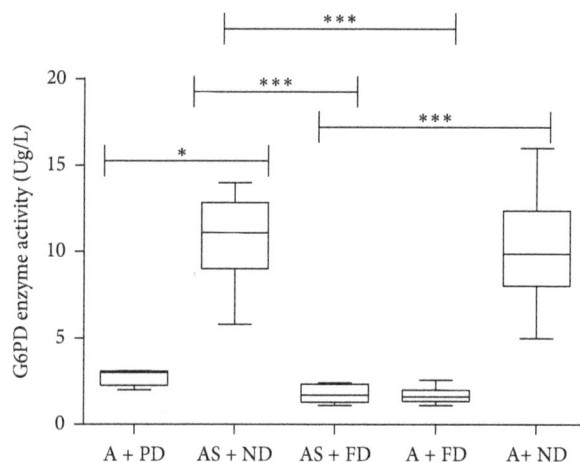

FIGURE 2: Comparison of red blood cell G6PD enzyme activity levels of blood donors. G6PD activities of red cells were measured using quantitative G6PD kit from Trinity Biotech and calculated against the donor haemoglobin levels. Statistical differences between G6PD enzyme activities were estimated using Kruskal-Wallis test with Dunn's posttest for multiple comparisons. A: haemoglobin A; S: haemoglobin S; ND: no qualitative G6PD activity; FD: full qualitative G6PD defect; PD: partial qualitative G6PD defect ($^*p < 0.05$; $^{***}p < 0.0001$).

or full qualitative defect when compared to donors with no qualitative enzyme defect (Figure 1; $p < 0.05$ (A + PD versus AS + ND); $p < 0.001$ (AS + ND versus AS + FD; AS + ND versus A + FD; AS + FD versus A + ND); A: haemoglobin A; S: haemoglobin S; ND: no qualitative G6PD activity; FD: full qualitative G6PD defect; PD: partial qualitative G6PD defect). However, this reduced G6PD enzyme activity was independent of the haemoglobin phenotype of the donor (Figure 2; $p = $ ns (AS + ND versus A + ND; AS + FD versus A + FD)).

TABLE 5: % G6PD enzyme activity calculated from the adjusted male median of study participants.

% G6PD activity	A + PD ($n = 4$)	A + FD ($n = 21$)	AS + FD ($n = 14$)	A + N ($n = 136$)	AS + N ($n = 25$)
Median (range)	29.41 (19.61–30.39)	15.69 (10.78–25.49)	16.67 (10.78–23.53)	97.06 (49.02–156.9)	108.8 (56.86–137.3)
Mean (95% CI)	27.21 (19.11–35.3)	16.53 (14.63–18.42)	17.23 (14.43–20.02)	99.79 (95.77–103.8)	105.4 (95.82–114.9)

A and S represent haemoglobin A and haemoglobin S, respectively; N: no qualitative red cell G6PD enzyme defect; PD: partial qualitative red cell G6PD enzyme defect; FD: full qualitative red cell G6PD enzyme defect.

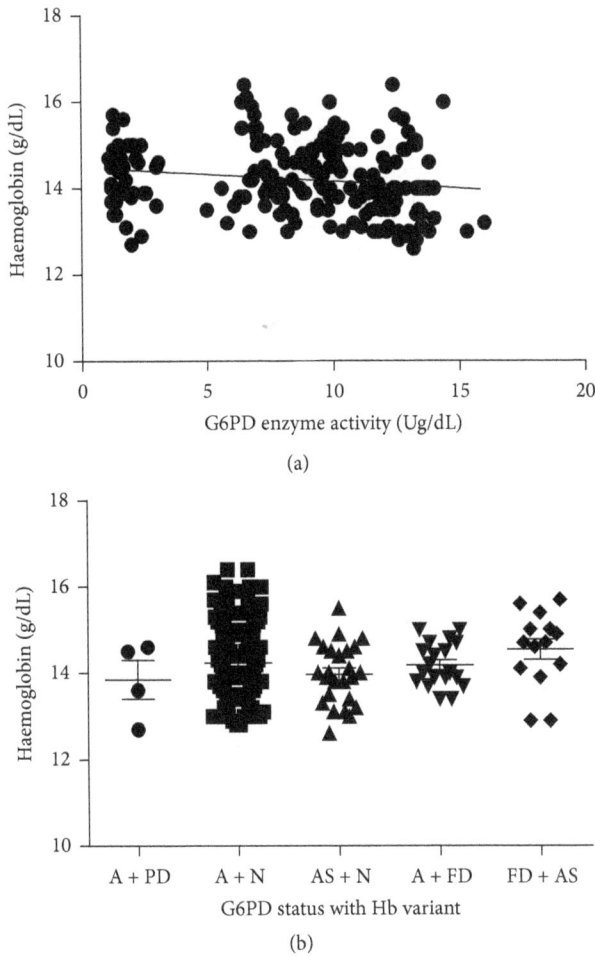

(a)

(b)

FIGURE 3: G6PD enzyme activity levels in relation to participant haemoglobin levels. (a) A scatter plot showing an inverse correlation between the participant haemoglobin levels and G6PD enzyme activity (Spearman correlation coefficient, $r = -0.2023$; $p = 0.0041$). (b) Comparing the haemoglobin levels of the participants with regard to the haemoglobin variant and/or G6PD enzymopathy status (A: haemoglobin A; S: haemoglobin S; ND: no qualitative G6PD activity; FD: full qualitative G6PD defect; PD: partial qualitative G6PD defect).

The study also found a weak but statistically significant inverse relationship between donor haemoglobin levels and red cell G6PD enzyme activity (Figure 3(a); $r = -0.2023$; $p = 0.0041$). However, when the data were stratified into the various haemoglobin variants, there was no significant difference in the haemoglobin levels between these groups (Figure 3(b)).

TABLE 6: Logistic regression of factors associated with sickle haemoglobin variant (AS).

Parameters	OR (95% CI)	P value
Age group		
18–29	0.229 (0.014–3.826)	0.305
30–39	0.250 (0.015–4.217)	0.336
40–49	0.231 (0.011–4.838)	0.345
50–59	Reference	
Sex		
Male	0.711 (0.183–2.758)	0.621
Female	Reference	
G6PD status		
Normal	Reference	
Partial defect	5.029 (5.029)	
Full defect	3.627 (1.630–8.067)	**0.002**
G6PD activity		
Mild deficiency	2.410 (1.049–5.534)	**0.038**
Nondeficient	0.676 (0.273–1.676)	0.398
Increased activity	Reference	—
Donor type		
Commercial	5.609 (1.309–24.035)	**0.020**
Voluntary	2.404 (1.071–5.397)	**0.034**
Replacement	Reference	—

OR: odds ratio; CI: confidence interval.

The 100% G6PD enzyme activity was calculated based on the adjusted G6PD-normal male median of the study participants as previously recommended [17] and is summarised in Table 5. As per the WHO recommendations, 39 (19.5%) of the participants with G6PD enzymopathy had mild G6PD deficiency, that is, 10–60% activity (Table 5) [11]. However, none had severe enzyme deficiency, that is, <10% enzyme activity.

Our study also revealed that, in our donor population, having a sickle cell trait was significantly associated with higher chance of having full qualitative red cell G6PD defect ($p = 0.002$, OR: 3.627, CI (1.630–8.067)) and mild red cell G6PD enzyme activity level ($p = 0.038$, OR: 2.410, CI (1.049–5.534)). Additionally, there was a significantly higher chance of commercial ($p = 0.020$, OR: 5.609, CI (1.309–24.035)) or voluntary donors ($p = 0.034$, OR: 2.404, CI (1.071–5.397)) having the sickle cell trait (Table 6; see also Supplementary Tables S1 and S2 in Supplementary Material available online at http://dx.doi.org/10.1155/2016/7302912).

4. Discussion

In the blood donor preselection protocol, prospective donors are screened using haemoglobin levels and a battery of serological tests that focusses mainly on transfusion-transmitted diseases. However, this study argues a case for the widening of the predonation screening protocol to include screening for other red cell pathologies in populations in which inheritance of such pathologies is inherently high. In this study, we show that coinheritance of sickle cell haemoglobin variant and red cell G6PD enzymopathy could be as high as 7%. Moreover, we found that 19.5% of the donor blood units are prone to stressor-induced haemolysis in any prospective recipient as a consequence of their inherent G6PD enzymopathy.

Previous studies have estimated prevalence rates of sickle cell trait and/or G6PD status in various populations. For example, a study by Omisakin et al. and Jeremiah estimated prevalence of HbS trait of 26.1 and 19.68%, respectively [14, 18], in blood donors. Egesie et al. also found SCT prevalence of 20.8% in a study that involved males in Jos in Nigeria [13]. Others have also reported SCT prevalence ranging from 20 to 40% for Ghanaian populace [12, 19]. The 19.5% prevalence rate found in our blood donors is consistent with these previous works. However, a similar work done in Ghana found a comparatively lower SCT prevalence of 11.3% in a group of 150 blood donors [20]. Also, in this study, only 3% of the participants had knowledge of their sickle cell status and haemoglobin phenotype, which agrees with a study by Lippi et al., who stated that most blood donors, especially those with SCT, were not aware of their sickle cell status [21].

With regard to G6PD enzymopathy, the WHO estimates a 15–26% prevalence rate in Ghana [11]. The 19.5% prevalence of G6PD deficiency recorded in this study confirms the prevalence rate suggested by the WHO [11] for the Ghanaian populace. Moreover, prevalence of G6PD deficiency in this study was comparable to estimated G6PD enzymopathy prevalence rates in blood donors in Osogbo, Osun State, Nigeria [22], and in Yasuj, Iran [23], that reported G6PD deficiency prevalence rates of 19.5% and 14.17%, respectively. Our prevalence rate also falls within the population-based G6PD deficiency predicted by Howes et al., for Nigeria (2%–31%), Sudan (1%–29%), and Democratic Republic of Congo (4%–32%) [10]. However, a previous cross-sectional study in Nigeria reported a relatively higher prevalence rate of 25.5% in blood donors [24]. The variance may be due to the different sample sizes (200 in the present study versus 314 in that study) and/or demographics of the studied population. In spite of the fact that G6PD enzymopathy is sex-linked and has a higher frequency in males, 93% of the blood donors in the present study were males (compared to 7% females). This is interesting as in areas with high prevalence of sex-linked enzymopathies one would expect a higher proportion of female donors to reduce the likelihood of transfusing blood with red cell enzyme deficiencies. This agrees favourably with previous studies that were undertaken in Ghana [20] and Riyadh, Saudi Arabia [25], which, respectively, found 92% and 98.7% of blood donors being males. Others have

suggested such reasons as pregnancy, low body weight, and/or potential low iron levels due to menstrual cycle for the lower proportion of donors being females [26].

Presently, haemoglobin levels ≥12 g/dL are used as the threshold for predonation screening [4]. While this is necessary in ensuring that prospective donors are protected, it does not give any indication of inherited red cell haemoglobinopathies or enzymopathies. Our data shows that there is no correlation between the donor haemoglobin levels and G6PD enzyme activity or sickle cell haemoglobin trait (HbS) inheritance as well as no significant differences in the haemoglobin levels of donors with HbS trait and G6PD enzymopathy. It is estimated that most of the transfusions are used to correct malaria-induced severe anaemia [1]. Most of these cases are managed with such drugs as primaquine that can induce acute red cell haemolysis in G6PD deficient individuals with its consequent detrimental outcomes. Our study therefore strongly argues for the need to include screening for haemoglobinopathies and sickle cell trait in the predonation selection protocol in areas where genetic pressure due to malaria endemicity has led to selection of inheritance of SCT and/or G6PD enzymopathy as these offer survival advantages [5]. This is particularly important considering that prevalence of coinheritance of G6PD enzymopathy and sickle cell haemoglobin variant is estimated to be 7% in participants who donated blood at our study centre. This agrees with a previous study by Egesie et al., in Jos, Nigeria, that also found a prevalence of coinheritance of both G6PD enzymopathy and HbS variant to be 5.4% [27]. The differences in the prevalence rates could be due to the different sample sizes in the two studies; 130 blood donors in the study by Egesie et al. compared to 200 blood donors in the present study. Additionally, whereas Egesie et al. recruited donors aged between 20 and 49 years, this study recruited donors aged between 18 and 59 years. This could have also accounted for our slightly higher G6PD enzymopathy as 50.5% of our study participants were in the 18–24 years' category.

Moreover, we also found 19.5% of the donors had mild enzyme deficiency (10–60% enzyme activity). Individuals with this enzyme activity are known to undergo haemolysis when subjected to stressors like infection and/or drug therapy [11, 17]. As most of the recipients of blood in our study population may usually be suffering from severe malaria and on drug therapy, this calls for some urgency in the inclusion of G6PD and/or HbS status in all prospective donors so as to protect the potential recipients.

Our study has some limitations which include our inability to screen our G6PD deficient donors for their G6PD genotypes as these are known to impact the G6PD enzyme activity levels. Also, we acknowledge that, compared to the fluorescence spot test, the methaemoglobin reduction assay has low sensitivity with regard to heterozygous females who may have relatively high G6PD enzyme activity. Additionally, we did not make an estimate for reticulocyte counts in our study participants, although reticulocytes having remnants of RNA have higher G6PD enzyme activity. This potential confounding effect of reticulocytosis was not accounted for in our study.

5. Conclusion

The high prevalence of SCT and G6PD enzymopathy coinheritance demonstrated in this study suggests that screening for these inherited conditions must be incorporated into existing protocols. Individuals with rare blood groups, who might necessarily donate in spite of their haemoglobin variant and/or G6PD enzymopathy, must have their donated units appropriately labelled to minimise complications in high-risk recipients.

Competing Interests

The authors have no competing interests to declare.

Authors' Contributions

Patrick Adu, David Larbi Simpong, and Godfred Takyi were involved in the conception and design of the research; Patrick Adu, David Larbi Simpong, and Richard K. D. Ephraim were involved in the interpretation of data and writing the manuscript; Patrick Adu was involved in the statistical analysis of the data; Godfred Takyi performed all experimental procedures in this paper.

Acknowledgments

The authors are grateful to the entire management and laboratory staff of the Holy Trinity Hospital, Berekum, for their support.

References

[1] M. Cheeseborough, *District Laboratory Practice in Tropical Countries 2*, vol. 2, Cambridge University Press, Cambridge, UK, 2nd edition, 2006.

[2] NBSG, *National Guidelines for the Clinical use of Blood and Blood products in Ghana*, WHO Country Office, Accra, Ghana, 2013.

[3] F. Mimouni, S. Shohat, and S. H. Reisner, "G6PD-deficient donor blood as a cause of hemolysis in two preterm infants," *Israel Journal of Medical Sciences*, vol. 22, no. 2, pp. 120–122, 1986.

[4] J. Stanley, "Blood collection and processing," in *Immunohematology Principles & Practice*, pp. 3–15, Lippincott Williams & Wilkins, Baltimore, Md, USA, 2011.

[5] A. Mehta, P. J. Mason, and T. J. Vulliamy, "Glucose-6-phosphate dehydrogenase deficiency," *Best Practice and Research: Clinical Haematology*, vol. 13, no. 1, pp. 21–38, 2000.

[6] C. Ruwende and A. Hill, "Glucose-6-phosphate dehydrogenase deficiency and malaria," *Journal of Molecular Medicine*, vol. 76, no. 8, pp. 581–588, 1998.

[7] M. S. Santana, W. M. Monteiroa, A. M. Siqueiraa et al., "Glucose-6-phosphate dehydrogenase deficient variants are associated with reduced susceptibility to malaria in the Brazilian Amazon," *Transactions of the Royal Society of Tropical Medicine and Hygiene*, vol. 107, no. 5, pp. 301–306, 2013.

[8] E. Beutler, "G6PD deficiency," *Blood*, vol. 84, no. 11, pp. 3613–3636, 1994.

[9] H. G. Klein and D. J. Anstee, *Mollison's Blood Transfusion in Clinical Medicine*, Blackwell, Oxford, UK, 11th edition, 2005.

[10] R. E. Howes, F. B. Piel, A. P. Patil et al., "G6PD deficiency prevalence and estimates of affected populations in malaria endemic countries: a geostatistical model-based map," *PLoS Medicine*, vol. 9, no. 11, Article ID e1001339, 2012.

[11] WHO, *Glucose-6-Phosphate Dehydrogenase Deficiency*, WHO, Geneva, Switzerland, 1989.

[12] K. Ohene-Frempong, J. Oduro, H. Tetteh, and F. Nkrumah, "Screening newborns for sickle cell disease in Ghana," *Pediatrics*, vol. 121, supplement 2, pp. S120–S121, 2008.

[13] O. J. Egesie, D. E. Joseph, I. Isiguzoro, and U. G. Egesie, "Glucose-6-phosphate dehydrogenase (G6PD) activity and deficiency in a population of Nigerian males resident in Jos," *Nigerian Journal of Physiological Sciences*, vol. 23, no. 1-2, pp. 9–11, 2008.

[14] C. T. Omisakin, A. J. Esan, A. A. Ogunleye, O. Ojo-Bola, M. F. Owoseni, and D. P. Omoniyi, "Glucose-6-phosphate dehydrogenase (G6pd) deficiency and sickle cell trait among blood donors in Nigeria," *American Journal of Public Health Research*, vol. 2, no. 2, pp. 51–55, 2014.

[15] D. S. Young, L. C. Pestaner, and V. Gibberman, "Effects of drugs on clinical laboratory tests," *Clinical Chemistry*, vol. 21, no. 5, pp. 1D–432D, 1975.

[16] B. J. Bain, M. A. Laffan, and S. Mitchell Lewis, *Dacie and Lewis Practical Haematology*, Elsevier Churchill Livingstone, 2011.

[17] G. J. Domingo, A. W. Satyagraha, A. Anvikar et al., "G6PD testing in support of treatment and elimination of malaria: recommendations for evaluation of G6PD tests," *Malaria Journal*, vol. 12, article 391, 2013.

[18] Z. A. Jeremiah, "Abnormal haemoglobin variants, ABO and Rh blood groups among student of African descent in Port Harcourt, Nigeria," *African Health Sciences*, vol. 6, no. 3, pp. 177–181, 2006.

[19] WHO, *Management of Haemoglobin Disorders*, World Health Organization, Nicosia, Cyprus, 2008.

[20] S. Antwi-Baffour, R. O. Asare, J. K. Adjei, R. Kyeremeh, and D. N. Adjei, "Prevalence of hemoglobin S trait among blood donors: a cross-sectional study," *BMC Research Notes*, vol. 8, article 583, 2015.

[21] G. Lippi, M. Mercadanti, C. Alberta, and M. Franchini, "An unusual case of a spurious, transfusion-acquired haemoglobin S," *Blood Transfusion*, vol. 8, no. 3, pp. 199–202, 2010.

[22] E. O. Akanni, B. S. A. Osenil, V. O. Agbona et al., "Glucose-6-phosphate dehydrogenase deficiency in blood donors and jaundiced neonates in Osogbo, Nigeria," *Medical Laboratory and Diagnosis*, vol. 1, no. 1, pp. 1–4, 2010.

[23] S. H. Nabavizadeh and A. Anushiravani, "The prevalence of G6PD deficiency in blood transfusion recipients," *Hematology*, vol. 12, no. 1, pp. 85–88, 2007.

[24] C. T. Omisikan, A. J. Esan, A. A. Ogunleye, O. Ojo-Bola, M. F. Owoseni, and D. P. Omoniyi, "Glucose-6-phosphate dehydrogenase (G6pd) deficiency and sickle cell trait among blood donors in Nigeria," *American Journal of Public Health Research*, vol. 2, no. 2, pp. 51–55, 2014.

[25] M. K. Alabdulaali, K. M. Alayed, A. F. Alshaikh, and S. A. Almashhadani, "Prevalence of glucose-6-phosphate dehydrogenase deficiency and sickle cell trait among blood donors in Riyadh," *Asian Journal of Transfusion Science*, vol. 4, no. 1, pp. 31–33, 2010.

[26] M. Bani and B. Giussani, "Gender differences in giving blood: a review of the literature," *Blood Transfusion*, vol. 8, no. 4, pp. 278–287, 2010.

[27] O. J. Egesie, U. G. Egesie, E. D. Jatau, I. Isiguzoro, and D. B. Ntuhun, "Prevalence of sickle cell trait and glucose 6 phosphate dehydrogenase deficiency among blood donors in a Nigerian tertiary hospital," *African Journal of Biomedical Research*, vol. 16, no. 2, pp. 143–147, 2013.

23

Seroprevalence of Hepatitis C, Hepatitis B, Cytomegalovirus, and Human Immunodeficiency Viruses in Multitransfused Thalassemic Children in Upper Egypt

Ramadan A. Mahmoud,[1] Abdel-Azeem M. El-Mazary,[2] and Ashraf Khodeary[3]

[1]*Department of Pediatrics, Faculty of Medicine, Sohag University, Sohag 82524, Egypt*
[2]*Department of Pediatrics, Faculty of Medicine, Minia University, Minia 61111, Egypt*
[3]*Department of Clinical Pathology, Faculty of Medicine, Sohag University, Sohag 82524, Egypt*

Correspondence should be addressed to Ramadan A. Mahmoud; ramadan.aboelhassan@yahoo.com

Academic Editor: Meral Beksac

Background. Frequent blood transfusions in thalassemia major children expose them to the risk of transfusion-transmitted infections (TTIs). The aim of this study was to estimate the prevalence of hepatitis C virus (HCV), hepatitis B virus (HBV), human immunodeficiency virus (HIV), and cytomegalovirus (CMV) in thalassemic children attending the Pediatrics Departments of both Sohag and Minia Universities of Upper Egypt, during the period from May 2014 to May 2015. *Methods.* Serum samples were screened for hepatitis B surface antigen (HBsAg), anti-HCV, anti-CMV, and anti-HIV type 1 and type 2 using the Vitek Immunodiagnostic Assay System. *Results.* The frequencies of anti-HCV, HBsAg, anti-CMV, and anti-HIV type 1 and type 2 were found to be 37.11%, 4.12%, 4.12%, 0.00%, and 0.00%, respectively. Seropositivity for anti-HCV, HBsAg, and anti-CMV increased with increasing age of the patients, duration of the disease, serum ferritin level (ng/mL), and liver enzymes (U/L), while it was not significantly associated with gender, frequency of blood transfusion, or the status of splenectomy operation ($P > 0.05$). *Conclusion.* The frequency of TTIs, especially HCV, is considerably high among Egyptian children with thalassemia major. It is therefore important to implement measures to improve blood transfusion screening, such as polymerase chain reaction, in order to reduce TTIs from blood donor units.

1. Introduction

Thalassemias are the commonest monogenic disorders in the world [1], and the incidence rate is higher in the Middle East [2]. β-thalassemia constitutes a major health problem in Egypt with an estimated carrier rate of 9-10% [3]. It is an autosomal recessive disorder of hemoglobin synthesis caused by a direct downregulation in the synthesis of structurally normal β-globin chains. Due to the excess α-globin chains relative to the β-globin chains, α-globin tetramers ($\alpha 4$) are formed and interact with the red cell membrane, leading to hemolytic anemia and increased erythroid production [4].

Survival of the patients mainly depends upon regular blood transfusions, which may lead to further complications, such as absorptive iron overload and transfusion-transmitted infections (TTIs), and this may contribute to the morbidity and mortality of patients with thalassemia major [5].

Screening of donor blood through national protocols for possible infections, including hepatitis B virus (HBV), hepatitis C virus (HCV), cytomegalovirus (CMV), and human immunodeficiency virus (HIV), is considered the optimal preventive method. There is a constant need to explore the effect of currently used protocols of blood donor screening by determining the burden of TTIs in multitransfused patients [6].

In Egypt the lack of a central surveillance system for disease epidemiology is a major obstacle regarding the assessment of the current situation of infectious diseases, including TTIs, and, therefore, regional and periodic studies are the only option to monitor recent developments. There are only a few studies about TTIs in thalassemic children in Egypt [3, 7–9]. To our knowledge, no study has described the situation of TTIs in thalassemic children in Upper Egypt. These areas had low social economic income compared to other parts in Egypt [10]. The objective of this study was to evaluate the seroprevalence of HBV, HCV, CMV, and HIV. Furthermore, TTI-associated clinical and laboratory risk factors were investigated in this study including gender, family history, duration of the illness, frequency of blood transfusions, splenectomy, hemoglobin, ferritin level, creatinine levels, and liver enzymes.

2. Materials and Methods

In this cross-sectional study, we analyzed blood samples taken from 97 transfusion-dependent thalassemic children during the period from May 2014 to May 2015 in the Pediatrics Departments, Faculty of Medicine, in both Sohag and Minia Universities of Upper Egypt. Ethical approval for the study was obtained from the Research Committee of the Medical Faculty, Sohag and Minia Universities, and written informed consents were obtained from all guardians/parents of the children prior to data and sample collection.

Inclusion criteria included all known cases of β-thalassemia major according to hemoglobin electrophoresis data. Complete information regarding clinical profile and family history of patients was also mandatory for inclusion criteria.

Hemophilic children, as well as children with other types of hemolytic anemias, such as α-thalassemia, sickle cell anemia, and spherocytosis were excluded from the study.

Thalassemic children were subjected to a detailed history and thorough clinical examination. Special emphasis was given on personal history (age, gender, and location), family history (parent consanguinity, and family history of similar conditions), clinical data (age of diagnosis and number of blood transfusions), and clinical examination (pallor, jaundice, hepatomegaly, cirrhotic manifestations, splenomegaly, splenectomy, and murmur on the heart) and laboratory data (hemoglobin, serum ferritin levels, serum creatinine, and liver enzymes) were recorded.

For laboratory assessments, 7 mLs of blood was obtained by venipuncture with strict sterile measures into a sterile plane tube and pediatric EDTA vacationer tube. In children receiving blood transfusions, samples were drawn before packed-RBC transfusion. Serum was collected in two tubes: one for serological testing and the other for the HCV-RT-PCR. The serum was kept at −20°C until the time of the assay.

For the serological tests, HBsAg, HCV antibodies, CMV IgM antibodies, and HIV type 1 and type 2 antibodies were measured by the Vitek Immunodiagnostic Assay System (VIDAS-BioMerieux, France) which is an enzyme-linked fluorescent assay, and it was performed according to the manufacturer's instructions. Briefly, the instrument uses a disposable pipette tip called the solid-phase receptacle, which is coated with antigens and also acts as a pipetting device. All the ready-to-use reagents are contained in a sealed strip. The specimen (serum or plasma) is added to the reagent strip, and all the following steps of the test are done automatically, without any further manipulation.

The positive HCV cases were confirmed and tested for viral load by reverse transcriptase polymerase chain reaction (RT-PCR) [11]. RNA extraction was carried out using the Qiagen RNA extraction kit according to the kit manual. PCR was performed using the Applied Biosystems® TaqMan® Universal PCR master mix and the Applied Biosystems StepOne™ Real-Time PCR System according to the manufacturer's instructions.

A complete blood count (CBC) was performed with all samples using a Celtic autocounter after calibration. Pretransfusion samples were considered for patients requiring blood transfusions at the time of study. Serum ferritin levels, alanine transaminase level (ALT), aspartate aminotransferase (AST), and creatinine levels were measured using VIDAS.

2.1. Statistical Analysis. Data was analyzed using SPSS (Statistical Package of Social Science) version 16. Quantitative data are represented as the mean (standard deviation) or median (range). Data were analyzed using the Mann-Whitney test as they were not normally distributed. Qualitative data are presented as number and percentage and were compared using either the Chi-square test or the Fisher exact test. Graphs were produced using Excel software. The P value was considered significant at $P < 0.05$.

3. Results

In the study with a total of 97 thalassemic children, 36.08% of patients were female and 63.92% were male. The mean age at the time of study was 8.89 (5.07) years (range: 6–18 years). The mean age at diagnosis was 11.40 (13.18) months. The mean duration of the disease was 7.94 (4.90) years. The mean ferritin level was 2875 (1764) (ng/mL). Complete history and clinical examination was done for all the children included in the study as shown in Table 1.

A total of 36 patients (37.11%) were found to be anti-HCV antibody- (anti-HCV-) positive (Table 2). All positive cases were confirmed by HCV-RT-PCR. There were only 4 (4.12%) patients that were found to be positive for HBsAg and anti-CMV IgM. There were no cases that were positive for anti-HIV type 1 or type 2. Three patients had two infectious diseases simultaneously (two had HBV and HCV, and one had HCV and CMV).

The risk factors for hepatitis C virus are shown in Table 3 and include age of the patients [7.69 (5.01) years in negative cases compared to 12.63 (4.96) years in positive cases ($P = 0.04$)], mean ferritin level [2416 (1283) ng/mL in negative cases compared to 3652 (2173) ng/mL in positive cases ($P = 0.006$)], serum ALT [48 (7.4) U/L in negative cases compared to 65 (5.1) U/L in positive cases ($P = 0.001$)], serum AST [47 (9.44) U/L in negative cases compared to 61 (8.9) U/L in positive cases ($P = 0.02$)], and duration of the disease [7.75 (4.62) years in negative cases compared to 10.56 (5.48) years for positive cases ($P = 0.02$)]. With a total of 97 patients included in the study there were 6 patients (6.18%) who had manifestations of liver cirrhosis, two were HBV and HCV positive, two were HCV positive, and two were serologically free of viruses.

For hepatitis B virus infection, risk factors are shown in Table 4 and included the age of patients [7.77 (4.08%) years

TABLE 1: Demographic characteristics of beta thalassemia major children.

Characteristics		Summary statistics
Age/years	Mean (SD)	8.89 (5.07)
	Median (range)	10 (6–18)
Gender	Females	35 (36.08%)
	Males	62 (63.92%)
Age at diagnosis/months	Mean (SD)	11.40 (13.18)
	Median (range)	6 (3–72)
Frequency of blood transfusion/months	Mean (SD)	1.09 (0.42)
Duration of disease/years	Mean (SD)	7.94 (4.90)
Family history	No	42 (43.30%)
	Yes	55 (56.70%)
Ferritin level (ng/mL)	Mean (SD)	2875 (1764)
Alanine transaminase (ALT) (U/L)	Mean (SD)	55 (15.4)
Aspartate aminotransferase (AST) (U/L)	Mean (SD)	62 (9.44)
Creatinine (mg/dL)	Mean (SD)	0.6 (0.54)
Hb level (g/dL)	Mean (SD)	6.77 (1.87)
Hepatomegaly	No	9 (9.27%)
	Yes	88 (90.73%)
Splenomegaly	No	3 (3.09%)
	Yes	94 (96.9%)
Splenectomy	No	56 (57.73%)
	Yes	41 (42.27%)
Age at splenectomy/years	Mean (SD)	8.39 (2.47)
Pallor	No	11 (11.34%)
	Yes	86 (88.66%)
Jaundice	No	80 (82.47%)
	Yes	17 (17.53%)
Murmur	No	56 (57.73%)
	Yes	41 (42.27%)

TABLE 2: Prevalence of transfusion transmitted infections (TTIs) in thalassemic children.

Transfusion transmitted infections (TTIs)		Numbers (percentage)
Hepatitis C virus	Negative	61 (62.89%)
	Positive	36 (37.11%)
Hepatitis B virus	Negative	93 (95.88%)
	Positive	4 (4.12%)
CMV	Negative	93 (95.88%)
	Positive	4 (4.12%)
HIV	Negative	97 (100%)

in negative cases compared to 13.5 (1.73) years in positive cases ($P = 0.04$)], mean ferritin level [2809 (1750) ng/mL in negative cases compared to 4407 (1541) ng/mL in positive cases ($P = 0.04$)], serum ALT [43 (4.4) U/L in negative cases compared to 58 (3.5) U/L in positive cases ($P = 0.03$)], serum AST [42 (9.44) U/L in negative cases compared to 63 (6.3) U/L in positive cases ($P = 0.04$)], and duration of the disease [7.71 (4.86) years in negative cases compared to 13.25 (1.73) years in positive cases ($P = 0.02$)].

CMV risk factors are shown in Table 5 and include age of the patients [8.69 (6.01) years in negative cases compared to 13.63 (4.21) years in positive cases ($P = 0.03$)], mean ferritin level [2894 (1770) ng/mL in negative cases compared to 4735 (1789) ng/mL in positive cases ($P = 0.04$)], and mean duration of the disease [7.82 (4.92) years in negative cases compared to 13.69 (3.79) years in positive cases ($P = 0.03$)]. The distribution of disease status (thalassemia and hepatitis B, hepatitis C, CMV, and HIV) was not significantly associated with gender, frequency of blood transfusion, hemoglobin level, creatinine level, or splenectomy operations ($P > 0.05$).

4. Discussion

Thalassemia major is one of the most common autosomal single-gene thalassemic disorders. It is prevalent in more than 60 countries of the world with a carrier population of up to 150 million worldwide [12]. In order to reduce the complications of severe anemia in β-thalassemic patients,

TABLE 3: Risk factors for HCV.

Risk factors		HCV		P value*
		No (n = 61)	Yes (n = 36)	
Age/years	Mean (SD)	7.69 (5.01)	12.63 (4.96)	0.04
	Median (range)	9 (1–19)	14 (6.5–18)	
Gender	Females	26 (42.62%)	9 (25.00%)	0.08
	Males	35 (57.38%)	27 (75.00%)	
Duration of the disease/years	Mean (SD)	7.75 (4.62)	10.56 (5.48)	0.02
Frequency of blood transfusion/months	Mean (SD)	1.11 (0.48)	1.04 (0.30)	0.57
Splenectomy	No	36 (59.02%)	20 (55.56%)	0.74
	Yes	25 (40.98%)	16 (44.44%)	
Ferritin level (ng/dL)	Mean (SD)	2416 (1283)	3652 (2173)	0.006
Alanine transaminase (ALT) (U/L)	Mean (SD)	48 (7.4)	65 (5.1)	0.001
Aspartate aminotransferase (AST) (U/L)	Mean (SD)	47 (9.44)	61 (8.9)	0.02

* P values were obtained by using Mann-Whitney test or Chi-square test.

TABLE 4: Risk factors for HBV.

Risk factors		HBV		P value*
		No (n = 93)	Yes (n = 4)	
Age/years	Mean (SD)	7.77 (4.08%)	13.5 (1.73)	0.04
	Median (range)	8 (1–20)	13.5 (12–15)	
Gender	Females	34 (36.56%)	1 (25.00%)	0.08
	Males	59 (63.44%)	3 (75.00%)	
Duration of the disease/years	Mean (SD)	7.71 (4.86)	13.25 (1.73)	0.02
Frequency of blood transfusion/months	Mean (SD)	1.09 (0.43)	1 (0)	0.77
Splenectomy	No	56 (60.22%)	2 (50%)	1.00
	Yes	37 (39.78%)	2 (50%)	
Ferritin level (ng/dL)	Mean (SD)	2809 (1750)	4407 (1541)	0.04
Alanine transaminase (ALT) (U/L)	Mean (SD)	43 (4.4)	58 (3.5)	0.03
Aspartate aminotransferase (AST) (U/L)	Mean (SD)	42 (9.44)	63 (6.3)	0.04

* P values were obtained by using Mann-Whitney test or Chi-square test percentage.

early and regular blood transfusion therapy is mandatory. Thalassemic patients had a risk for iron overload and for TTIs, such as HBV, HCV, CMV, and HIV [13]. The current study focuses on the prevalence of these viruses in children attending the Pediatrics Departments of both Sohag and Minia Universities of Upper Egypt.

In Egypt, the screening tests for the blood donors include HCV antibodies, HBsAg, and HIV antibodies. Moreover, in the 2000 some blood bank added CMV antibody and syphilis antibodies to the blood donor screening [8]. These tests were done by ELISA or immunofluorescence based methods in national and governmental blood banks which have high sensitivity and specificity [14]. However, many nongovernmental and private hospitals sometimes used rapid and cheap immunochromatographic methods for blood donors screening which have lower sensitivity and specificity, which contribute to the increased rates of TTIs [15]. Furthermore, the diagnosis of viral hepatitis in the window phase is still an obstacle in Egypt, because of Egypt's constrained economy which limits the implementation of sensitive screening techniques as RT-PCR for all cases [16].

Egypt has one of the highest prevalence rates of the virus in the world; an estimated 10–15% of the population, about 8–10 million people, is carrying hepatitis C antibodies. Five million of those are actively infected. The iatrogenic role of parenteral antischistosomal therapy campaigns carried out until the 1980s may have contributed to such high incidence of HCV. Sharing razors, piercing, and tattooing were also suggested as possible explanations [17].

The implementation of routine blood donor screening tests for HCV in the early 1990s led to a reduction in the transfusion of HCV to blood recipients [18], from about 70% in one cohort study [19] to 37% in this present study. Furthermore, the introduction of advanced screening methods, such as RT-PCR, has led to a further decline in transfusion-related viral hepatitis [11]. RT-PCR technologies can detect viremia earlier than the existing screening tests. Blood centers in some developed countries as the United States have implemented RT-PCR routinely for all blood donations since 1999. This strategy has reduced the window period for HCV detection by 50–60 days and decreased the risk for HCV transmission from 1 in 103,000 to 1 in 2,000,000 transfused units [20].

TABLE 5: Risk factors for CMV.

Risk factors		No ($n = 93$)	Yes ($n = 4$)	P value*
		CMV		
Age/years	Mean (SD)	8.69 (6.01)	13.63 (4.21)	0.03
	Median (range)	10 (1–21)	15 (6.5–18)	
Gender	Females	32 (34.41%)	3 (75.00%)	0.14
	Males	61 (65.59%)	1 (25.00%)	
Duration of the disease/years	Mean (SD)	7.82 (4.92)	13.69 (3.79)	0.03
Frequency of blood transfusion/months	Mean (SD)	1.09 (0.43)	0.88 (0.25)	0.21
Splenectomy	No	55 (59.14%)	1 (25.00%)	0.31
	Yes	38 (40.86%)	3 (75.00%)	
Ferritin level (ng/dL)	Mean (SD)	2894 (1770)	4735 (1789)	0.04
Alanine transaminase (ALT) (U/L)	Mean (SD)	55 (3.4)	56 (3.7)	0.43
Aspartate aminotransferase (AST) (U/L)	Mean (SD)	50 (6.44)	54 (6.8)	0.14

* P values were obtained by using Mann-Whitney test, Chi-square test, or Fisher exact test.

However, despite these efforts, posttransfusion transmission of HCV has remained a major health problem in multitransfused patients, leading to increased morbidity and mortality. In the present study, more than 37% of patients were positive for anti-HCV. These results can be compared with previously conducted studies from other regions of Egypt, such as anti-HCV in one Egyptian report of about 34% [7], and in another study of about 24% [8]. Moreover, in other countries, anti-HCV-positive cases were about 40.5% in Jordan [21], 30% in India [22], and 35% in Pakistan [23].

Furthermore, the severity of liver cirrhosis due to HCV in patients with thalassemia may be greater because of concomitant iron overload. It has been demonstrated that iron and HCV infection are independent but mutually reinforcing risk factors for the development of liver fibrosis and cirrhosis. It appears therefore that patients with thalassemia, particularly those with poor control of iron overload, face an increased risk of developing cirrhosis [24].

In the present study, four patients were HCV positive and had manifestations of liver cirrhosis. Ardalan et al. found that the rate of liver fibrosis accelerated in patients with iron overload and HCV when compared to patients with thalassemia major alone [25]. Moreover, Zurlo et al. found that advanced liver fibrosis is one of the most common causes of death in transfusion-dependent thalassemia patients over 15 years old [26].

Children with thalassemia major are particularly susceptible to HBV because they receive multiple blood transfusions. These children have higher infection rates than normal children. Egypt has adopted a universal hepatitis B vaccine service for infants since 1992. The primary objective of vaccination is to eliminate chronic HBV infections and ultimately reduce the reservoir for new infections [17]. In the present study, about 4% were positive for HBV, and in another Egyptian study [8], about 3% were positive for HBV. These results were slightly higher than a recent North Indian study, in which out of the 462 thalassemic children 13 cases (2.8%) were positive for HBsAg by ELISA [27], and also higher than an Iranian study in which only 1.5% were HBsAg positive [28].

Screening in most Egyptian blood banks is performed for HBsAg but not for core antibody (anti-HBc). Anti-HBc appears at the onset of acute HBV infection and may also indicate chronic infection. The routine implementation of anti-HBc testing was recommended to reduce the risk of transfusion-transmitted HBV. In a previous Egyptian study, 7.8% of blood samples were anti-HBc positive, of which 6.25% were HBV DNA positive [29]. In another Egyptian study by Said et al., they found that the prevalence of anti-HBc among HBsAg negative blood donors was 14.2% [30]. Furthermore, HBV can also be transmitted through components that are HBsAg negative but HBV DNA positive. Altindis et al. recommended routine screening of blood units by sensitive PCR-based methods, to detect possible occult HBV infections [31].

For CMV, only 4% of thalassemic patients were CMV positive, and these results were slightly higher than the Jamal et al. study in Malaysia [32], which found that the incidence of CMV was about 1.8%. Transfusion-transmitted HIV is, fortunately, not a major cause for concern, owing to advanced testing techniques, such as the recent generation of ELISA screening tests, as well as decreasing prevalence of such diseases, which is less than 0.02% in Egyptian population [33], conservative culture, and increasing awareness about this infection in the general population. Therefore, in this study, we did not find any positive cases for HIV type 1 or type 2. These results corroborate other studies [28, 32] that also found no positive cases for HIV in thalassemic patients. Nevertheless, an Indian study found that the seroprevalence of HIV was about 1.5% [34].

As shown in the present study, patients with thalassemia have a high prevalence of hepatitis B and hepatitis C infections. Furthermore, HCV and HBV infected patients had significantly higher liver enzymes than noninfected patients. Chronic hepatitis C virus infection has been associated with liver iron loading. The cause of elevated serum iron indices in some HCV-infected individuals is not clear. The concomitant increase of serum AST and ALT levels suggests that iron and ferritin are released from damaged hepatocytes as a result of hepatic necroinflammation [35]. In addition, increased iron has been shown to enhance HCV replication in vitro [36].

In the current study, splenomegaly was observed in 96.9% of patients, whereas 90.73% of patients had hepatomegaly. The distribution of HCV, HBV, CMV, and HIV was studied by considering different clinical parameters related to thalassemia. In this study, we found that older age of the patients, longer duration of the disease in years, elevated liver enzymes (U/L), and increasing ferritin level (ng/mL) are associated with higher seroprevalence of TTIs. Similar findings were reported by other studies [37–39]. Though the standardized blood screening procedures were outlined in the 1990s for blood-related products and were subsequently implemented in various countries, higher prevalence of TTIs, especially HCV, among thalassemic patients requires greater attention from a public health perspective. Screening of blood donors by advanced ELISA screening tests and RT-PCR could detect HCV in early stages of diseases and will provide better opportunities for risk assessment.

5. Conclusion

A total of 97 homozygous β-thalassemia patients were included in this study. The seroprevalence of HCV was the highest TTI in thalassemic children, with a lower percentage for HBV and CMV cases but there were no HIV cases. These seroprevalence-positive cases were significantly associated with older age, longer duration of diseases, increased liver enzymes, and higher ferritin levels. Recent solid-blood screening programs including advanced ELISA screening tests, liver enzymes, and RT-PCR will hopefully reduce the risk of TTIs associated with blood transfusions.

Conflict of Interests

The authors had no conflict of interests.

Acknowledgment

The authors thank proof-reading-services.com for linguistic editing.

References

[1] S. L. Thein, "Genetic modifiers of β-thalassemia," *Haematologica*, vol. 90, no. 5, pp. 649–660, 2005.

[2] S. H. Ansari, T. S. Shamsi, M. Ashraf et al., "Molecular epidemiology of β-thalassemia in Pakistan: far reaching implications," *International Journal of Molecular Epidemiology and Genetics*, vol. 2, no. 4, pp. 403–408, 2011.

[3] A. El-Beshlawy, N. Kaddah, A. Moustafa, G. Mouktar, and I. Youssry, "Screening for β-thalassaemia carriers in Egypt: significance of the osmotic fragility test," *Eastern Mediterranean Health Journal*, vol. 13, no. 4, pp. 780–786, 2007.

[4] S. L. Schrier, "Pathophysiology of thalassemia," *Current Opinion in Hematology*, vol. 9, no. 2, pp. 123–126, 2002.

[5] C. Skarmoutsou, I. Papassotiriou, J. Traeger-Synodinos et al., "Erythroid bone marrow activity and red cell hemoglobinization in iron-sufficient β-thalassemia heterozygotes as reflected by soluble transferrin receptor and reticulocyte hemoglobin

content. Correlation with genotypes and HB A2 levels," *Haematologica*, vol. 88, no. 6, pp. 631–636, 2003.

[6] S. Aziz, J. Rajper, and W. Noorulain, "Treatment outcome of HCV infected paediatric patients and young adults at Karachi, Pakistan," *Journal of Ayub Medical College, Abbottabad*, vol. 24, no. 3-4, pp. 56–58, 2012.

[7] F. Said, A. E. Beshlawy, M. Hamdy et al., "Intrafamilial transmission of hepatitis C infection in Egyptian multitransfused thalassemia patients," *Journal of Tropical Pediatrics*, vol. 59, no. 4, pp. 309–313, 2013.

[8] E. Hussein, "Evaluation of infectious disease markers in multi-transfused Egyptian children with thalassemia," *Annals of Clinical and Laboratory Science*, vol. 44, no. 1, pp. 62–66, 2014.

[9] A. A. Adly and F. S. Ebeid, "Cultural preferences and limited public resources influence the spectrum of thalassemia in Egypt," *Journal of Pediatric Hematology/Oncology*, vol. 37, no. 4, pp. 281–284, 2015.

[10] B. S. Buckner and E. B. Buckner, "Post-revolution Egypt: the Roy adaptation model in community," *Nursing Science Quarterly*, vol. 28, no. 4, pp. 300–307, 2015.

[11] C. Velati, L. Romanò, L. Fomiatti et al., "Impact of nucleic acid testing for hepatitis B virus, hepatitis C virus, and human immunodeficiency virus on the safety of blood supply in Italy: a 6-year survey," *Transfusion*, vol. 48, no. 10, pp. 2205–2213, 2008.

[12] L. A. Quratul-Ain, M. Hassan, S. M. Rana, and F. Jabeen, "Prevalence of β-thalassemic patients associated with consanguinity and anti-HCV-antibody positivity—a cross sectional study," *Pakistan Journal of Zoology*, vol. 43, no. 1, pp. 29–36, 2011.

[13] A. H. Mollah, N. Nahar, A. Siddique, K. S. Anwar, T. Hassan, and G. Azam, "Common transfusion-transmitted infectious agents among thalassaemic children in Bangladesh," *Journal of Health Population and Nutrition*, vol. 21, no. 1, pp. 67–71, 2003.

[14] J. M. Barrera, B. Francis, G. Ercilla et al., "Improved detection of anti-HCV in post-transfusion hepatitis by a third-generation ELISA," *Vox Sanguinis*, vol. 68, no. 1, pp. 15–18, 1995.

[15] A. A. Adeyemi, O. A. Omolade, and R. R. Raheem-Ademola, "Immunochromatographic testing method for hepatitis B, C in blood donors," *Journal of Antivirals & Antiretrovirals*, vol. 3, no. 10, pp. 4172–4175, 2013.

[16] H. Zaghloul and M. El-Shahat, "Recombinase polymerase amplification as a promising tool in hepatitis C virus diagnosis," *World Journal of Hepatology*, vol. 6, no. 12, pp. 916–922, 2014.

[17] E. Hussein, "Blood donor recruitment strategies and their impact on blood safety in Egypt," *Transfusion and Apheresis Science*, vol. 50, no. 1, pp. 63–67, 2014.

[18] J. G. Donahue, A. Muñoz, P. M. Ness et al., "The declining risk of post-transfusion hepatitis C virus infection," *The New England Journal of Medicine*, vol. 327, no. 6, pp. 369–373, 1992.

[19] K. Al-Naamani, I. Al-Zakwani, S. Al-Sinani, F. Wasim, and S. Daar, "Prevalence of hepatitis C among multi-transfused thalassaemic patients in Oman, single centre experience," *Sultan Qaboos University Medical Journal*, vol. 15, no. 1, pp. e46–e51, 2015.

[20] S. L. Stramer, S. A. Glynn, S. H. Kleinman et al., "National heart, lung, and blood institute nucleic acid test study group. Detection of HIV-1 and HCV infections among antibody negative blood donors by nucleic acid-amplification testing," *The New England Journal of Medicine*, vol. 351, no. 8, pp. 760–768, 2004.

[21] M. Al-Sheyyab, A. Batieha, and M. El-Khateeb, "The prevalence of hepatitis B, hepatitis C and human immune deficiency

virus markers in multi-transfused patients," *Journal of Tropical Pediatrics*, vol. 47, no. 4, pp. 239–242, 2001.

[22] M. Irshad and S. Peter, "Spectrum of viral hepatitis in thalassemic children receiving multiple blood transfusions," *Indian Journal of Gastroenterology*, vol. 21, no. 5, pp. 183–184, 2002.

[23] M. Rahman and Y. Lodhi, "Prospects and future of conservative management of beta thalassemia major in a developing country," *Pakistan Journal of Medical Sciences*, vol. 20, no. 2, pp. 105–112, 2004.

[24] E. Angelucci, P. Muretto, A. Nicolucci et al., "Effects of iron overload and hepatitis C virus positivity in determining progression of liver fibrosis in thalassemia following bone marrow transplantation," *Blood*, vol. 100, no. 1, pp. 17–21, 2002.

[25] F. A. Ardalan, M. R. F. Osquei, M. N. Toosi, and G. Irvanloo, "Synergic effect of chronic hepatitis C infection and beta thalassemia major with marked hepatic iron overload on liver fibrosis: a retrospective cross-sectional study," *BMC Gastroenterology*, vol. 4, article 17, 2004.

[26] M. Zurlo, P. De Stefano, C. Borgna-Pignatti et al., "Survival and causes of death in thalassaemia major," *The Lancet*, vol. 334, no. 8653, pp. 27–30, 1989.

[27] R. N. Makroo, J. S. Arora, M. Chowdhry, A. Bhatia, U. K. Thakur, and A. Minimol, "Red cell alloimmunization and infectious marker status (human immunodeficiency virus, hepatitis B virus and hepatitis C virus) in multiply transfused thalassemia patients of North India," *Indian Journal of Pathology and Microbiology*, vol. 56, no. 4, pp. 378–383, 2013.

[28] S. Mirmomen, S.-M. Alavian, B. Hajarizadeh et al., "Epidemiology of hepatitis B, hepatitis C, and human immunodeficiency virus infections in patients with beta-thalassemia in Iran: a multicenter study," *Archives of Iranian Medicine*, vol. 9, no. 4, pp. 319–323, 2006.

[29] W. Antar, M. H. El-Shokry, W. A. Abd El Hamid, and M. F. Helmy, "Significance of detecting anti-HBc among Egyptian male blood donors negative for HBsAg," *Transfusion Medicine*, vol. 20, no. 6, pp. 409–413, 2010.

[30] Z. N. Said, M. H. El Sayed, I. I. Salama et al., "Occult hepatitis B virus infection among Egyptian blood donors," *World Journal of Hepatology*, vol. 5, no. 2, pp. 64–73, 2013.

[31] M. Altindis, I. Uslan, Z. Cetinkaya et al., "Investigation of hemodialysis patients in terms of the presence of occult hepatitis B," *Mikrobiyoloji Bülteni*, vol. 41, no. 2, pp. 227–233, 2007.

[32] R. Jamal, G. Fadzillah, S. Z. Zulkifli, and M. Yasmin, "Seroprevalence of hepatitis B, hepatitis C, CMV and HIV in multiply transfused thalassemia patients: results from a thalassemia day care center in Malaysia," *Southeast Asian Journal of Tropical Medicine and Public Health*, vol. 29, no. 4, pp. 792–804, 1998.

[33] D. Oraby, "Harm reduction approach in Egypt: the insight of injecting drug users," *Harm Reduction Journal*, vol. 10, article 17, 2013.

[34] S. Manisha, K. Sanjeev, N. Seema, C. Dilip, and D. Rashmi, "A cross-sectional study on burden of hepatitis C, hepatitis B, HIV and syphilis in multi-transfused thalassemia major patients reporting to a Government Hospital of Central India," *Indian Journal of Hematology and Blood Transfusion*, vol. 31, no. 3, pp. 367–373, 2015.

[35] J. E. Nelson and K. V. Kowdley, "Iron and hepatitis C," *Current Hepatitis Reports*, vol. 3, no. 4, pp. 140–147, 2004.

[36] S. Kakizaki, H. Takagi, N. Horiguchi et al., "Iron enhances hepatitis C virus replication in cultured human hepatocytes," *Liver*, vol. 20, no. 2, pp. 125–128, 2000.

[37] H. Hussain, R. Iqbal, M. H. Khan et al., "Prevalence of hepatitis C in β thalassaemia major," *Gomal Journal of Medical Sciences*, vol. 6, no. 2, pp. 87–90, 2008.

[38] M. A. Shah, M. T. Khan, Z. Ullah, and Y. Ashfaq, "Prevalence of hepatitis B and C virus infection in multiple transfused thalassemic patients in North West Frontier Province," *Pakistan Journal of Medical Sciences*, vol. 21, no. 4, pp. 281–283, 2005.

[39] M. R. Uddin, M. Rana, M. Islam et al., "Seroprevalence of hepatitis C virus in thalassemic patients," *Journal of Dhaka Medical College*, vol. 18, no. 2, pp. 115–119, 2009.

24

Regulatory T Cells and Profile of FOXP3 Isoforms Expression in Peripheral Blood of Patients with Myelodysplastic Syndromes

Galina A. Dudina ⓘ,[1] Almira D. Donetskova,[2,3] Marina M. Litvina ⓘ,[2] Alexander N. Mitin ⓘ,[2] Tatiana A. Mitina,[4] and Sergey A. Polyakov[5]

[1]*Loginov Moscow Clinical Center of the Moscow Health Department, 111123 Moscow, Russia*
[2]*National Research Center–Institute of Immunology Federal Medical-Biological Agency of Russia, 115522 Moscow, Russia*
[3]*Pirogov Russian National Research Medical University, 117997 Moscow, Russia*
[4]*Moscow Regional Research Clinical Institute Named after MF Vladimirsky, 129110 Moscow, Russia*
[5]*Celgene International Holdings Corporation, 125047 Moscow, Russia*

Correspondence should be addressed to Galina A. Dudina; 4ex@inbox.ru

Academic Editor: Meral Beksac

We have investigated the frequencies of regulatory T cells and the level of FOXP3 isoforms expression in peripheral blood of patients with myelodysplastic syndromes and found the significant reduction of regulatory T cells at all stages of the disease. At the same time in untreated patients, we observed the shift in the FOXP3 isoforms expression profile towards the full-length molecule possibly due to inflammation. Based on the already known information about the potentially higher functional activity of FOXP3 molecule lacking exon 2, we have also hypothesized that our finding may explain the high risk of autoimmune disorders in this disease.

1. Introduction

Myelodysplastic syndrome (MDS) is a heterogeneous group of diseases, caused by clonal stem cell disorders, with the specific sign of peripheral cytopenia due to ineffective hemopoiesis with normal or increased cellularity of the bone marrow. The clinical manifestations, course, and outcome of MDS are highly diverse, and the median survival varies from 6 months to 5 years [1]. MDS has always been viewed through the prism of clonal expansion of hematopoietic progenitor cell with further risk of transformation into acute myeloid leukemia (AML) in approximately 30–40% of patients [2]. Despite the existence of prediction scales with a well-defined prognostic structure based on cytological and cytogenetic laboratory parameters the course of the disease and the progression of leukemic infiltration are often very unpredictable. The problems of predicting acute leukemia, in turn, make it difficult to select the treatment tactics. The number of clinical studies aimed at investigating new approaches to stratifying the risk of the disease progression is growing every year.

Considering that the immune system plays an active role in the pathogenesis of MDS, one can assume that some immunological parameters, for example, the number of regulatory T cells (Treg), can be used as prognostic criteria. To some extent participation of Treg in MDS pathogenesis can explain the association of this disease with both autoimmune disorders [3] and tumor transformation [1], considering that low quantity and decreased function of Treg lead to weak suppression of excessive immune response, while a high number and increased function of Treg can lead to disruption of the immune surveillance of tumor growth.

Most of the conducted studies link increased Treg frequencies with an unfavorable MDS prognosis [4–7]. Despite a similar conclusion in these studies, the data obtained on the number of Treg in MDS were rather contradictory, probably relating to different sample preparation protocols and gating strategies used in flow cytometry analysis [8]. This assumption is indirectly confirmed by differences in Treg frequencies in the age-matched healthy donors.

Attempts to use functional Treg characteristics as a prognostic criterion for MDS have also been made. Mailloux et al.

TABLE 1: Groups of patients with MDS.

Group	MDS-primary, $n=21$	E-MDS, $n=27$	L-MDS, $n=28$	Age control, $n=26$
Age, years	72 (64–76.5)	71.5 (64-76)	68.5 (63-73)	72 (48-79)
p	0.53	0.67	0.96	-
Sex				
Male	7 (33.3%)	12 (44.4%)	16 (57.1%)	11 (42.3%)
Female	14 (66.7%)	15 (55.6%)	12 (42.9%)	15 (57.7%)
p	0.56	1.0	0.41	-

Note: p value is pointed relatively to age control group (two-tailed Fisher's exact test for sex, Mann-Whitney U test for age).

have demonstrated that an increased number of Treg with the effector memory T-cells phenotype correlated with a poor prognosis of MDS, such as transformation into acute myeloid leukemia and low survival [9]. However, the obtained results may not be so much a prognostic criterion but the reflection of a specific stage of the disease.

Before considering the functional Treg characteristics as a prognostic criterion for MDS, one must take into account that the main regulator of Treg differentiation and function is the FOXP3 transcription factor [10]. So the features of its expression should have a significant effect on the Treg function. In the studies of the molecular structure of FOXP3, it has been determined that alternative splicing in humans results in four mRNA variants and four isoforms of FOXP3: the full-length molecule (FOXP3-FL); with exon 2 deletion (FOXP3Δ2); with exon 7 deletion (FOXP3Δ7); and with simultaneous deletion of exons 2 and 7 (FOXP3Δ2Δ7) [11–13]. In a recently published review [14], Mailer R. analyzes in detail the biology of FOXP3 alternative splicing and the specific functions of FOXP3 isoforms. Functional significance of the regions encoded by the deleted exons is different. In brief, exon 2 encodes the FOXP3 domain responsible for binding transcription factors of RORα and RORγt families [15, 16] that determine the proinflammatory Th17 polarization of the immune response; exon 7 encodes the sequence responsible for FOXP3 dimerization, and its absence disrupts the Treg suppressor function [13, 17]. An essential feature of FOXP3 molecules lacking exon 2 and 7 products is their preferential localization within the nucleus: Magg et al. have shown that they lose nuclear export signal (NES) sequences located in the regions encoded by exons 1/2 and 6/7 [18]. This group has also demonstrated that FOXP3 expression is mainly detected in the cytoplasm upon activation of naive $CD4^+CD25^-$ T cells, in contrast to a predominant localization in the nucleus in $CD4^+CD25^+$ Treg [18]. Localization of FOXP3 within the nucleus is very crucial for its function as a transcriptional activator and suppressor. Therefore, we can assume that FOXP3Δ2, which has a suppressor function and is located predominantly in the nucleus, is the dominant isoform that determines Treg functional activity.

Considering the inconsistency of the available data on the number of Treg, their potentially important role in MDS pathogenesis, and functional differences between expressed FOXP3 isoforms, we decided to evaluate not only the number and percentage of Treg in this disease but also the level of

FOXP3 isoforms expression in patients with MDS at different stages of the disease.

2. Materials and Methods

Seventy-six MDS patients were enrolled in the study (Table 1). They were divided into three groups: primary (MDS-primary), early-stage (E-MDS), and late-stage MDS (L-MDS). Patients before treatment (any stage of disease) represented the MDS-primary group. E-MDS and L-MDS groups consisted of pretreated patients. They were divided according to the International Prognostic Scoring System (IPSS). Using blast percentage, karyotype, and number of cytopenias, this scoring system reliably estimates survival and risk of leukemic transformation [1]. In the IPSS, cytopenias were defined as hemoglobin < 10 g/dL, absolute neutrophil count < 1.83×10^9/L, and platelet count < 100×10^9/L. Cytogenetic categories were as follows: good (normal, -Y, del (20q), del (5q)), poor (chromosome 7 abnormalities, and complex which is defined as 3 or more abnormalities), and intermediate (all other abnormalities). Pretreated patients who scored less than or equal to 1.0 according to IPSS (low and intermediate-1 risk groups) were assembled into E-MDS group. Pretreated patients who scored 1.5 and more according to IPSS (intermediate-2 and high-risk groups) were assembled into L-MDS group. MDS-primary group included 21 patients (14 women, 7 men) and age median was 72.0 (64–76.5) years. E-MDS group included 27 patients (15 women, 12 men), age median was 71.5 (64–76) years. L-MDS group included 28 patients (12 women, 16 men), age median was 68.5 (63–73) years. Twenty-six age-matched healthy donors (15 women, 11 men), age median of 72 (48–79) years, were enrolled as an age control group (Table 1). Thus, the patient characteristics were similar to each other in the age and sex and corresponded to the age control group. All patients from the E-MDS and L-MDS groups were red blood cell (RBC) transfusion dependent. The blood transfusion burden ranged from 2–3 to 5–6 packed RBC units per month. Patients had been receiving RBC transfusions from 4 months to 5 years. The study was conducted before prescription of hypomethylating or cytostatic therapy even in the L-MDS group.

MDS patients (up to 20% blasts) of any IPSS risk aged 18 years and more who signed informed consent form were included in the study. Patients with other malignancies, with severe uncontrolled cooccurring chronic and recurrent

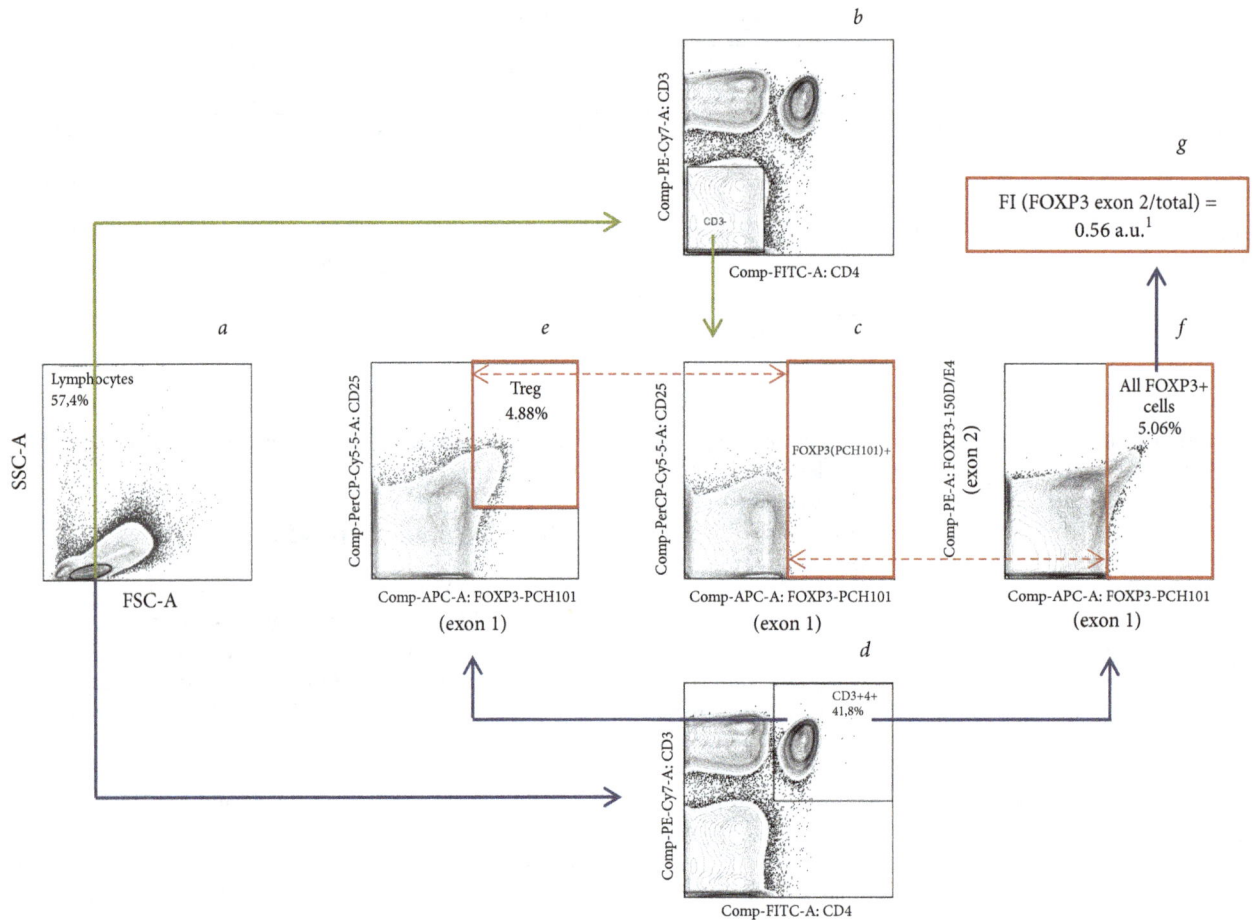

FIGURE 1: Flow cytometry. The algorithm of regulatory T cells gating using PBMCs[2] of the 74-year-old healthy donor. (a) Lymphocytes among PBMCs. (b–c) Establishing FOXP3[+] gate using CD3[−] cells known not to express FOXP3: CD3[−] cells among lymphocytes (b); establishing FOXP3 (exon 1)[+] gate using CD3[−] cells (c). (d–e) Detection of Treg: CD4[+] T cells among lymphocytes (d); CD25[+] FOXP3 (exon 1)[+] – Treg among CD4[+] T cells (e). (f–g) Analysis of FOXP3 isoform expression: all FOXP3[+] cells among CD4[+] T cells (f); calculation of FI (FOXP3 exon 2/total) parameter in all FOXP3[+] cells = [(FOXP3 exon 2 MFI)/(FOXP3 exon 1 MFI)] (g). The solid arrows show the gating algorithm. The dashed bidirectional arrows show the alignment of the established gates for CD3[−] and CD3[+]CD4[+] cells. [1]a.u.: arbitrary units; [2]PBMCs: peripheral blood mononuclear cells.

diseases, pregnant or breastfeeding women, and patients with psychiatric disorders making the patient unable to sign informed consent were excluded.

The study material was peripheral blood. Blood samples were collected into the test tubes with an anticoagulant. Cells were counted on a hematology analyzer according to the conventional technique. Isolation of peripheral blood mononuclear cells (PBMCs) and their subsequent analysis were carried out within the next 6 hours.

PBMCs were isolated by centrifugation in a Ficoll density gradient (1.077 g/cm^3), suspended in PBS with 1% BSA and 0.01% NaN$_3$ (washing and incubation buffer), and incubated with monoclonal antibodies (MAbs) against surface markers for 30 min at 4°C. Then cells were washed and permeabilized for 40 min in Foxp3 Fixation/Permeabilization Buffer (eBioscience) according to the company's methodological guidelines, washed again and incubated for 90 min at 4°C in the dark with anti-FOXP3 MAbs, washed for the last time, and analyzed immediately using a flow cytometer. As Treg is a minor population, at least 2×10^5 cells entering the

lymphocyte gate were analyzed, and this made it possible to reduce the error. Flow cytometry was performed on a BD FACSCanto™ II flow cytometer (Becton Dickinson) in the standard mode. The data were analyzed using FlowJo software (Treestar).

MAbs labeled with different fluorophores, i.e., FITC (fluorescein isothiocyanate), PE (phycoerythrin), APC (allophycocyanin), PerCP-eFluor 710 (peridinin-chlorophyll-protein-eFluor 710), and PE-Cy7 (phycoerythrin-cyanin7), were used. The following combination of MAbs manufactured by eBioscience was used (isotype controls from the same company): CD3-PE-Cy7, CD4-FITC, CD25-PerCP-eFluor710, FOXP3 (PCH101)-APC, and FOXP3 (150D/E4)-PE. The peculiarity of this technique is the epitope specificity of anti-FOXP3 MAbs. The PCH101 MAbs recognize the FOXP3 epitope encoded by exon 1; in other words, all FOXP3 isoforms, and the 150D/E4 MAbs recognize the epitope encoded by exon 2, i.e., FOXP3-FL and FOXP3Δ7 exclusively. The gating algorithm for discrimination of Treg is presented in Figure 1, a, d, e, and all FOXP3[+] cells are presented in Figure 1, a, d, *f*. Previous studies have shown that it is impossible to divide the FOXP3$^+$ population according to the level of FOXP3 isoforms expression and it is useful to estimate the ratio of the appropriate fluorescent intensities in the total FOXP3$^+$ population [19, 20]. Thus we determined the mean fluorescent intensities (MFI) of fluorophore-conjugated MAbs binding to FOXP3 exon 2 (FOXP3 exon 2 MFI) and exon 1 (FOXP3 exon 1 MFI) in all CD3$^+$CD4$^+$FOXP3$^+$ cells to derive parameter FI (FOXP3 exon 2/total) = [(FOXP3 exon 2 MFI)/(FOXP3 exon 1 MFI)] (Figure 1, f, g), as it was described previously [19]. CD3$^-$ cells that do not express FOXP3 were used as a negative control for the establishment of the gate for FOXP3$^+$ cells (see Figure 1, *a–c*).

The statistical analysis was performed using nonparametric statistics. The parameters were presented as *Me* (*L-H*), where *Me* is the median, *L* is the lower quartile, and *H* is the upper quartile. We used Kruskal-Wallis test to analyze four groups. In case of statistically significant differences between groups, we used Mann–Whitney *U* test to compare the quantitative characteristics of the two groups. The relative frequencies were presented using 95% confidence intervals as X [X1; X2], where X was a frequency and X1 and X2 were the lower and upper confidence limits, respectively. We used two-tailed Fisher's exact test for comparing two independent binomial proportions. A p value less than 0.05 was considered statistically significant. Data analysis was performed with StatSoft Statistica v.12.0.

3. Results

Seventy-six patients with the verified diagnosis of MDS were examined in accordance with the World Health Organization classification for tumors of the hematopoietic and lymphoid tissues (2008) (Table 2). 14 patients had refractory anemia (RA), six had an isolated deletion of the long arm of chromosome 5 (del(5q)), 5 had refractory anemia with ring sideroblasts (RARS), 17 had refractory cytopenia with multilineage dysplasia (RCMD), 15 had refractory anemia with excess blasts 1 (RAEB-1), and 19 had RAEB-2. 48 patients had no karyotype changes, and 28 had the following chromosomal abnormalities: 6 patients, del(5q); 4 patients, del(7q); 2 patients, del(20q); 2 patients, del(Y); 8 had abnormalities of two chromosomes, and 6 had more than three clonal chromosome rearrangements. In accordance with IPSS all MDS population was classified into low-risk (19 patients), intermediate-1 risk (12 patients), intermediate-2 risk (19 patients), and high-risk groups (26 patients). Pretreated patients divided by this criterion in the two groups (E-MDS and L-MDS) were represented as follows: low-risk, 13 patients; intermediate-1 risk, patients 14; intermediate-2 risk, patients 10; and high-risk groups, 18 patients. It should be noted beforehand that all the results obtained for the E-MDS and L-MDS groups had no statistically significant differences, so in the text below the significance of the differences is mentioned only in the context of a comparison with the MDS-primary or age control groups. However, we did not join E-MDS and L-MDS groups to emphasize the absence of these differences in our study, despite previous findings

TABLE 2: The characteristics of patients with MDS.

Parameter	Patients with MDS, *n*=76	Frequency, %
Age, years	69 (63–76)	-
Sex		
Male	35	46.1 [34.8; 57.3]
Female	41	53.9 [42.7; 65.2]
MDS variant (WHO2008)		
RA[1]	14	18.4 [9.7; 27.1]
MDS associated with isolated	6	7.9 [1.8; 14.0]
del(5q)	5	6.6 [1.0; 12.2]
RARS[2]	17	22.4 [13.0; 31.7]
RCMD[3]	15	19.7 [10.8; 28.7]
RAEB[4]-1	19	25.0 [15.3; 34.7]
RAEB-2		
Karyotype		
Normal	48	63.2 [52.3; 74.0]
Abnormal*	28	36.8 [26.0; 47.7]
IPSS		
Low	19	25.0 [15.3; 34.7]
Intermediate-1	12	15.8 [7.6; 24.0]
Intermediate-2	19	25.0 [15.3; 34.7]
High	26	34.2 [23.5; 44.9]

Note: *The karyotype changes are described in the text. [1]RA, refractory anemia; RARS, refractory anemia with ring sideroblasts; RCMD, refractory cytopenia with multilineage dysplasia; RAEB, refractory anemia with excess blasts.

linking a poor prognosis of the disease with increased Treg frequencies [4–7].

In all MDS groups, the absolute number of leukocytes, lymphocytes, and CD4$^+$ T cells in peripheral blood was reduced in comparison with the age control group (Table 3), which is typical for MDS. In pretreated patients (E-MDS and L-MDS groups), the decrease in the number of leukocytes and lymphocytes became more notable in comparison with the primary patients. In addition, there was a significant decrease in the number of CD4$^+$ T cells in the L-MDS group. However, in contrast to the previously published data on the possible increase in the number of Treg in certain cases of MDS [3–6], we observed an approximately twofold decrease in the absolute number of Treg in all MDS groups compared to the age control group (Table 4). It is necessary to clarify that only cells with CD3$^+$CD4$^+$CD25$^+$FOXP3$^+$ phenotype were considered as Treg. FOXP3 expression, in this case, was determined by the binding of cells with PCH101 MAbs (Figure 1, *e*) which detect all FOXP3 molecules. The quantitative decrease of Treg was proportional to the degree of leukopenia and somewhat more notable than the reduction in the number of lymphocytes and all CD4$^+$ T cells, which is evident in the graphs with the absolute number of cell populations in the peripheral blood of MDS patients (Figure 2). The more notable Treg reduction in comparison with all CD4$^+$ T cells was due to a decrease in the percentage of Treg among

TABLE 3: The absolute number of cell populations in the peripheral blood of patients with MDS and age-matched healthy donors (10^9 cells/L).

Group	Leukocytes	Lymphocytes	CD4$^+$T cells
Age control, n=26	6.15 (5.4–7.7)	2.0 (1.7–2.4)	0.8 (0.6–1.0)
MDS-primary[1], n=21	4.1* (3.0–5.8)	1.6 (1.2–2.6)	0.5* (0.4–0.9)
E-MDS[2], n=27	3.1**† (2.0–3.9)	1.2**† (0.9–1.5)	0.4** (0.3–0.6)
L-MDS[3], n=28	2.6**† (1.7–3.9)	1.1*† (0.8–2.1)	0.4*† (0.2–0.6)

Note: *$p<0.05$ rel. to age control; **$p<0.001$ rel. to age control; $^†p<0.05$ rel. to MDS-primary. [1]MDS-primary, primary myelodysplastic syndrome; [2]E-MDS, early-stage myelodysplastic syndrome; [3]L-MDS, late-stage myelodysplastic syndrome.

TABLE 4: The absolute number and percentage of regulatory T cells in the peripheral blood of patients with MDS and age-matched healthy donors.

Group	Treg, 10^6 cells/L	Percentage of Treg among CD4$^+$ T cells, %
Age control, n=26	29.8 (23.3–40.2)	4.1 (3.4–4.3)
MDS-primary[1], n=21	17.0** (12.0–19.7)	3.2* (2.7–4.0)
E-MDS[2], n=27	13.6** (7.9–19.9)	3.1* (1.8–4.7)
L-MDS[3], n=28	12.6** (8.0–17.3)	3.6 (2.8–5.8)

Note: *$p<0.05$ rel. to age control; **$p<0.001$ rel. to age control. [1]MDS-primary, primary myelodysplastic syndrome; [2]E-MDS, early-stage myelodysplastic syndrome; [3]L-MDS, late-stage myelodysplastic syndrome.

CD4$^+$ T cells (Table 4). In MDS-primary and E-MDS groups, the Treg percentage reduction was statistically significant, suggesting a higher probability of developing autoimmune disorders in these MDS groups. In general, the decrease in the number of Treg, regardless of the stage of disease, reflects an overall decline in the number of cells of bone marrow origin in the periphery and is a sign of disrupted hemopoiesis in MDS.

Assuming that disturbance of lymphopoiesis as part of hemopoiesis affects not only the quantity but also the function of the cells, we investigated the level of FOXP3 isoforms expression in Treg, which has different functional properties, as we noted above. To this end, we analyzed the MFI of FOXP3 exon 2 and FOXP3 exon 1 in all CD3$^+$CD4$^+$FOXP3$^+$ cells and calculated the parameter FI (FOXP3 exon 2/total) as have been described in Materials and Methods. We have found that MFI of FOXP3 exon 2 in the MDS-primary group increased in comparison with the age control group. This difference of exon 2 fluorescent intensities between primary MDS patient and healthy age-matched donor is clearly visible on the flow cytometry plots reflecting exon 1 and exon 2 coexpression in CD3$^+$CD4$^+$ cells (Figure 3). After calculation of FI (FOXP3 exon 2/total) parameter (Table 5) we have found that the ratio of FOXP3-FL to all FOXP3 was significantly increased in the MDS-primary group relative to the age control group, but after treatment, in E-MDS and L-MDS groups, the ratio returned to normal. Thus, the diminished frequency of Treg in MDS is accompanied by the relative accumulation of FOXP3-FL, and this FOXP3 isoforms imbalance disappears after the treatment, although the amount of Treg remains unchanged.

4. Discussion

Our study has revealed the decrease in frequency and likely functional activity of Treg in MDS. We suppose that the reduction of Treg functional activity in MDS patients

is associated with changing the ratio of FOXP3 isoforms expression in favor of FOXP3-FL. The likely reason for the relative accumulation of FOXP3-FL is the inability of Treg to suppress excessive immune response and inflammation that develop in primary MDS patients. Our speculation is based on the following. First, Wang et al. have shown that FOXP3 can be transiently expressed in stimulated nonregulatory CD4$^+$ T cells [21]. Second, Lundberg et al. have shown that T cell receptor stimulation induced FOXP3-FL expression in CD4$^+$ T cells in vitro [19]. Additionally, they have determined that the coronary artery disease, one of the chronic inflammatory diseases, is associated with the aforementioned FOXP3 isoforms expression pattern defined in PBMCs of the patients with this diagnosis [19]. Third, in our study, the relative increase of FOXP3-FL in primary patients with MDS was abrogated by treatment. In other words, this increase was transient.

Another explanation for the possible decrease in the functional activity of Treg cannot be ruled out. It is based on the already known information about the functional properties of different FOXP3 isoforms [13–18]. Assuming that FOXP3-FL predominant pattern is intrinsic for Treg in MDS and its correction in treated patients is associated with the direct effect of treatment on Treg, we can hypothesize that it is the altered FOXP3 isoforms expression that determines the functional activity of Treg.

Indirectly, the relationship of Treg functional activity and FOXP3 isoforms expression is confirmed by data on the level of FOXP3 isoforms expression in Treg during their differentiation in the human thymus [22], as well as in multiple myeloma [23] and chronic inflammatory bowel diseases [20]. A similar technique using MAbs specific to the exon 1 and the exon 2 was employed in those studies to determine the FOXP3 isoforms expression. Here we need to make a significant remark. In our previous studies, we classified Treg subpopulations as FOXP3 exon 2$^+$ and exon 2$^-$ [22, 23] as some other investigators did [24–26]. Now we consider that

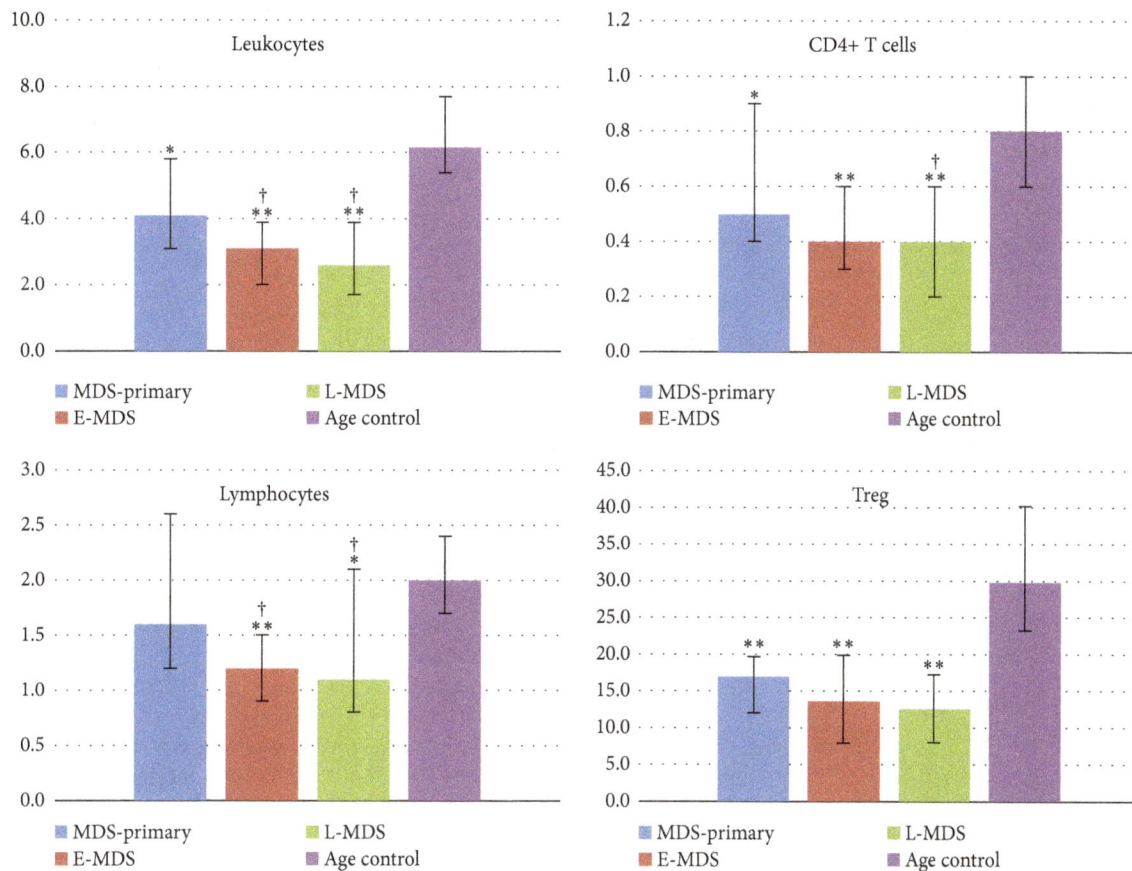

FIGURE 2: The absolute number of cell populations in the peripheral blood of MDS patients and age-matched healthy donors (10^9 cells/L, and Treg: 10^6 cells/L). Note: $*p<0.05$ rel. to age control; $**p<0.001$ rel. to age control; $^\dagger p<0.05$ rel. to MDS-primary. MDS-primary: primary myelodysplastic syndrome; E-MDS: early-stage myelodysplastic syndrome; L-MDS: late-stage myelodysplastic syndrome groups.

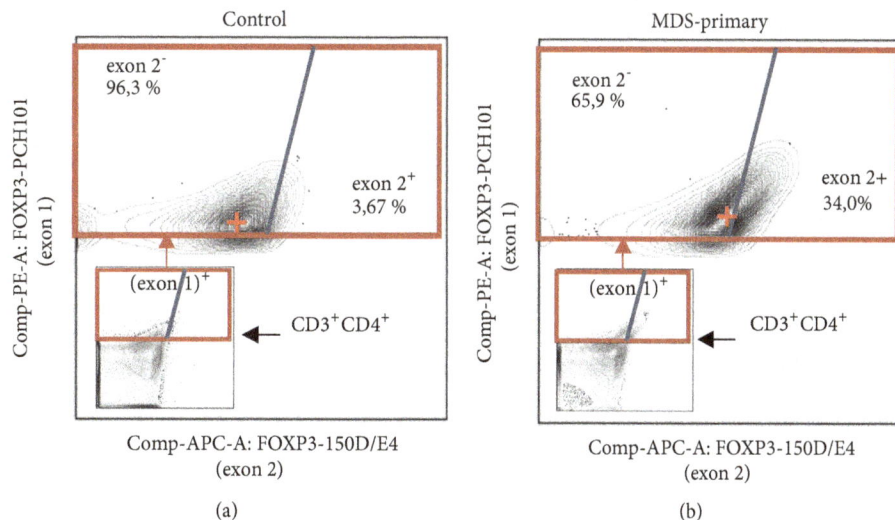

FIGURE 3: Flow cytometry. Contour plots reflecting FOXP3 exon 1 and exon 2 coexpression in CD3+CD4+ cells (small plots) and CD3+4+FOXP3+ cells (large plots) from PBMC[1] of healthy age-matched donor (a) and primary patient with MDS (b). The red cross marks the medians of the corresponding fluorescent intensities in the total FOXP3+ gate. [1]PBMCs: peripheral blood mononuclear cells.

TABLE 5: The ratio of FOXP3 exon 2 fluorescence intensity to FOXP3 total fluorescence intensity in CD3$^+$CD4$^+$FOXP3$^+$ cells from the peripheral blood of the patients with MDS and age-matched healthy donors.

Group	FI (FOXP3 exon 2/total), a.u.[4]
Age control, n=26	0.52 (0.48–0.56)
MDS-primary[1], n=21	0.68* (0.59–0.75)
E-MDS[2], n=27	0.56[†] (0.47–0.65)
L-MDS[3], n=28	0.54[††] (0.47–0.62)

[1]MDS-primary: primary myelodysplastic syndrome; [2]E-MDS: early-stage myelodysplastic syndrome; [3]L-MDS: late-stage myelodysplastic syndrome; [4]a.u.: arbitrary units. Note: *$p<0.001$ rel. to age control; [†]$p<0.05$ rel. to MDS-primary; [††]$p <0.001$ rel. MDS-primary.

it was incorrect. In this discussion, we will try to reinterpret those data. With the formal setting of the gates for the FOXP3 exon 2$^+$ and exon 2$^-$ cells, as shown in Figure 3, increase in the percentage of the FOXP3 exon 2$^+$ cells is accompanied by the increase in the corresponding MFI predominantly in the channel reflecting the FOXP3-FL expression. This fact allows us to interpret the rise in the percentage as the relative accumulation of FOXP3-FL in the FOXP3$^+$ cells.

According to the published data, during differentiation in the thymus, the percentage of Treg precursors expressing FOXP3-FL declined as they matured from 65% in the double-positive CD25$^+$ thymocytes to 33% in the single-positive CD4$^+$ Treg [22]. A new interpretation allows us to think that FOXP3-FL dominates in CD4$^+$CD8$^+$CD25$^+$ FOXP3$^+$ thymocytes and FOXP3Δ2 predominates in CD3$^+$ CD4$^+$CD25$^+$FOXP3$^+$ thymocytes. Thereby the functional maturation of Treg in the human thymus is accompanied by the accumulation of FOXP3Δ2.

The further accumulation of FOXP3Δ2 most likely accompanies oncological diseases. For instance, previously we have demonstrated a twofold increase in the number of Treg in the peripheral blood of primary patients with multiple myeloma [23]. Accumulation of FOXP3Δ2 in Treg, maintained even in the remission after Treg quantity normalization, accompanied this increase [23]. These data indicate that FOXP3Δ2 is involved in the pathogenesis of multiple myeloma and, possibly, has a higher functional activity than FOXP3-FL.

Another indirect confirmation of the high functional activity of the FOXP3Δ2 was obtained in the study of chronic inflammatory bowel diseases (IBD) [20]. Initially, the authors have assumed that Th17 polarization of the immune response in IBD may be caused by the accumulation of Treg expressing exclusively FOXP3Δ2 because of an inability of FOXP3Δ2 to bind RORγt. Nevertheless, no difference in the expression pattern of FOXP3Δ2 relative to FOXP3-FL was seen in the *lamina propria* of patients with Crohn's disease and nonspecific ulcerative colitis versus non-IBD controls. Against a background of a general increase in the quantity of Treg and Th17 polarization in IBD, the absence of FOXP3Δ2 accumulation indicates that the accompanying inflammation is not associated with this isoform. Thus, the opportunity of FOXP3Δ2 to accumulate in the nucleus is more significant when suppressing the immune response than the inability to restrict IL-17 expression.

At the end of the discussion, it is necessary to clarify the discrepancy between our and the earlier obtained data

on the Treg amount in MDS. It is possible that, in addition to the differences in sample preparation protocols and flow cytometry strategy, we evaluated the results differently. We did not attempt to link individual fluctuations in the Treg population that were also present in our study with the disease prognosis but used the already available IPSS evaluation system to divide the patients into groups. Therefore, we have demonstrated a trend common for all groups, including the primary patients, towards a decrease in the number and possibly functional impairment of Treg. The results obtained earlier undoubtedly indicate a poor disease prognosis with an increase in the Treg number but are more likely to be a particular case rather than a general trend. These differences can be explained by heterogeneity of diseases united under the common name of MDS that are often manifested by secondary immunodeficiency due to impaired hemopoiesis in the altered bone marrow niche. The nature of the developing dysplasia, which leads to disruption of the well-defined interactions between cells of bone marrow origin, especially those related to the immune system, determines the pathogenesis and clinical symptoms of the disease. The vector of these disorders is determined by what the differentiation stage was initially affected. It is possible that a detailed study of the mechanisms underlying the MDS pathogenesis will lead to an isolation of individual diseases with characteristic clinical features and outcome.

5. Conclusion

We have shown the decrease in the absolute number and the percentage of Treg among CD4$^+$ T cells in the peripheral blood of all patients with MDS. In untreated patients, the Treg number reduction was accompanied by the relative accumulation of FOXP3-FL that could reflect the presence of inflammation and a decrease in the functional activity of Treg. These observations could explain the high risk of autoimmune disorders in this disease and would be useful for further understanding the role of Treg and FOXP3 isoforms in the pathogenesis of MDS.

Conflicts of Interest

The authors declare that there are no conflicts of interest regarding the publication of this paper.

Acknowledgments

This research was supported by Celgene International Holdings Corporation.

References

[1] N. Gangat, M. M. Patnaik, and A. Tefferi, "Myelodysplastic syndromes: Contemporary review and how we treat," *American Journal of Hematology*, vol. 91, no. 1, pp. 76–89, 2016.

[2] S. Semochkin, T. Tolstykh, G. Dudina, and O. Fink, "Clinical and epidemiological characteristics of myelodysplastic syndromes in adults," *Georgian Medical News*, no. 252, pp. 108–115, 2016.

[3] T. Braun and P. Fenaux, "Myelodysplastic Syndromes (MDS) and autoimmune disorders (AD): cause or consequence?" *Best Practice & Research Clinical Haematology*, vol. 26, no. 4, pp. 327–336, 2013.

[4] S. Y. Kordasti, W. Ingram, J. Hayden et al., "Wlodarski M.W., Maciejewski J.P., Farzaneh F., Mufti G.J. CD4$^+$CD25^{high} Foxp3$^+$ regulatory T cells in myelodysplastic syndrome (MDS)," *Blood*, vol. 110, no. 3, pp. 847–850, 2007.

[5] W. Hamdi, H. Ogawara, H. Handa, N. Tsukamoto, Y. Nojima, and H. Murakami, "Clinical significance of regulatory T cells in patients with myelodysplastic syndrome," *European Journal of Haematology*, vol. 82, no. 3, pp. 201–207, 2009.

[6] I. Kotsianidis, I. Bouchliou, E. Nakou et al., "Kinetics, function and bone marrow trafficking of CD4$^+$CD25$^+$FOXP3$^+$ regulatory T cells in myelodysplastic syndromes (MDS)," *Leukemia*, vol. 23, no. 3, pp. 510–518, 2009.

[7] J. D. Kahn, M. E. D. Chamuleau, T. M. Westers et al., "Regulatory T cells and progenitor B cells are independent prognostic predictors in lower risk myelodysplastic syndromes," *Haematologica*, vol. 100, no. 6, pp. e220–e222, 2015.

[8] E. Balaian, C. Schuster, C. Schönefeldt et al., "Selective expansion of regulatory T cells during lenalidomide treatment of myelodysplastic syndrome with isolated deletion 5q," *Annals of Hematology*, vol. 95, no. 11, pp. 1805–1810, 2016.

[9] A. W. Mailloux, C. Sugimori, R. S. Komrokji et al., "Expansion of effector memory regulatory T cells represents a novel prognostic factor in lower risk myelodysplastic syndrome," *The Journal of Immunology*, vol. 189, no. 6, pp. 3198–3208, 2012.

[10] S. Sakaguchi, T. Yamaguchi, T. Nomura, and M. Ono, "Regulatory T cells and immune tolerance," *Cell*, vol. 133, no. 5, pp. 775–787, 2008.

[11] S. E. Allan, L. Passerini, R. Bacchetta et al., "The role of 2 FOXP3 isoforms in the generation of human CD4$^+$ Tregs," *The Journal of Clinical Investigation*, vol. 115, no. 11, pp. 3276–3284, 2005.

[12] G. Kaur, J. C. Goodall, L. B. Jarvis, and J. Hill Gaston, "Characterisation of Foxp3 splice variants in human CD4+ and CD8+ T cells—Identification of Foxp3Δ7 in human regulatory T cells," *Molecular Immunology*, vol. 48, no. 1-3, pp. 321–332, 2010.

[13] R. K. Mailer, K. Falk, O. Rötzschke, and D. Unutmaz, "Absence of Leucine Zipper in the Natural FOXP3Δ2Δ7 Isoform Does Not Affect Dimerization but Abrogates Suppressive Capacity," *PLoS ONE*, vol. 4, no. 7, p. e6104, 2009.

[14] R. K. Mailer, "Alternative Splicing of FOXP3—Virtue and Vice," *Frontiers in Immunology*, vol. 9, 2018.

[15] J. Du, C. Huang, B. Zhou, and S. F. Ziegler, "Isoform-Specific Inhibition of ROR -Mediated Transcriptional Activation by Human FOXP3," *The Journal of Immunology*, vol. 180, no. 7, pp. 4785–4792, 2008.

[16] K. Ichiyama, H. Yoshida, Y. Wakabayashi et al., "Foxp3 inhibits RORγt-mediated IL-17A mRNA transcription through direct interaction with RORγt," *The Journal of Biological Chemistry*, vol. 283, no. 25, pp. 17003–17008, 2008.

[17] W.-J. Chae, O. Henegariu, S.-K. Lee, and A. L. M. Bothwell, "The mutant leucine-zipper domain impairs both dimerization and suppressive function of Foxp3 in T cells," *Proceedings of the National Acadamy of Sciences of the United States of America*, vol. 103, no. 25, pp. 9631–9636, 2006.

[18] T. Magg, J. Mannert, J. W. Ellwart, I. Schmid, and M. H. Albert, "Subcellular localization of FOXP3 in human regulatory and nonregulatory T cells," *European Journal of Immunology*, vol. 42, no. 6, pp. 1627–1638, 2012.

[19] A. K. Lundberg, L. Jonasson, G. K. Hansson, and R. K. W. Mailer, "Activation-induced FOXP3 isoform profile in peripheral CD4+ T cells is associated with coronary artery disease," *Atherosclerosis*, vol. 267, pp. 27–33, 2017.

[20] J. D. Lord, K. Valliant-Saunders, H. Hahn, R. C. Thirlby, and S. F. Ziegler, "Paradoxically increased FOXP3+ T cells in IBD do not preferentially express the isoform of FOXP3 lacking exon 2," *Digestive Diseases and Sciences*, vol. 57, no. 11, pp. 2846–2855, 2012.

[21] J. Wang, A. Ioan-Facsinay, E. I. H. van der Voort, T. W. J. Huizinga, and R. E. M. Toes, "Transient expression of FOXP3 in human activated nonregulatory CD4$^+$ T cells," *European Journal of Immunology*, vol. 37, no. 1, pp. 129–138, 2007.

[22] A. N. Mitin, M. M. Litvina, N. I. Sharova et al., "FOXP3 expression and its isoform ratio during T cells differentiation," *Immunologiya*, vol. 33, no. 4, pp. 172–176, 2012 (Russian).

[23] A. N. Mitin, M. M. Litvina, T. A. Mitina, A. K. Golenkov, and A. A. Yarilin, "Flow cytometry analysis of FOXP3 and its isoforms expression by CD4+ T cells from peripheral blood in various forms of multiple myeloma," *Immunologiya*, vol. 35, no. 4, pp. 215–219, 2014.

[24] C. Miyabe, Y. Miyabe, K. Strle et al., "An expanded population of pathogenic regulatory T cells in giant cell arteritis is abrogated by IL-6 blockade therapy," *Annals of the Rheumatic Diseases*, vol. 76, no. 5, pp. 898–905, 2017.

[25] M. E. Free, D. O. Bunch, J. A. McGregor et al., "Patients with antineutrophil cytoplasmic antibody-associated vasculitis have defective Treg cell function exacerbated by the presence of a suppression-resistant effector cell population," *Arthritis & Rheumatology*, vol. 65, no. 7, pp. 1922–1933, 2013.

[26] B. Jakiela, T. Iwaniec, H. Plutecka, M. Celinska-Lowenhoff, S. Dziedzina, and J. Musial, "Signs of impaired immunoregulation and enhanced effector T-cell responses in the primary antiphospholipid syndrome," *Lupus*, vol. 25, no. 4, pp. 389–398, 2016.

25

Myeloablative Conditioning with PBSC Grafts for T Cell-Replete Haploidentical Donor Transplantation Using Posttransplant Cyclophosphamide

Scott R. Solomon, Melhem Solh, Lawrence E. Morris, H. Kent Holland, and Asad Bashey

Blood and Marrow Transplant Program at Northside Hospital, Atlanta, GA 30342, USA

Correspondence should be addressed to Scott R. Solomon; ssolomon@bmtga.com

Academic Editor: Franco Aversa

Relapse is the main cause of treatment failure after nonmyeloablative haploidentical transplant (haplo-HSCT). In an attempt to reduce relapse, we have developed a myeloablative (MA) haplo-HSCT approach utilizing posttransplant cyclophosphamide (PT/Cy) and peripheral blood stem cells as the stem cell source. We summarize the results of two consecutive clinical trials, using a busulfan-based (n = 20) and a TBI-based MA preparative regimen (n = 30), and analyze a larger cohort of 64 patients receiving MA haplo-HSCT. All patients have engrafted with full donor chimerism and no late graft failures. Grade III-IV acute GVHD and moderate-severe chronic GVHD occurred in 23% and 30%, respectively. One-year NRM was 10%. Predicted three-year overall survival, disease-free survival, and relapse were 53%, 53%, and 26%, respectively, in all patients and 79%, 74%, and 9%, respectively, in patients with a low/intermediate disease risk index (DRI). In multivariate analysis, DRI was the most significant predictor of survival and relapse. Use of TBI (versus busulfan) had no significant impact on survival but was associated with significantly less BK virus-associated hemorrhagic cystitis. We contrast our results with other published reports of MA haplo-HSCT PT/Cy in the literature and attempt to define the comparative utility of MA haplo-HSCT to other methods of transplantation.

1. Introduction

Seventy percent of patients who urgently need an allogeneic hematopoietic stem cell transplantation (HSCT) do not have an available HLA-matched sibling donor. In such patients, a search for an HLA-matched unrelated donor (MUD) can identify an 8/8 HLA-identical donor for approximately 30% to 40% of transplant recipients. The probability of finding an acceptable MUD varies by ethnic groups, ranging from 75% in the white Europeans, to 30% to 40% in the Mexican and Central/South Americans, to 15% to 20% for the African Americans and black Caribbeans [1]. In addition, MUD transplantation is also complicated by the amount of time it takes from search initiation to transplantation, causing some patients to relapse or physically deteriorate while waiting for transplantation. In contrast, a haploidentical family member (haplo) can be identified and rapidly utilized in nearly all cases.

Historically, HSCT from a partially HLA-mismatched relative has been complicated by unacceptably high incidences of graft rejection, severe graft-versus-host disease (GVHD), and nonrelapse mortality (NRM) [2, 3]. To address the risk of graft rejection and GVHD, extensive T cell depletion has been utilized in association with antithymocyte globulin (ATG) and high peripheral blood stem cell (PBSC) dose [4]; however, NRM from infectious complications remains a challenge. More recently, the investigators at Johns Hopkins University have pioneered a method to selectively deplete alloreactive cells in vivo by administering high doses of cyclophosphamide (Cy) in a narrow window after transplantation [5]. After nonmyeloablative (NMA) conditioning, this approach has resulted in low NRM (4% and 15% at 1 and 2 years, resp.), because of low rates of GVHD and infectious complications. Immune reconstitution was promising with low risk of cytomegalovirus (CMV) or invasive mold infections. Using high-dose, posttransplantation cyclophosphamide (PT/Cy), crossing the HLA barrier in HSCT is now feasible without the need for extensive T cell depletion or serotherapy.

Studies of NMA haplo-HSCT with PT/Cy show remarkable tolerability of this approach with low rates of GVHD, infection, and NRM. Relapse of malignancy remains the predominant cause of treatment failure, occurring in approximately 45% to 51% of patients [5, 6]. NMA haplo-HSCT with PT/Cy has also been associated with an approximately 10% rate of engraftment failure resulting in autologous recovery. The use of more intense/myeloablative (MA) preparative regimens and PBSC grafts may potentially reduce the rate of relapse and graft rejection following haplo-HSCT PT/Cy transplants. However, only a limited number of such studies have been reported. In this paper, we report our experience with MA conditioning and PBSC allografts for T-replete haplo-HSCT using PT/Cy. We define the major predictors of outcome following this strategy. We also describe other published reports of MA haplo-HSCT PT/Cy in the literature. Finally, we compare the outcomes of MA and NMA haplo-HSCT using PT/Cy and attempt to define the comparative utility of MA haplo-HSCT in relation to MUD transplantation.

2. Busulfan-Based MA Haplo-HSCT (NSH 864 Protocol)

In a proof-of-principle study of MA haplo-HSCT, twenty patients with high risk hematologic malignancies were treated with a preparative regimen of fludarabine (125–180 mg/m^2), i.v. busulfan (440–520 mg/m^2) and Cy (29 mg/kg) before transplant, a G-CSF-mobilized PBSC graft, and posttransplant GVHD prophylaxis comprised of Cy 50 mg/kg/d on d +3 and +4, MMF 15 mg/kg three times daily d +5–+35, and tacrolimus (target 5–15 ng/mL) days +5 to +180 [7]. The median age of patients was 44 years (range: 25–56 years). Eleven patients (55%) underwent HSCT with relapsed/refractory disease (acute myelogenous leukemia [AML] 5, chronic myelogenous leukemia-blast crisis [CML-BC] 1, acute lymphoblastic leukemia 2, non-Hodgkin lymphoma 1, Hodgkin's disease 1, and chronic lymphocytic leukemia/Richters 1). The remaining patients had either AML CR1 with poor-risk cytogenetics and/or induction failure or chronic myelogenous leukemia resistant to all tyrosine kinase inhibitors.

All patients engrafted and demonstrated 100% donor chimerism in both peripheral blood T cell and myeloid cells from day +30. Cumulative incidence of one-year NRM was 10% and that of grade III-IV acute GVHD and severe chronic GVHD was 10% and 5%, respectively. Relapse was acceptable, occurring in 40% of patients, despite the fact that the majority had relapsed/refractory disease at time of transplant. With a median follow-up of 20 months, estimated probabilities of overall and disease-free survival (DFS) were 69% and 50%, respectively.

There were no cases of invasive mold infections or EBV-related PTLD. Only one patient had CMV disease and only one patient died of a viral infection (parainfluenza 3) suggesting that anti-infection immunity was preserved with this approach. However, nonfatal BK virus-associated hemorrhagic cystitis (HC) was seen in 75% of patients at a median of

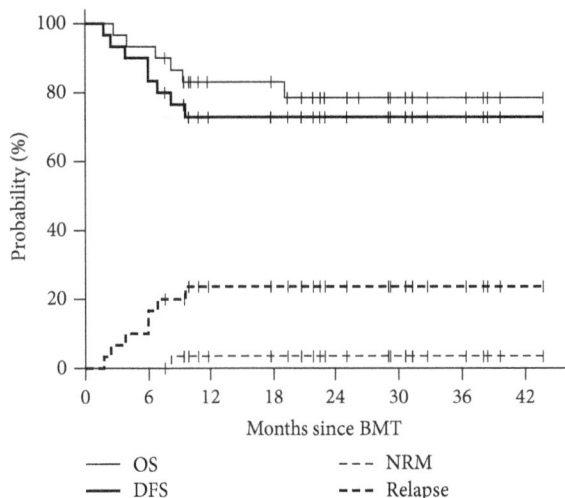

FIGURE 1: Kaplan-Meier analysis of overall survival, disease-free survival, and nonrelapse mortality and following TBI-based MA haplo-HSCT.

38 days after transplant. Although it is not a life-threatening complication, it was a source of significant morbidity for some patients. We hypothesized that HC was predisposed to by the combined effect of high-dose busulfan and PT/Cy.

3. Total-Body Irradiation-Based Haplo-HSCT (NSH 922 Protocol)

In an attempt to reduce the risk of BK virus-associated HC, thirty patients were enrolled on prospective phase II trial utilizing a TBI-based myeloablative preparative regimen (fludarabine 25 mg/m^2/d × 3 d and TBI 150 cGy bid on d −4 to −1 [total dose 1200 cGy]) followed by infusion of unmanipulated peripheral blood stem cells from a haploidentical family donor [8]. Postgrafting immunosuppression again consisted of Cy 50 mg/kg/day on days 3 and 4, MMF through d 35, and tacrolimus through d 180. Median patient age was 46.5 years (range 24–60). Transplant diagnosis included AML [9], ALL [6], CML [5], MDS [1], and NHL [2]. Using the revised Dana-Farber/CIBMTR disease risk index (DRI), patients were classified as having low [4], intermediate [10], high [11], and very high [3] risk.

All patients engrafted with a median time to neutrophil and platelet recovery of 16 and 25 days, respectively. All evaluable patients achieved sustained complete donor T cell and myeloid chimerism by day +30. Acute GVHD, grades II–IV and III-IV, was seen in 43% and 23%, respectively. The cumulative incidence of moderate-to-severe chronic GVHD was 22% (severe in 10%). Nonrelapse mortality (NRM) at 2 years was 3%, which consisted of one death due to noninfectious respiratory failure/ARDS 8 months after transplant in a patient with chronic GVHD. Estimated two-year survival, DFS, and relapse were 78%, 73%, and 24%, respectively (Figure 1). Two-year DFS and relapse rate in patients with low/intermediate disease risk, determined by the DRI, were

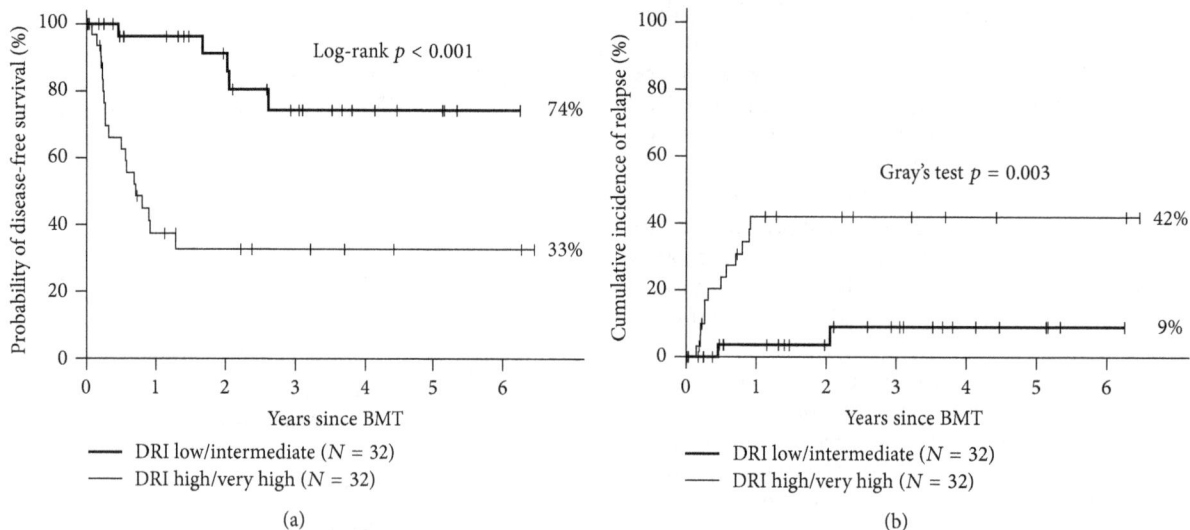

FIGURE 2: Effect of disease risk index on (a) disease-free survival and (b) relapse following MA haplo-HSCT.

100% and 0%, respectively, compared with 39% and 53% for patients with high/very high risk disease.

As noted in our prior experience with busulfan-based MA haplo-HSCT, posttransplant fever was common and occurred in the first 5 posttransplant days in nearly all patients. Fevers resolved in all patients following administration of PT/Cy. CMV reactivation (≥400 copies/mL) occurred in 15/26 (58%) of at-risk patients (either donor or recipient with CMV positive serostatus) at a median of day +43 after transplant (range 11–157). CMV disease did not occur. There were no episodes of invasive mold infection or infectious death in the first 100 days after transplant. There were no cases of EBV reactivation. BK virus-associated HC of any grade occurred in 30% of patients and was severe (grade ≥ 3) in 7%. As compared with our previous experience with busulfan-based MA haplo-HSCT, HC occurred significantly less often following TBI-based MA haplo-HSCT (any grade: 30% versus 75%, p = 0.005; severe HC: 7% versus 30%, p = 0.037).

4. Predictors of Outcome following MA Haplo-HSCT and PT/Cy

In order to determine predictors of outcome following MA haplo-HSCT and PT/Cy, we evaluated that sixty-four consecutive patients have been transplanted following either busulfan-based (n = 20; NSH 864) or TBI-based (n = 44; including 30 patients on NSH 922 and the remaining 14 patients treated identically after completion of the trial) MA conditioning, T cell-replete PBSC infusion, PT/Cy, and tacrolimus/mycophenolate mofetil. Median age of the cohort was 43 years (range 21–60). Patient characteristics included a high/very high disease risk by the Dana-Farber/CIBMTR disease risk index (DRI) in 32 patients (50%), KPS <90 in 69%, and comorbidity index (CMI) of ≥2 in 58% of patients. The most common indications for transplant were AML, ALL, and advanced-phase CML in 55%, 20%, and 12% of patients,

respectively. Median follow-up for surviving patients was 24 months.

All patients engrafted with full donor chimerism and no late graft failures. Grade II–IV, III-IV acute GVHD and moderate-severe chronic GVHD occurred in 46%, 23%, and 30%, respectively. One-year NRM was 10%. Predicted three-year overall survival (OS), disease-free survival (DFS), and relapse are 53%, 53%, and 26%, respectively. In the 32 patients with standard risk disease (low/intermediate DRI), outcomes were significantly improved with one-year NRM of 0% and predicted 3-year OS, DFS, and relapse of 79%, 74%, and 9%, respectively (Figure 2).

In multivariate analysis, high/very high DRI was the most significant negative predictor of OS (HR 13.26, p < 0.001), followed by CMI ≥2 (HR 3.54, p = 0.01) and age (HR 1.26, p = 0.038, per 5-year increase in age). DRI was also significantly associated with DFS (HR 10.84, p < 0.001), NRM (HR 15.0, p = 0.004), and relapse (HR 8.85, p = 0.004) (Table 1). Conditioning regimen (TBI versus busulfan) had no significant impact on OS, DFS, NRM, or relapse.

5. Additional Published Experience with MA Haplo-HSCT and PT/Cy

Several other groups have published similar experiences with MA haplo-HSCT with PT/Cy. Grosso et al. [12] reported a "two-step" strategy where a defined dose of haploidentical T cells (2×108/kg) was infused after MA doses of TBI. Patients then received 60 mg/kg of CY on two consecutive days, followed later by infusion of highly purified CD34+ cells from the donor. All patients engrafted and the cumulative incidence of grade III-IV acute GVHD and NRM was 7.4% and 22.5%, respectively, for the 27 patients treated. With a median follow-up of 40 months, overall survival was 48%. A second study from the same group [13], which included only patients in remission at the time of transplant, demonstrated

TABLE 1: Predictors of transplant outcomes following MA haplo HSCT.

	OS		DFS		NRM		Relapse	
	HR	p	HR	p	HR	p	HR	p
DRI (high versus low/int)	**13.26**	*<0.001*	**10.84**	*<0.001*	**15.0**	*0.004*	**8.85**	*0.004*
CMI (≥2 versus <2)	**3.54**	*0.010*	**3.09**	*0.018*	**13.6**	*0.007*	—	—
Age (<50 versus ≥50)	**1.26**	*0.038*	**1.31**	*0.015*	**1.43**	*0.055*	—	—

The following variables were considered in Cox analysis: age, diagnosis, Karnofsky performance status (KPS), comorbidity index (CMI), revised Dana-Farber disease risk index (DRI), conditioning regimen (busulfan versus TBI), year of transplant, acute GVHD, and chronic GVHD. Variables were selected by 10% threshold. Acute and chronic GVHD were modeled as time-dependent variables.

a 2 yr NRM, relapse, and PFS of 4%, 19%, and 74%, respectively. The requirement for stringent ex vivo T depletion of the hematopoietic cell product differentiates this approach and may limit its widespread applicability. Furthermore, given the resistance of hematopoietic stem cells to Cy, such delayed infusion of selected CD34+ cells may be unnecessary.

Symons et al. [11] reported on 97 patients with either leukemias in complete remission or lymphoma with chemosensitive disease. Patients received MA haplo-HSCT PT/Cy utilizing bone marrow grafts. The preparative regimen consisted of IV busulfan (pharmacokinetically adjusted) on days −6 to −3 and Cy (50 mg/kg/day) on days −2 and −1, except for patients with acute lymphocytic leukemia or lymphoblastic lymphoma who received Cy (50 mg/kg/day) on days −5 and −4 and TBI (200 cGy twice daily) on days −3 to −1. Donor engraftment occurred in 73/82 (89%) patients. Estimated probabilities of NRM and grade III-IV acute GVHD at 100 days were 11% and 7%, respectively. The cumulative incidence of relapse was 44%. With a median follow-up of surviving patients of 474 days, estimated 2 yr overall and disease-free survival is 57% and 49%, respectively.

Raiola et al. [10] reported on 50 patients receiving a MA haplo-HSCT PT/Cy utilizing bone marrow grafts. The regimens used were thiotepa, busulfan, and fludarabine (n = 35) or TBI and fludarabine (n = 15). Forty-five patients (90%) engrafted with an 18-month cumulative incidence of NRM, relapse, and PFS of 18%, 22%, and 51%, respectively. PFS was 67% for patients transplanted in remission versus 37% for patients with active disease. Reported incidences of acute and chronic GVHD were low. As in our experience, HC was more common in patients receiving busulfan rather than TBI-based conditioning.

Whether PBSC or BM is the preferred stem cell source following MA haplo-HSCT remains unclear; however BM appears to be associated with a higher rate of graft failure, occurring in approximately 10% of patients in both the series by Raiola et al. [10] and the experience of Symons et al. [11]. Graft failure has not been reported with PBSC based myeloablative haplo-HSCT and PT/Cy.

6. Comparison of MA and NMA Haplo-PT/Cy

The overall risk of relapse associated with MA haplo-HSCT in the majority of studies is 20–25% [7, 8, 10, 13] and compares favorably with that reported for NMA haplo-HSCT (45–51%) [5, 6]. In our analysis of 64 patients receiving MA haplo-HSCT, relapse risk in patients with low (n = 7) or

intermediate (n = 25) DRI was 9%, compared with 42% relapse rate in high (n = 24) or very high (n = 8) DRI patients. This compares favorably to that seen in the NMA setting, where relapse risk according to DRI was recently analyzed in 372 consecutive patients by the group from Johns Hopkins University [14]. In this analysis, the risk of relapse was also highly correlated with DRI, with relapse occurring in approximately 75%, 50%, and 20% of patients in the high/very high, intermediate, and low DRI groups, respectively. The finding of higher relapse following NMA conditioning parallels what has been seen following matched related or unrelated donor transplantation [9, 15–17].

7. Comparison of MA Haplo-PT/Cy with MA MUD Transplants

In order to evaluate the comparative efficacy of MA haplo-HSCT, we have compared outcomes of patients receiving TBI-based MA haplo-HSCT with PT/Cy (n = 30) with a contemporaneously treated cohort of consecutive patients at our institution receiving HLA-matched (8/8 HLA-A, HLA-B, HLA-C, and HLA-DR) MA T cell-replete MUD transplantation (n = 48) [8]. Haplo- and MUD transplant patients were well matched according to age, diagnosis, disease risk, CMV serostatus, and comorbidity index. The groups did differ in the use of PBSC as the stem cell source which was utilized in all haplotransplant recipients compared with 32 of 48 MUD transplants recipients. When compared with recipients of MA MUD transplants, outcomes after MA haplo-HSCT were statistically similar to 2 yr OS and DFS being 78% and 73%, respectively, after haplotransplant versus 71% and 64%, respectively, after MUD transplants. Grade II–IV acute GVHD was seen less often following haplotransplantation compared with MUD transplantation (43% versus 63%, p = 0.049), as was moderate-to-severe chronic GVHD (22% versus 58%, p = 0.003). The lower incidence of chronic GVHD occurred despite the greater use of PBSC in the haplo-HSCT group.

Similarly, a Center for International Blood and Marrow Transplant Research (CIBMTR) analysis [18] compared outcomes of adults with acute myeloid leukemia (AML) after haplo- (n = 192) and MUD (n = 1982) transplantation, including 104 MA haplotransplants and 1245 MA MUD transplants. In this large analysis, there were no significant differences in 1 yr NRM (12% versus 14%), 3 yr relapse (44% versus 39%), or 3 yr OS (46% versus 44%), comparing MA haplo- and MA MUD transplants, respectively. Grade II–IV acute GVHD (16% versus 33%), grade III-IV acute GVHD (7% versus 13%), and chronic GVHD (30% versus 53%) were all statistically lower in haplopatients compared with MUD patients.

8. Immune Recovery following MA Haplo-PT/Cy

Historically, MA haplotransplantation has been associated with considerable infectious morbidity and mortality. In contrast, our experience and others suggest that MA haplo-PT/Cy may significantly reduce the risk of infectious complications. In a published series of thirty patients undergoing TBI-based MA haplo-PT/Cy [8], CMV reactivation (≥400 copies/mL) occurred in only 15/26 (58%) of at-risk patients (either donor or recipient with CMV positive serostatus), and CMV disease did not occur. There were no episodes of invasive mold infection or infectious death in the first 100 days after transplant. Furthermore, there were no cases of EBV, HHV6, or adenovirus infections.

The reduced risk of infectious complications following MA haplo-PT/Cy has translated into low NRM, approximately 10% in the first year after transplant. Our experience compares favorably to the results reported with T cell-depleted (TCD) MA haplo, where NRM of approximately 40% have been seen, with much of this attributable to infectious mortality [4, 19–21]. Ciurea and colleagues at the MD Anderson Cancer Center analyzed their outcomes following MA haplo-PT/Cy following a preparative regimen of fludarabine, melphalan, and thiotepa, with historical results of TCD MA haplo using the same preparative regimen [20]. In this analysis, one-year NRM favored PT/Cy (16% versus 42%) as did death directly attributable to infection (9% versus 24%), with significantly less viral and fungal infections seen in PT/Cy versus TCD patients. T cell subset analysis demonstrated significant improvements in T cell recovery in PT/Cy versus TCD patients, with more rapid reconstitution noted in multiple T cell subsets (CD4, CD8, naïve, and memory).

Immune reconstitution following haplo-PT/Cy is characterized by a diverse T cell receptor repertoire and appears dependent on T memory stem cells maturing from naïve T cells [22, 23]. These cells are adoptively transferred in the donor graft and have been shown to survive cyclophosphamide-induced deletion. Furthermore, regulatory T cells also are preferentially preserved following PT/Cy, likely due to higher aldehyde dehydrogenase in these cells [24]. Finally, murine studies have demonstrated that PT/Cy relatively spares pathogen and cancer-specific T cells [25]. The selective elimination of alloreactive donor T cells with relative preservation of non-alloreactive donor T cell clones provides a mechanistic understanding of the surprisingly low infectious mortality following MA haplo-PT/Cy.

9. Discussion

In the past decade, there has been a growing interest in the use of haplo-HSCT due to the rapid and nearly universal availability of donors, which is a critical issue in patients with advanced hematologic malignancies. A major advance in the success of haplo-HSCT is the use of properly timed PT/Cy, a technique pioneered by investigators at Johns Hopkins University [5, 26]. Using a NMA approach, this strategy has resulted in low rates of GVHD, infection, and NRM. However, relapse remains the major cause of treatment failure, occurring in approximately half of transplant recipients. One explanation for the high rate of relapse, as in other NMA HSCT trials, is that the transplantation conditioning was not intense enough to achieve sufficient tumor cytoreduction.

In order to reduce the risk of relapse in patients with high risk hematologic malignancies, our group and others have demonstrated the feasibility of performing MA haplo-HSCT utilizing PT/Cy. In 64 consecutive patients transplanted at our institution following either busulfan-based ($n = 20$) or TBI-based ($n = 44$) MA conditioning, we have noted universal engraftment with rapid donor chimerism, acceptable rates of GVHD (grade III-IV acute GVHD and moderate-severe chronic GVHD occurred in 23% and 30%, resp.), and a low one-year NRM of 10%. Predicted three-year overall survival (OS), disease-free survival (DFS), and relapse were 53%, 53%, and 26%, respectively, and in the 32 patients with standard risk disease (low/intermediate DRI), outcomes were very favorable (3-year OS, DFS, and relapse of 79%, 74%, and 9%, resp.).

Relapse appears less following MA conditioning with relapse rates in the majority of studies of 20–25% [7, 8, 10, 13], compared with that reported for NMA haplo-BMT (45–51%) [5, 6]. However, truly defining the influence of the preparative regimen intensity on relapse risk will likely require a randomized controlled trial. When comparing our results with the other published experiences of MA haplo-HSCT using PT/Cy, it becomes evident that disease risk, as defined by either the DRI or disease status at the time of transplant, is the primary driver of outcomes, with 2 yr DFS being approximately 67–74% [8, 10, 13] in patients transplanted in remission without high risk disease defined by the DRI. Whether PBSC or BM is the preferred stem cell source following myeloablative haplo-HSCT remains unclear; however BM appears to be associated with a higher rate of graft failure, occurring in approximately 10% of patients [10, 11] receiving marrow grafts, and is obviously more consequential following MA conditioning.

Although there have been no randomized studies to date, there is now compelling evidence regarding the equivalent efficacy and safety of haplo-HSCT PT/Cy and MUD transplantation, in both the NMA and MA setting [8, 18, 27–29]. When considering the optimal transplant donor type, MUD versus haplo-HSCT, one must consider the inherent advantages of haplodonors including near universal and rapid availability, as well as lower costs related to donor searching and graft acquisition, whereas as almost all patients have an available haplomatched family member, the availability of an 8/8 matched unrelated donor varies according to ethnic background, ranging from 75% for white patients of European descent to less than 20% for the African Americans. Furthermore, given the complexities inherent in registry searching, time from initiation of donor searching to transplant can be significant, averaging around 3 months.

In conclusion, our results show that MA haplo-HSCT results in favorable engraftment, acceptable rates of GVHD, and low nonrelapse mortality. Relapse rates appear lower than that reported with NMA haplo-HSCT. DRI represents the strongest predictor of outcome following MA haplo-HSCT and PT/Cy. Disease-free and overall survival is equivalent to recipients of MA MUD transplants. Therefore, in younger patients without contraindications to standard intensity conditioning, MA haplo-HSCT is a valid option for patients with advanced hematologic malignancies who lack timely access to a conventional donor.

Conflict of Interests

The authors declare that there is no conflict of interests regarding the publication of this paper.

References

[1] L. Gragert, M. Eapen, E. Williams et al., "HLA match likelihoods for hematopoietic stem-cell grafts in the U.S. registry," The New England Journal of Medicine, vol. 371, no. 4, pp. 339–348, 2014.

[2] P. G. Beatty, R. A. Clift, E. M. Mickelson et al., "Marrow transplantation from related donors other than HLA-identical siblings," The New England Journal of Medicine, vol. 313, no. 13, pp. 765–771, 1985.

[3] R. Szydlo, J. M. Goldman, J. P. Klein et al., "Results of allogeneic bone marrow transplants for leukemia using donors other than HLA-identical siblings," Journal of Clinical Oncology, vol. 15, no. 5, pp. 1767–1777, 1997.

[4] F. Aversa, A. Terenzi, A. Tabilio et al., "Full haplotype-mismatched hematopoietic stem-cell transplantation: a phase II study in patients with acute leukemia at high risk of relapse," Journal of Clinical Oncology, vol. 23, no. 15, pp. 3447–3454, 2005.

[5] L. Luznik, P. V. O'Donnell, H. J. Symons et al., "HLA-haploidentical bone marrow transplantation for hematologic malignancies using nonmyeloablative conditioning and high-dose, posttransplantation cyclophosphamide," Biology of Blood and Marrow Transplantation, vol. 14, no. 6, pp. 641–650, 2008.

[6] C. G. Brunstein, E. J. Fuchs, S. L. Carter et al., "Alternative donor transplantation after reduced intensity conditioning: results of parallel phase 2 trials using partially HLA-mismatched related bone marrow or unrelated double umbilical cord blood grafts," Blood, vol. 118, no. 2, pp. 282–288, 2011.

[7] S. R. Solomon, C. A. Sizemore, M. Sanacore et al., "Haploidentical transplantation using T cell replete peripheral blood stem cells and myeloablative conditioning in patients with high-risk hematologic malignancies who lack conventional donors is well tolerated and produces excellent relapse-free survival: results of a prospective phase II trial," Biology of Blood and Marrow Transplantation, vol. 18, no. 12, pp. 1859–1866, 2012.

[8] S. R. Solomon, C. A. Sizemore, M. Sanacore et al., "Total body irradiation-based myeloablative haploidentical stem cell transplantation is a safe and effective alternative to unrelated donor transplantation in patients without matched sibling donors," Biology of Blood and Marrow Transplantation, vol. 21, no. 7, pp. 1299–1307, 2015.

[9] O. Ringdén, M. Labopin, G. Ehninger et al., "Reduced intensity conditioning compared with myeloablative conditioning using unrelated donor transplants in patients with acute myeloid leukemia," Journal of Clinical Oncology, vol. 27, no. 27, pp. 4570–4577, 2009.

[10] A. M. Raiola, A. Dominietto, A. Ghiso et al., "Unmanipulated haploidentical bone marrow transplantation and posttransplantation cyclophosphamide for hematologic malignancies after myeloablative conditioning," Biology of Blood and Marrow Transplantation, vol. 19, no. 1, pp. 117–122, 2013.

[11] H. J. Symons, A. Chen, C. Gamper et al., "Haploidentical BMT using fully myeloablative conditioning, T cell replete bone marrow grafts, and post-transplant cyclophosphamide (PT/Cy) has limited toxicity and promising efficacy in largest reported experience with high risk hematologic malignancies," Biology of Blood and Marrow Transplantation, vol. 21, no. 2, p. S29, 2015.

[12] D. Grosso, M. Carabasi, J. Filicko-O'Hara et al., "A 2-step approach to myeloablative haploidentical stem cell transplantation: a phase 1/2 trial performed with optimized T-cell dosing," Blood, vol. 118, no. 17, pp. 4732–4739, 2011.

[13] D. Grosso, S. Gaballa, O. Alpdogan et al., "A two-step approach to myeloablative haploidentical transplantation: low nonrelapse mortality and high survival confirmed in patients with earlier stage disease," Biology of Blood and Marrow Transplantation, vol. 21, no. 4, pp. 646–652, 2015.

[14] S. R. McCurdy, J. A. Kanakry, M. M. Showel et al., "Risk-stratified outcomes of nonmyeloablative HLA-haploidentical BMT with high-dose posttransplantation cyclophosphamide," Blood, vol. 125, no. 19, pp. 3024–3031, 2015.

[15] M. Aoudjhane, M. Labopin, N. C. Gorin et al., "Comparative outcome of reduced intensity and myeloablative conditioning regimen in HLA identical sibling allogeneic haematopoietic stem cell transplantation for patients older than 50 years of age with acute myeloblastic leukaemia: a retrospective survey from the Acute Leukemia Working Party (ALWP) of the European group for Blood and Marrow Transplantation (EBMT)," Leukemia, vol. 19, no. 12, pp. 2304–2312, 2005.

[16] M. Mohty, M. Labopin, L. Volin et al., "Reduced-intensity versus conventional myeloablative conditioning allogeneic stem cell transplantation for patients with acute lymphoblastic leukemia: a retrospective study from the European Group for Blood and Marrow Transplantation," Blood, vol. 116, no. 22, pp. 4439–4443, 2010.

[17] A. Shimoni, I. Hardan, N. Shem-Tov et al., "Allogeneic hematopoietic stem-cell transplantation in AML and MDS using myeloablative versus reduced-intensity conditioning: the role of dose intensity," Leukemia, vol. 20, no. 2, pp. 322–328, 2006.

[18] S. O. Ciurea, M.-J. Zhang, A. A. Bacigalupo et al., "Haploidentical transplant with posttransplant cyclophosphamide vs matched unrelated donor transplant for acute myeloid leukemia," Blood, vol. 126, no. 8, pp. 1033–1040, 2015.

[19] F. Ciceri, M. Labopin, F. Aversa et al., "A survey of fully haploidentical hematopoietic stem cell transplantation in adults with high-risk acute leukemia: a risk factor analysis of outcomes for patients in remission at transplantation," Blood, vol. 112, no. 9, pp. 3574–3581, 2008.

[20] S. O. Ciurea, V. Mulanovich, R. M. Saliba et al., "Improved early outcomes using a T cell replete graft compared with T cell depleted haploidentical hematopoietic stem cell transplantation," Biology of Blood and Marrow Transplantation, vol. 18, no. 12, pp. 1835–1844, 2012.

[21] B. Federmann, M. Bornhauser, C. Meisner et al., "Haploidentical allogeneic hematopoietic cell transplantation in adults using CD3/CD19 depletion and reduced intensity conditioning: a

phase II study," *Haematologica*, vol. 97, no. 10, pp. 1523–1531, 2012.

[22] N. Cieri, G. Oliveira, R. Greco et al., "Generation of human memory stem T cells after haploidentical T-replete hematopoietic stem cell transplantation," *Blood*, vol. 125, no. 18, pp. 2865–2874, 2015.

[23] A. Roberto, L. Castagna, V. Zanon et al., "Role of naive-derived T memory stem cells in T-cell reconstitution following allogeneic transplantation," *Blood*, vol. 125, no. 18, pp. 2855–2864, 2015.

[24] C. G. Kanakry, S. Ganguly, M. Zahurak et al., "Aldehyde dehydrogenase expression drives human regulatory T cell resistance to posttransplantation cyclophosphamide," *Science Translational Medicine*, vol. 5, no. 211, Article ID 211ra157, 2013.

[25] D. Ross, M. Jones, K. Komanduri, and R. B. Levy, "Antigen and lymphopenia-driven donor T cells are differentially diminished by post-transplantation administration of cyclophosphamide after hematopoietic cell transplantation," *Biology of Blood and Marrow Transplantation*, vol. 19, no. 10, pp. 1430–1438, 2013.

[26] P. V. O'Donnell, L. Luznik, R. J. Jones et al., "Nonmyeloablative bone marrow transplantation from partially HLA-mismatched related donors using posttransplantation cyclophosphamide," *Biology of Blood and Marrow Transplantation*, vol. 8, no. 7, pp. 377–386, 2002.

[27] A. Bashey, X. Zhang, K. Jackson et al., "Comparison of outcomes of hematopoietic cell transplants from T-replete haploidentical donors using post-transplantation cyclophosphamide with 10 of 10 HLA-A, -B, -C, -DRB1, and -DQB1 allele-matched unrelated donors and HLA-identical sibling donors: a multivariable analysis including disease risk index," *Biology of Blood and Marrow Transplantation*, vol. 22, no. 1, pp. 125–133, 2016.

[28] A. Bashey, X. Zhang, C. A. Sizemore et al., "T-cell-replete HLA-haploidentical hematopoietic transplantation for hematologic malignancies using post-transplantation cyclophosphamide results in outcomes equivalent to those of contemporaneous HLA-matched related and unrelated donor transplantation," *Journal of Clinical Oncology*, vol. 31, no. 10, pp. 1310–1316, 2013.

[29] A. Di Stasi, D. R. Milton, L. M. Poon et al., "Similar transplantation outcomes for acute myeloid leukemia and myelodysplastic syndrome patients with haploidentical versus 10/10 human leukocyte antigen-matched unrelated and related donors," *Biology of Blood and Marrow Transplantation*, vol. 20, no. 12, pp. 1975–1981, 2014.

Permissions

List of Contributors

Mohammad Faizan Zahid
Aga Khan University, Karachi 74800, Pakistan

David Alan Rizzieri
Division of Hematologic Malignancies and Cellular Therapy, Duke Cancer Institute, Durham, NC 27710, USA

Ivor Wilson and Fredericka Sey
Ghana Institute of Clinical Genetics, Korle-Bu, Accra, Ghana

Eugenia V. Asare
Ghana Institute of Clinical Genetics, Korle-Bu, Accra, Ghana
Department of Haematology, Korle-Bu Teaching Hospital, Accra, Ghana

Yvonne Dei-Adomakoh and Edeghonghon Olayemi
Ghana Institute of Clinical Genetics, Korle-Bu, Accra, Ghana
Department of Haematology, College of Health Sciences, University of Ghana, Accra, Ghana

Amma A. Benneh-Akwasi Kuma
Department of Haematology, College of Health Sciences, University of Ghana, Accra, Ghana

Kevon Parmesar
Department of Haematology, Kings College Hospital NHS Foundation Trust, Denmark Hill, London SE5 9RS, UK
Kings College London, Kings College Hospital NHS Foundation Trust, Denmark Hill, London SE5 9RS, UK

Kavita Raj
Department of Haematology, Kings College Hospital NHS Foundation Trust, Denmark Hill, London SE5 9RS, UK
Department of Haematology, Guys and St. Thomas' NHS Foundation Trust, Great Maze Pond, London SE1 9RT, UK

Cesar Mauricio Rodr-guez Barrero and Lyle Alberto Romero Gabalan
KINESTASIS Seedlings of Research, University of Cundinamarca, Fusagasug´a, Colombia

Edgar Eduardo Roa Guerrero
KINESTASIS Seedlings of Research, University of Cundinamarca, Fusagasugá, Colombia

GITEINCO Research Group, University of Cundinamarca, Fusagasugá, Colombia

Fekri Samarah and Kamal Dumaidi
Department of Medical Technology, Faculty of Allied Health Sciences, Arab American University in Jenin, State of Palestine

Mahmoud A. Srour
Department of Biology and Biochemistry, Faculty of Science, Birzeit University, Birzeit, State of Palestine

Dirgham Yaseen
Rafidia Governmental Hospital, Ministry of Health, Nablus, State of Palestine

Sarita Rani Jaiswal and Suparno Chakrabarti
Department of Blood and Marrow Transplantation, Dharamshila Hospital and Research Centre, Vasundhara Enclave, New Delhi 110096, India
Manashi Chakrabarti Foundation, Kolkata, India

Brandi Anders
Department of Pharmacy, West Virginia University Medicine, Morgantown, WV, USA

Alexandra Shillingburg and Aaron Cumpston
Department of Pharmacy, West Virginia University Medicine, Morgantown, WV, USA
Osborn Hematopoietic Malignancy and Transplantation Program, MBRCC, West Virginia University, Morgantown, WV, USA

Lauren Veltri
Section of Hematology/Oncology, Department of Internal Medicine, West Virginia University, Morgantown, WV, USA

Abraham S. Kanate, Nilay Shah and Michael Craig
Osborn Hematopoietic Malignancy and Transplantation Program, MBRCC, West Virginia University, Morgantown, WV, USA

Amr Hanbali, Mona Hassanein, Walid Rasheed, Mahmoud Aljurf and Fahad Alsharif
King Faisal Specialist Hospital and Research Center, Riyadh, Saudi Arabia

Kamel Ait-Tahar, Amanda P. Anderson, Alison H. Banham and Karen Pulford
Nuffield Division of Clinical Laboratory Sciences, Radcliffe Department of Medicine, University of Oxford, Oxford, UK

Martin Barnardo
Transplant Immunology & Immunogenetics, Oxford Transplant Centre, Churchill Hospital, Oxford, UK

Graham P. Collins and Chris S. R. Hatton
Department of Clinical Haematology, Churchill Hospital, Oxford, UK

Angesom Gebreweld
Department of Medical Laboratory Sciences, College of Medicine and Health Science, Wollo University, Dessie, Ethiopia

Aster Tsegaye
Department of Medical Laboratory Sciences, College of Health Science, Addis Ababa University, Ethiopia

Tarek Owaidah
Department of Pathology and Laboratory Medicine, King Faisal Specialist Hospital and Research Centre, Riyadh, Saudi Arabia
Center of Excellence inThrombosis and Hemostasis, King Saud University, Riyadh, Saudi Arabia

Abdulmajeed Albanyan, Khalid Al Saleh and Abdulkareem Al Momen
Center of Excellence inThrombosis and Hemostasis, King Saud University, Riyadh, Saudi Arabia

Mahasen Saleh
Pediatric Hematology, King Faisal Specialist Hospital and Research Centre, Riyadh, Saudi Arabia

Hazzah Alzahrani and Mahmood Abu-Riash
Oncology Center, King Faisal Specialist Hospital and Research Centre, Riyadh, Saudi Arabia

Ali Al Zahrani, Ayman Alsulaiman and Khawar Siddiqui
Research Center, King Faisal Specialist Hospital and Research Centre, Riyadh, Saudi Arabia

Mohammed Almadani
Ministry of Education, Riyadh, Saudi Arabia

Devi Subbarayan, Chidambharam Choccalingam and Chittode Kodumudi Anantha Lakshmi
Department of Pathology, Chettinad Health City and Research Institute, Kelambakkam, Chennai, Tamil Nadu, India

Stefan O. Ciurea
Department of Stem Cell Transplant and Cellular Therapy, The University of Texas MD Anderson Cancer Center, Houston, TX 77030, USA

Piyanuch Kongtim
Department of Stem Cell Transplant and Cellular Therapy, The University of Texas MD Anderson Cancer Center, Houston, TX 77030, USA
Division of Hematology, Department of Internal Medicine, Faculty of Medicine, Thammasat University, Pathumthani 12120, Thailand

Kai Cao
Department of Laboratory Medicine,The University of Texas MD Anderson Cancer Center, Houston, TX 77030, USA

B. F. Faye, D. Sow, M. Seck, N. Dieng, S. A. Toure, M. Gadji, A. Sall, T. N. Dieye, A. O. Toure and S. Diop
Hematology, Cheikh Anta Diop University, BP 5005, Dakar, Senegal

A. B. Senghor, Y. B Gueye and D. Sy
Centre National de Transfusion Sanguine, BP 5002, Dakar, Senegal

William A. Fabricius and Muthalagu Ramanathan
Division of Hematology-Oncology, Bone Marrow Transplant Service, Department of Medicine, University of Massachusetts Medical School, 55 Lake Avenue N., Worcester, MA 01655, USA

Mona Hamdy, Niveen Salama and Amira Elrefaee
Department of Pediatrics, Faculty of Medicine, Cairo University, Cairo, Egypt

Ghada Maher
Department of Chemical Pathology, Faculty of Medicine, Cairo University, Cairo, Egypt

Shatha Farhan, Edward Peres and Nalini Janakiraman
Stem Cell Transplant Program, Henry Ford Hospital, Detroit, MI 48202, USA

Victor V. Revin, Antonina A. Ushakova, Natalia V. Gromova, Larisa A. Balykova, Elvira S. Revina, Vera V. Stolyarova, Tatiana A. Stolbova, Ilya N. Solomadin, Alexander Yu. Tychkov and Nadezhda V. Revina
Federal State-Financed Academic Institution of Higher Education "National Research Ogarev Mordovia State University", Saransk 430005, Russia

Oksana G. Imarova
GBUZ RM "National Hospital forWar Veterans", Saransk 430005, Russia

Alexandros Makis, Athanasios Gkoutsias, Theodoros Palianopoulos and Nikolaos Chaliasos
Department of Pediatrics, University Hospital of Ioannina, Ioannina, Greece

Eleni Pappa
Department of Internal Medicine, University Hospital of Ioannina, Ioannina, Greece

Evangelia Papapetrou and Christina Tsaousi
Hematology Laboratory, University Hospital of Ioannina, Ioannina, Greece

Eleftheria Hatzimichael
Hematology Department, University Hospital of Ioannina, Ioannina, Greece

Eléonore Kafando
University Ouaga I Professor Joseph KI-ZERBO, 03 BP 7021 Ouagadougou 03, Burkina Faso

Salam Sawadogo and Koumpingnin Nebie
University Ouaga I Professor Joseph KI-ZERBO, 03 BP 7021 Ouagadougou 03, Burkina Faso
National Blood Transfusion Centre, 01 BP 5372 Ouagadougou, Burkina Faso

Sonia Sontie, Ashmed Nana, Honorine Dahourou and Dieudonné Yentema Yonli
National Blood Transfusion Centre, 01 BP 5372 Ouagadougou, Burkina Faso

Tieba Millogo
African Institute of Public Health, 12 BP 199 Ouagadougou, Burkina Faso

Jean-Baptiste Tapko
African Society for Blood Transfusion, Cameroon

Jean-Claude Faber
Association Luxembourgeoise des H'emophiles, 33 rue Albert Ier, 1117, Luxembourg

Véronique Deneys
CHU UCL Namur asbl, 15 place L. Godin, 5000 Namur, Belgium

Shatha Farhan, Edward Peres and Nalini Janakiraman
Stem Cell Transplant Program, Henry Ford Hospital, 2799W. Grand Blvd, Detroit, MI 48202, USA

Michael Bazydlo
Division of Biostatistics, Henry Ford Hospital, 2799W. Grand Blvd, Detroit, MI 48202, USA

Klodiana Neme and Nancy Mikulandric
Division of Pharmacy, Henry FordHospital, 2799W. Grand Blvd, Detroit, MI 48202, USA

Patrick Adu, David Larbi Simpong and Richard K. D. Ephraim
Department of Medical Laboratory Technology, School of Allied Health Sciences, University of Cape Coast, Cape Coast, Ghana

Godfred Takyi
Holy Family Hospital, Berekum, Brong-Ahafo Region, Ghana

Ramadan A. Mahmoud
Department of Pediatrics, Faculty of Medicine, Sohag University, Sohag 82524, Egypt

Abdel-Azeem M. El-Mazary
Department of Pediatrics, Faculty of Medicine, Minia University, Minia 61111, Egypt

Ashraf Khodeary
Department of Clinical Pathology, Faculty of Medicine, Sohag University, Sohag 82524, Egypt

Galina A. Dudina
Loginov Moscow Clinical Center of the Moscow Health Department, 111123 Moscow, Russia

Marina M. Litvina and Alexander N. Mitin
National Research Center–Institute of Immunology FederalMedical-Biological Agency of Russia, 115522 Moscow, Russia

Almira D. Donetskova
National Research Center–Institute of Immunology FederalMedical-Biological Agency of Russia, 115522 Moscow, Russia
Pirogov Russian National ResearchMedical University, 117997 Moscow, Russia

Tatiana A. Mitina
Moscow Regional Research Clinical Institute Named after MF Vladimirsky, 129110 Moscow, Russia

Sergey A. Polyakov
Celgene International Holdings Corporation, 125047 Moscow, Russia

Scott R. Solomon, Melhem Solh, Lawrence E. Morris, H. Kent Holland and Asad Bashey
Blood and Marrow Transplant Program at Northside Hospital, Atlanta, GA 30342, USA

Index